MODERN ADMINISTRATIVE PRACTICES IN PHYSICAL EDUCATION AND ATHLETICS

MODERN ADMINISTRATIVE PRACTICES IN PHYSICAL EDUCATION AND ATHLETICS

Third Edition

MATTHEW C. RESICK, *Kent State University*
BEVERLY L. SEIDEL, *Kent State University*
JAMES G. MASON, *The University of Texas at El Paso*

ADDISON-WESLEY PUBLISHING COMPANY
Reading, Massachusetts • Menlo Park, California
London • Amsterdam • Don Mills, Ontario • Sydney

This book is in the
ADDISON-WESLEY SERIES IN PHYSICAL EDUCATION

Consulting Editor
Paul Hunsicker

 Printed in the United States of America. Published simultaneously in Canada.

Library of Congress Catalog Card No. 78-67946.

ISBN 0-201-06249-6
ABCDEFGHIJK-MA-79

PREFACE TO THIRD EDITION

The administration of the educational system is, indeed, a controversial subject today, regardless of the level of the system (nursery school through higher education) or the particular subject-matter area within the system (physical education, mathematics, or vocational education). The general public is taking an ever greater interest in how schools are managed and in the politics behind such operation. As an indication of this, one need only look at the feminist movement and its insistence on, for example, a commitment to athletics for girls and women. Teachers, too, are exhibiting greater concern about the climate in which they work, as evidenced by the increasing number of governance issues which are a part of professional negotiations.

As theorists attempt to deal with such issues, there is a growing trend to use a systems analysis approach, with an attendant emphasis on quantitative methods, to study the complex problems of educational administration. At the same time, other theorists are more interested in defining personal traits necessary for effective leadership. Although research in the latter area has been notably unsuccessful, there is rather general agreement that a humanistic concept that places a premium on the quality of personal interrelationships among all those who together make up the educational enterprise is a significant factor in the success or failure of the venture. These two movements seem to be mutually exclusive, if not contradictory; however, it is probable that truly effective and efficient administration demands attention to both quantity and quality factors. Any management system that pursues efficiency without considering values such as the role of the staff in the decision-making process is ultimately self-destructive. Likewise, attention to personnel concerns can conceivably become so demanding of time that administrative efficiency is lost. Thus it would seem that the practicing administrators, whether superintendents of schools or heads of physical education departments, need to keep abreast of the literature in both areas and try to make research findings compatible if they are to avoid an insoluble value dilemma.

Administrators must recognize the tremendous impact their actions have on those working under them; likewise, subordinates need to recognize that even in democratic administration, a hierarchical organization which attends to management functions is necessary. Although it is recognized that some value conflict is not only inevitable but probably healthy for the organization, it would seem that the less real the conflict, the better the administrative task will be discharged. If all concerned in the administrative process were to keep abreast of current theory and trends, the chances of serious conflict would be considerably minimized.

This third edition continues the original attempt to emphasize both administrative theory and practice. Given an acceptance of the democratic administrative stance avowed by the authors, instructors and students can, by the use of the case study approach, become more adept at working efficiently and well in groups, a necessary skill if democratic administration is to flourish. Since case studies are an integral part of every chapter, their continuous use ought to make possible a realization of whether deliberations and proposed solutions are not only compatible with theory but also consistent.

The implications of two recent pieces of federal legislation are included in this edition. Title IX of the Education Amendments of 1972 stipulates that sex discrimination is illegal in schools which receive federal assistance, and the Education for All Handicapped Children Act (P.L. 94–142) is designed to ensure that all handicapped children have available to them a free and appropriate public education in the least restrictive environment possible. Both of these acts have a great curricular and cocurricular impact on physical education and athletics. The implications of Title IX are by this time fairly well understood; however, implementation of the act has not been fully accepted. It is doubtful that the implications of the Education for All Handicapped Children Act for mainstreaming in physical education have completely surfaced. In addition, all chapter, references and case studies have been up-dated and revised, and the "Study Stimulators" have once again been expanded.

January 1979

M.C.R.
B.L.S.
J.A.M.

PREFACE TO FIRST EDITION

The focus of this book, as implied in the title, is on administrative practices in physical education, and not on theoretical concepts of program and curriculum. Therefore, no attempt has been made to define physical education or to discuss objectives for the program to any great degree. Such concepts are fairly well defined in the undergraduate's mind by the time he enrolls in a course in administration of physical education. Even if this were not true, instructors generally proceed within a framework of their own definitions and their own theory of the field.

There is considerable doubt in the minds of many educators whether administrative abilities of future teachers can be developed by means of curricular materials. The authors of this text do not claim to have the answers to the many diversified problems in physical education, intramurals, and athletics. Unfortunately, administrative problems do not come into focus in neat capsules with tidy chapter labels; rather, they generally cross unit lines. For example, a predominantly legal problem may also have budgetary implications.

Since, however, the material needs some system of organization, chapters are given traditional titles. In addition, case study problems are included at the end of each chapter which depict the latitude of a typical administrative problem. It is the hope of the authors that the readers may receive a better insight into administrative problems by seeing samples of them in case study form. Instructors may formulate their own additional problems, or they can obtain them from the authors. Case studies presuppose a concept of learning which

> . . . at least tolerates the notion that the study of concrete situations may yield significant insight and facets of knowledge which can elude even the most successful attempts to educate through communicating generalizations and presumed norms about administrative situations and behaviors.[1]

One can never be sure that all facets of the case have been discovered. New groups usually bring out new insights.

Another, hopefully fresh, approach to the area of administration is the use of *study stimulators,* a group of questions preceding each chapter which alert the student to some of the more pertinent areas discussed in the chapter. These replace the traditional discussion and test questions found at the end of most texts. The chapters on democratic administration and interscholastic athletics are vastly different from those found in other texts; the chapters on legal liability and public and human relations bring the reader sound, pertinent and usable ideas.

This book is written primarily for the undergraduate student. It does not attempt to cover all the problems which he will encounter. No book can. Emphasis is given to those areas which should aid the student and teacher to grow professionally while on the job.

---

[1] Cyril Sargent and Eugene L. Belisle, *Educational Administration: Cases and Concepts,* (Boston: Houghton Mifflin, 1955): p. 5.

CONTENTS

PART I / GENERAL

PART I
GENERAL

1

THEORY OF ADMINISTRATION

STUDY STIMULATORS

1. Why should students study administration? Aren't administrators mostly trained on the job?
2. Have there really been any noted changes in administration in schools in the last quarter-century?
3. What different types of administration are possible within the framework of a department of physical education?
4. What are the specific functions of a department head in the fields of physical education and athletics?
5. What factors should be considered in a good definition of administration?
6. What purposes are served by the line charts of departments such as those depicted in this chapter?
7. Why do circular organization charts seem less threatening to teachers?
8. Should some administrative positions be sex-linked?

Theory has no practical presuppositions, but practice always presupposes some theory. Ultimate values, for example, must first be simply seen and understood before we can do anything about them. Practical reason alone, in the absence of pure insight, is left without any stable grounds and must fall prey to random desires and interests.

JOHN WILD

INTRODUCTION

Administration or "administrivia," person-oriented or report-oriented, management by objectives or management by task—all of these are questions with which modern administrators continually wrestle. Although they may truly wish to employ a science of administration based on the latest theoretical constructs, they always seem to be confronted with administrivia, which rears its ugly head and gets in the way of a person-oriented approach with its attendant emphasis on human resources.

Such value conflicts are indeed perplexing to the responsible administrator who is conscientious about getting the job done as well as dedicated to a humanism that suggests that a staff is comprised of *persons,* not merely people. An administrator who has been in that position over a period of time has watched the process of administration go from one extreme to the other as in, for example, decision making, a vital part of the process. Whereas at one time decisions were made only by the administrators, because of their elevated positions, now decisions seem to be made "by the crowd." This is especially true in the modern era increasingly characterized by unionized teachers who demand a voice in governance, an era in which the American school teacher has gone from "obedient servant" to "militant professional."

Neither of these extreme ends of an administrative continuum is desirable. The question is one of balance, and it would seem that an appropriate balance cannot be effected until everyone involved truly understands administrative theory. Only after such understanding is reached can we expect to be able to cope effectively with the changing nature of the educational process and emerging patterns of educational governance. Even though there is strong evidence that workers directly relate job satisfaction to the degree of control they have over their employment situation, perhaps if they better understood the theoretical underpinnings of the process of administration, they would be more willing to accept the reality of noncontrol in certain circumstances. Likewise, if administrators better understood the concept that the morale factor is more vital on occasion than the apparent need for an immediate decision, they would be more willing to accept the necessity for staff involvement in decision making. In other words, they may realize that process accomplishments in administration are more vital than the outcome or product.

It becomes apparent, then, that we must study administration from the perspective of a framework within education. An administrator who tries to use an industrial model and its attendant industrial-management techniques, with no consideration of the specific differences between education and industry, will almost certainly fail.

WHY STUDY ADMINISTRATION?

Students of physical education usually visualize administration as some vague, ill-defined concept which may be of some concern to them in the remote future. Nearly any teacher now in the field will quickly correct this assumption; many will no doubt add that, in fact, aspects of administration come into play even before the teacher starts on the job. The handling of the profusion of forms and records which need to be filled out, the advanced planning of course work, and the ordering of course materials are but a few examples of administration in its broadest sense. In addition, the study of administration seems mandatory for at least four reasons.

First, since physical education is a many-faceted field, the physical educator, male or female, is typically a person who plays many parts in his or her official capacity. Besides teaching, he or she may serve in the capacity of coach, athletic director, intramural director, or recreation consultant. Each of these duties carries with it specific administrative details. The more prepared one is for this aspect of the position, the less traumatic will be the actual discharge of one's responsibility.

A national trend toward consolidation of schools is a second factor that makes the study of administration mandatory. Since it is economically unfeasible to operate small schools, the chances for a one-person "department" have lessened considerably. The trend toward unified departments of physical education and away from traditional separate departments for girls and boys, encouraged and in a sense even mandated by Title IX of the Education Amendments of 1972, Public Law, 92–318, serves to compound this fact as does the public's demand for "accountability" in education. Unified departments would seem to guarantee some financial saving in that some duplication of facilities and equipment would be unnecessary. As departments become larger, the position of department head becomes more universal.[1] In all likelihood, beginning teachers will not assume positions as department heads; but they will work in more structured departments, and thus the administrative function takes on prime importance.

Third, the relative informality of the teaching situation in physical education leads the physical educator into more intimate contact with students—a closeness which seems to place the teacher in a position in which counseling and guidance aspects assume extreme importance. Many physical educators find themselves challenged by this aspect of their position and therefore seek additional training along these lines—training which will qualify them for positions as deans, guidance counselors, principals, or superintendents. It is unnecessary to list the administrative ramifications of positions such as these.

Last, since the authors advocate a type of democratic administration in which all teachers share, it is imperative that one understand administrative theory if one is to become a functional, contributing member.

In sum, the physical educator, perhaps more than any other teacher, is placed in a position in which administrative functions

---

[1] Donald C. Manlove and Robert Buser, "The Department Head: Myths and Reality," *Bulletin of the National Association of Secondary School Principals*, **50** (November 1966): 101.

are many and varied. Thus it is essential for him or her to become as familiar as possible with a general theory of administration and with particular roles played in the carrying out of administrative duties.

SCIENCE OF ADMINISTRATION

> . . . a science of administration consists of (1) a body of knowledge about the making and implementing of decisions by those who have responsibility for a total organization or for an important division, program, or function within it and (2) modes of inquiry which can add to this body of knowledge.[2]

The history of administrative thought in this country shows that it has undergone dramatic changes. As might be expected, many of these changes have occurred very recently, since research in the behavioral sciences has brought forth new and increased insight into the ways in which people function. The concept of administration has swung from the extreme of viewing employees as "cogs in the wheels of production"[3] to the necessity for viewing them as human beings worthy of humane consideration.

History

Gross[4] traces the study of administration as a science from the early 1900's when the key words were "administrative efficiency" and Gulick's famed POSDCORB (a manufactured word in which each initial stands for a facet of administration—P, programming; O, operating; S, staffing; D, directing; CO, coordinating; R, reporting; B, budgeting—and which still appears in many treatises dealing with administration) through an emphasis on human relationships per se to the present emphasis on the psycho-social aspects of administration in its relationship to administrative behavior. The concept of administrat*ive* behavior is much broader in scope than the term administrat*or* behavior, for it implies interrelationships and

---

[2] Jack A. Culbertson, "Trends and Issues in the Development of a Science of Administration," *Perspectives on Educational Administration and the Behavioral Sciences,* ed. W. W. Charters, et al. (Eugene, Oregon: University of Oregon, Center for the Advanced Study of Educational Administration, 1965): p. 3. Reprinted by permission.

[3] Jack A. Culbertson, "The Preparation of Administrators," in *Behavioral Science and Educational Administration,* ed. Daniel E. Griffiths (Chicago: University of Chicago Press, 1964): p. 304.

[4] Bertram M. Gross, "The Scientific Approach to Administration," *Behavioral Science and Educational Administration,* ed. Daniel E. Griffiths (Chicago: University of Chicago Press, 1964): pp. 33–72.

interactions between the officially designated leader and all the others involved in the administrative scheme. Gross cautions against contentment with the research which has been done, since the greatest advances in the area are yet to come. For example, those who view human relationships as the prime concern are prone to overlook the fact that, at least in its extreme form, this consideration may stifle creativity and foster conformity.

Values on which society places a premium are reflected in the genesis of administrative thought. Much of the study of administration has been under the aegis of business, engineering, psychology, and related fields. Administration *is* administration regardless of the field, and the preparation of educational administrators has therefore been based on this research as well as on research conducted by educators. However, Graff and Street[5] posit that educational administration as a distinct profession has characteristics peculiarly its own, namely:

1. The school is a unique institution charged with the responsibility of educating citizens.
2. The school takes its direction from all community institutions. "... education is a producer of people with knowledge and skill in all forms of problem solving to meet all problems of the community."
3. The school is concerned directly with people and the development of human potential.
4. The school is at the maelstrom of conflicting values since it deliberately brings people with different values together in the hope that they will find a common base for agreement.
5. The closeness of school and community interaction is unmatched in any other enterprise, public or private.

Insofar as the selection and qualifications of administrators in education are concerned, the literature can be roughly categorized into three periods.[6] The first, in which studies were restricted primarily to outlining duties of superintendents, covered the time span from the late 1800's to 1918. The second, in which studies focused

[5] Orin B. Graff and Calvin M. Street, "Developing a Value Framework for Education Administration," in *Administrative Behavior in Education,* eds. R. F. Campbell and R. T. Gregg (New York: Harper and Bros., 1957): pp. 122–125.

[6] John K. Hemphill, Daniel E. Griffiths, and Norman Fredericksen, *Administrative Performance and Personality* (New York: Bureau of Publications, Teachers College, Columbia University, 1962): pp. 2–5.

basically on the qualities needed by superintendents to be successful in the performance of their duties, occurred from 1918 to about 1948. And the third, characterized by an attempt to find new ways to understand the ramifications of the job of superintendent and to determine criteria for selection, began roughly around 1948. Present studies, focused on the behavioral sciences and the analysis of administrative situations, continue to encounter difficulties such as a lack of criteria by which to judge administrative behavior and a lack of concepts on which to base a description of the behavior that is observed. The doctrine of school administration as applied behavioral science does not have 100 percent acceptance but, according to Button,[7] it "probably will be fully accepted, and it seems unlikly it will be replaced soon." Button goes on to express the hope that education as a discipline will come of age and answer its own problems.

Litchfield,[8] in expressing the thought that the lack of an adequate theory of administration has hindered the integration of knowledge which is developing in the behavioral sciences as well as the embracing of a larger concept of social action, postulates five major propositions "which may provide at least the beginnings of a framework for a general theory of administrative action":

> 1. The administrative process is a cycle of action which includes the following specific activities: (a) decision making, (b) programming, (c) communicating, (d) controlling, (e) reappraising.
>
> 2. The administrative process functions in the areas of (a) policy, (b) resources, and (c) execution.
>
> 3. The administrative process is carried on in the context of a larger action system, the dimensions of which are (a) the administrative process, (b) the individual performing the administrative process, (c) the total enterprise within which the individual performs the process, (d) the ecology within which the individual and the enterprise function.
>
> 4. Administration is the performance of the administrative process by an individual or a group in the context of an enterprise functioning in its environment.
>
> 5. Administration and the administrative process occur in substantially the same generalized form in industrial, commercial, civil, educational, military, and hospital organizations.

---

[7] H. Warren Button, "Doctrines of Administration," *Education Digest,* **32** (March 1967): 44.

[8] Edward H. Litchfield, "Notes on a General Theory of Administration," *Administrative Science Quarterly,* **1** (June 1956): 12–28. Reprinted by permission.

Johnson[9] touches upon some of these points in discussing whether the prototype of a successful businessperson can be equally successful as an educational administrator. After discussing six traits of a typical successful businessperson (a moderate risk-taker, a hard-working innovator, an acceptor of responsibility, a seeker of feedback, a perceptive planner, and an organizer of human resources), and projecting them onto the educational administrative scene, he hypothesizes that an educational administrator who possesses such traits should also be successful. Johnson stresses, however, that there are some significant differences between the business enterprise and the educational enterprise and that, although theory suggests that persons who possess the enumerated traits ought to be successful as educational administrators, this cannot be guaranteed.

Present Trends

One of the most cogent and comprehensive works on administrative theory in education is that by Halpin.[10] This volume concentrates on the development of administrative theory in the third historical period mentioned above and cites three outstanding influences:

1. The establishment of 1947 of the National Conference for Professors of Educational Administration (NCPEA) facilitated communication among those who train educational administrators.

2. The Kellogg Foundation's financial support of the Cooperative Program in Educational Administration (CPEA) begun in 1950 facilitated interdisciplinary research, communication and respect.

3. The establishment in 1956 of the University Council for Educational Administration (UCEA) fostered research projects to measure the performance of school administrators. Although much has been done in detecting the *role* of a theory of educational administration including significant research along human relations and leadership lines, much remains to be done to develop a *theory* in educational administration.

Three main problems arise in this connection:

1. *The substantive problem.* The term "theory" carries too many meanings and thus is unclear. This is particularly true when some

---

[9] James J. Johnson, "Why Administrators Fail," *The Clearing House,* **48,** 1 (September 1973): 3–6.

[10] Andrew W. Halpin, *Theory and Research in Administration* (New York: Macmillan Co., 1966).

writers use the term to connote a value theory—a theory about how administrators *ought* to behave. According to Halpin, although normative standards are needed, such prescriptions do not constitute a theory, and therefore "the immediate purpose of research is to enable us to make more accurate predictions of events, not to prescribe preferential courses of human action." [11]

2. *The communicative problem.* Unfortunately, the background of practitioners and theorists is sometimes so diverse that on occasion they seem to be speaking a different language. Barriers between these two groups must be broken down if a science of research is ever to become practicable in any sense of the word.

3. *The motivative problem.* The task of pursuing a theory of educational administration is an important one, one that of itself should be sufficiently heuristic, and one that should be productive of much good. Therefore, Halpin warns against ulterior motives and pleads again for practitioners and theorists to get together and solve their problems with mutual respect for intellectual integrity.

Halpin defines what he considers to be the four components of administration as follows:

1. *The task.* "This is the purpose or mission of the organization as defined, whether formally or informally, by 'observers' of the organization proper." [12] It must be specified, readily recognizable and continuously evaluated.

2. *The formal organization.* "It is important that the formal organization not be forgotten. Yet discussions of 'democratic leadership' in education often overlook both the formal organization of the school and the responsibility that the administrator—and he alone—must discharge." [13]

3. *The work group.* "The work group is composed of individuals chosen to fill positions specified by the formal organization." [14] There may be many different work groups of different status assigned to different functions. If the leader creates a climate in which the members of a group can grow and develop through working on mutual problems, the work group will be a source of satisfaction to its members and thus a great morale booster.

---

[11] *Ibid.*, p. 8.
[12] *Ibid.*, p. 30.
[13] *Ibid.*, p. 32.
[14] *Ibid.*, p. 32.

4. *The leader.* "One member of the organization is formally charged with responsibility for the organization's accomplishment." [15] This does not preclude the selection of others to help lead, a concept which is developed further in the next chapter.

Halpin also devised a "Paradigm for Research on Administrative Behavior," [16] one that has been used with considerable frequency, in order to encourage and foster research on such behavior and thus to contribute to the eventual definition of a useful theory of administration.

Systems Analysis

Systems analysis is an organizational framework that incorporates within a theory of educational administration the research findings in the behavioral sciences. Milstein and Belasco, in a review of such research, state that systems analysis provides a "disciplined framework" within which the tasks of educational administration can be made more understandable through attention to the developing knowledges in the behavioral sciences.[17] They stress that there is no magic in systems analysis; in fact, in principle, such a framework is just good common sense. However, correctly employed, systems analysis provides an avenue by which problem solving can interrelate knowledges from the behavioral sciences to the practical needs of an organization.

The concept of systems analysis has generated a new vocabulary in administrative study. Such phrases as "management information systems" (MIS), "management by objectives" (MBO), and "software and hardware" are used with great currency in the literature. These terms are discussed briefly below.

Nearly 25 years ago systems analysts were claiming that machines would soon be making decisions; thus the administrator would be concerned only with such tasks as setting goals for the organization and dealing with employee relationships. Experienced administrators admitted the necessity for using computer data and other software and hardware components, but they insisted that they would continue, directly or indirectly through staff involvement, to make decisions. Today the conflict between humans and machines seems to have been resolved to the disadvantage of

---

[15] *Ibid.*, p. 34.

[16] *Ibid.*, p. 61.

[17] Mike M. Milstein and James A. Belasco, *Educational Administration and the Behavioral Sciences: A Systems Perspective* (Boston: Allyn and Bacon, 1973).

neither. Analysis of problems and related data and the prediction of solutions, with or without computers, can lead an educational enterprise at least part way toward the establishment and subsequent achievement of objectives. However, administrators with sound and accurate judgmental abilities must maintain leadership positions. It seems highly unlikely that machines can ever completely replace human beings, if for no other reason than the necessity to deal with human beings within the total system.

A *system* can be defined as a "multiplicity of parts, elements, or components that interact with one another and work together for some common purpose." [18] The educational enterprise that fails to systematize is shortsighted and is, in reality, asking for additional management problems. A *management information system* (MIS) is a comprehensive method of management in which "the needed information . . . is made available in the correct sequence, at the proper time, and in the most useful form." [19] Such needed information is furnished by hardware, "a functional component, such as a computer" [20] or other piece of equipment, and the "organized information used to make the hardware functional," [21] known as *software.*

Another type of system is the so-called *management by objectives* (MBO), in which "all management levels identify common goals, determine individual responsibilities, and then use these measures as operational guides." [22] Although MBO is currently extremely popular in management circles, it is essentially a person-to-person process which can work to the disadvantage of an organization if there is limited participation. Such problems as heavy paperwork, overemphasis on quantitative goals, and diminished incentives to improve performance often arise. In order to circumvent or counteract such problems, there must be a great amount of organizational tolerance along with concerted attention to all the human beings within the system. Likert and Fisher[23] propose that a group orientation be added, thus MBGO, which will allow managers and those under them to function as a team when developing objectives. Each member of the group then knows what is expected

---

[18] I. Carl Candoli *et al.*, *School Business Administration* (Boston: Allyn and Bacon, 1973), p. 117.

[19] *Ibid.*, p. 114.

[20] *Ibid.*, p. 113.

[21] *Ibid.*, p. 117.

[22] *Ibid.*, p. 114.

[23] Rensis Likert and M. S. Fisher, "MBGO: Puttinq Some Team Spirit into MBO," *Personnel,* **54** (January-February 1977): 40–47.

from each individual in order to effectuate team goals, and as a consequence, each can evaluate all individual team members. As discussed in Chapter 2, attention to the group process ought to culminate in increased problem-solving skills and greater loyalty among the team members. It would seem, however, that any MBO system, properly conceived and carried out, would indeed involve all team members from the start; if so, perhaps the concern of Likert and Fisher should be more appropriately laid at the doorstep of the managers within the system rather than the system itself.

Systems theory, if well defined, includes attention to a *model,* or a "representation of a system that is used to predict the effect of changes in certain aspects of the system on the performance of the system." [24] It is desirable to use a model because the suggested new system can then be tested by simulation, thus allowing for an evaluation of its impact before it is put into actual use.

In summary, a *system* is comprised of people, equipment, procedures, *people,* documents, PEOPLE, and communication; the collective task of these various elements is to collect, validate, transform, store, and retrieve data for use in the various administrative processes involved in POSDCORB (see p. 7).

The Role of Women in Administration

Landmark legal precedents, such as the 1964 Civil Rights Act, Title VII, as well as the Equal Rights Amendment and its attendant focus on an enlightened concept of the role of the female in society, have led to a burgeoning number of women in various administrative positions. However, because statistics show that unequal opportunities for and suppression of women in educational administration yet remain, women must continue to strive for full equality by better preparing themselves for administrative tasks via study in leadership and management theory. Likewise, those who are responsible for the employment of administrators must be willing to accept the fact, as stated by Reif, that "no significant differences exist between men and women that would limit the capacity of women to perform effectively in managerial roles." [25] As one example of this, Lied [26] studied the attitudes and behaviors of women physical education instructors, researchers, and administrators on the dimensions of

---

[24] Candoli, p. 115.

[25] W. E. Reif *et al.,* "Exploding Some Myths about Women Managers," *California Management Review,* **17** (Summer 1975): 72–79.

[26] Michael Lied, "Women as Leaders and Managers" (M.A. thesis, University of Illinois, 1977).

leadership ability and managerial competence. When he compared his results with those reported in the literature dealing with male subjects, he found that few, if any, significant differences exist between the leader behavior of males and females. Lied postulates, then, that there is no need for separate training of men and women to become leader-managers; rather, "once women have achieved positions of equality and can provide leader models for young women," study and training efforts can encompass all persons regardless of sex.

It seems that women physical educators may have a unique opportunity to fill leadership roles, since they have had a greater chance to serve as department heads because of their traditional one-sex departments. There is evidence that some colleges, in an attempt to comply with affirmative action standards, invaded departments of physical education for women in order to staff administrative positions at the upper-echelon level with females. If this is an advantage, it is likely to be a short-lived one, as departments of physical education for men and for women merge and as an increasing number of women from various academic disciplines prepare themselves through advanced study specifically for administrative positions.

Recent Studies in Physical Education

The complexity of the physical educator's task is perhaps responsible for the fact that, historically, the field has been more concerned with formal organization patterns than with research into all aspects of the administrative task. The little research that has been done has gone largely unnoticed. As graduate departments of physical education become more cognizant of the beneficial effects that can accrue from research that is person- as well as pattern-oriented, the number of scientific investigations into administrative concepts should increase.

Undoubtedly, one of the most comprehensive treatments of administrative research in physical education that has yet been done is that by Spaeth.[27] Her major purpose was "to analyze administrative research in physical education and athletics in relation to current approaches to behavioral research in educational administration." Spaeth theorized that any field must be aware of the increasing

---

[27] Marcia Jane Spaeth, "An Analysis of Administrative Research in Physical Education and Athletics in Relation to a Research Paradigm" (Ph.D. dissertation, University of Illinois, 1967).

amount of research in administrative thought and must incorporate workable aspects of such study into its own operation. After identifying the major emphases affecting research in educational administration and critically reviewing a sample of administrative research in physical education and athletics in relation to those identified emphases on Halpin's Research Paradigm, she made the following conclusions:

> 1. The behavioral approach to research in educational administration as reviewed in this investigation is relevant to the administration of physical education and athletics. This approach focuses on the interactions between people rather than on the technical aspects of administration.
>
> 2. The paradigm chosen as an organizing framework for the review of research was useful in selecting, classifying, and analyzing the individual research reports. A radical departure from the traditional ways of classifying administrative research in physical education and athletics was made possible by analyzing the research in terms of the relationships between the variables identified in the paradigm. Furthermore, by using the concepts defined in the paradigm, it was possible to relate the sample of research in physical education and athletics to other administrative research and to identify relationships between research within the field which might otherwise be overlooked.
>
> 3. There is an almost total lack of theoretical orientation in the design of research and interpretation of findings in the sample of administrative research in physical education and athletics reviewed in this investigation. . . . There also has been a tendency to use concepts of the social sciences without relating the findings of the investigations in physical education to the relevant findings or theoretical interpretation of the social sciences.
>
> 4. Due to a lack of theoretical orientation, no scientific hypotheses were stated in this sample of research. The few hypotheses stated were generally statements of belief which could neither be proved nor disproved rather than predictions of specific outcomes that are then tested empirically.
>
> 5. The administrative research in physical education and athletics reviewed in this investigation lacked the methodological rigor necessary for contributions to the development of scientific knowledge about administration. Evidences of this were found in inadequate sampling, lack of objective measurement in data collection, inadequate control of variables and statistical treatment of the data for the complexity of the problems, and the general lack of theoretical orientation.[28]

---

[28] *Ibid.*, pp. 144–146. Reprinted by permission.

A sad commentary, indeed, for the field of physical education! There is a great opportunity as well as need for this type of research. This fact is further established in a more recent research project which had for its purpose the study of similarities in meanings attached to selected concepts in administrative theory and research among three groups within Big Ten Universities: (1) practicing administrators in physical education, (2) graduate faculty teaching administrative courses in physical education, and (3) professors of educational administration. Among other conclusions, it was found that physical educators, whether administrators or graduate faculty members, do not associate the same meanings to administrative concepts as do professors of educational administration and that these differences revolve around the fact that professors of educational administration generally view the concepts as more contemporary and, potentially, more meaningful.[29]

It is perhaps only natural that administrators and the faculty under them view leadership differently. Among several studies conducted along this line, one in physical education by Allen,[30] which attempted among other purposes to identify and measure leadership style, concluded that administrators and faculty members differ significantly about their perceptions of administrators' behavior. This supports the same conclusion reached in a similar study conducted much earlier,[31] and in both instances such results can be attributed to a number of factors, not the least of which is the differing concept in these two groups of personnel about theories of administration. Perhaps a salient point is that ostensibly little progress has been made in resolving this problem.

FORMAL ORGANIZATION

Some type of line-staff pattern of organization has traditionally typified administrative structure in education as well as in military and business ventures. Current emphases on human relationships and research in the behavioral sciences seem to imply to some that such organizational patterns are not only no longer necessary, but are incompatible with new administrative theory. This is an incorrect

---

[29] William John Penny, "An Analysis of the Meanings Attached to Selected Concepts in Administration Theory" (Ph.D. dissertation, University of Illinois, 1968).

[30] Patricia Allen, "An Investigation of Administrative Leadership and Group Interaction in Departments of Physical Education for Women of Selected Colleges and Universities" (Ed.D. dissertation, University of Oregon, 1971).

[31] Beverly L. Seidel, "The Use of the Group Process in the Administration of Departmens of Physical Education in Selected Ohio Colleges and Universities" (Ed.D. dissertation, Case Western Reserve University, 1959).

assumption; in fact, since education is a function which the state delegates to the public along with the necessary *legal framework* within which to operate, some kind of hierarchical structure is necessary. *Someone* has to be responsible ultimately to the voters of the community for the proper functioning of the school as a public agency.

This legal power does not obviate attention to human relationships; in fact, sometimes the "extralegal" social power structure in the school may be used to influence the behavior of persons in the legal power structure. "The influence of the legal power structure tends to be visible to organization members. Less visible, but no less potent, is the influence of the extralegal power structure." [32] Although administrators may, and hopefully do, delegate decision making and other activities, they cannot delegate their ultimate *legal* responsibility.

As has been indicated, all administrative theory today is cognizant of the role of the individual in the overall administrative task and constant research is being carried on in an attempt to discover how best to utilize individual capacities. Therefore, there need be no conflict between "formal" and "informal" power structure advocates. Each has its place and each must function effectively for the other to be as productive as possible. The administrative structure of the school reflects the nature of the school's tasks and this structure can be shown by means of organizational charts. However, the key to effective line-staff relations lies in systems theory. A systems theorist is committed to examine line-staff interaction in terms of the consequences of such interaction on the total organization. Judgments about where and how decisions should be made are defined in terms of what is in the best interest of the organization. This concept requires, on occasion, inattention to line-staff positions.

Whereas vertical line and staff structural charts have been traditionally employed to give a graphic representation of superior to subordinate relationships and their attendant authority, recent attention to the personal feelings of personnel located on the lower levels of such charts has motivated a search for a method to chart organizational relationships which does not build into it a seemingly instinctive element of fear of power.

---

[32] Laurence Iannaccone, "An Approach to the Informal Organization of the School," *Behavioral Science and Educational Administration,* ed. Daniel E. Griffiths (Chicago: University of Chicago Press, 1964): p. 235.

> Accompanying this element of fear are several other sources of frustration to the faculty member. These are: (1) a sense of removal from the main authority, the boss; (2) a creation of an isolation concept with respect to job responsibility; and (3) a general feeling of frustration caused by the layering effect. It can be quickly pointed out that these deleterious effects are not an absolute outcome of the formal vertical line and staff organizational structure; however, a case can be made that the possible existence of these effects is great.[33]

Although circular organization charts are not new in administrative theory, their use seems to be steadily increasing as one means of circumventing some of the above cited negative feelings of staff members, while at the same time developing more positive attitudes toward the entire administrative scheme. The greatest advantage of circular organization lies in the fact that its outward flow in all directions obviates the necessity for any one person or program to be viewed as being at the bottom and thus less consequential to the total function of the administrative process. Factors which influence the school's function and thus the administrative line chart are such things as size of school, level of instruction, numbers of teachers, numbers and types of noninstructional personnel, program function, budget, and staff members' feelings and self-concepts. Since a theory of educational administration is developing which advocates the increasing release of the typical administrator's time for supervision and improvement of instruction, more and more "noninstructional" personnel, including administrators, are being employed.

In the figures given here, illustrating formal organization patterns in education, solid lines denote direct authority, while dashed lines denote advisory capacities only. Figures 1, 2, and 3 are examples of traditional line and staff charts while Figs. 4 and 5 are examples of circular organization.

Figure 1, although an example of a traditional line and staff chart at the secondary level, depicts more recent theory regarding the separation of that part of the administrative function which makes instruction possible from that part which is most concerned with actual instruction. Herman[34] carries this type of thinking one

---

[33] Martin McIntyre, "A Model for the 70's," *Journal of Health Physical Education Recreation,* **44,** 9 (November–December 1973): 29. (Reprinted by permission of the American Alliance for Health, Physical Education, and Recreation.)

[34] Jerry Herman, "A New Look at Organizing Administrative Functions," *The Clearing House,* **47** (January 1973): 273–276.

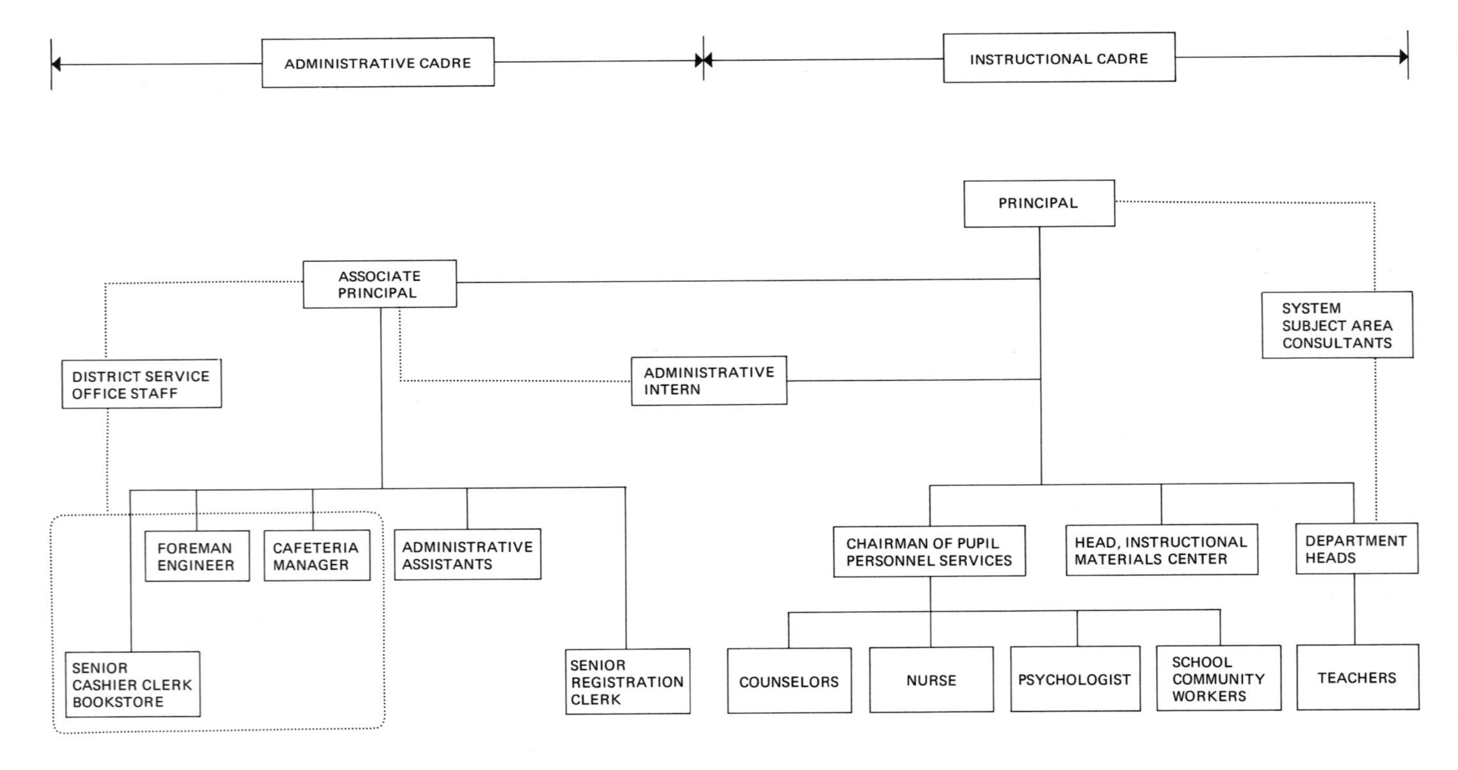

Fig. 1 High school organization chart, Phoenix Union High School system. (Courtesy of Phoenix, Arizona, Union High School System, Howard C. Seymour, Superintendent of Schools.)

step further by outlining the administrative tasks that need to be performed and then describing the type of individual he believes to be best suited to carry out such tasks. For example, "housekeeping chores" (those referred to, in part, as the Administrative cadre in Fig. 1) such as record-keeping and building and grounds maintenance can best be handled by a "Housekeeping Resources Manager," a person who needs good common sense but not necessarily a degree in education.

Figure 2 shows more specifically the place of a unified department of health, physical education, and athletics in a large city school system. Although health education is not discussed in this book, its obvious relationship to physical education and athletics is diagrammed. It is the belief of the authors that a unified department is the best arrangement for the following reasons:

1. All areas, properly conducted, have common objectives.
2. Common facilities and personnel are used.
3. If a problem concerning the use of facilities, equipment, and personnel arises, there is no delay of decision to a higher authority.
4. The superior administrative officer (e.g., principal or president) deals with only one unit rather than several interrelated areas.

A discussion of the administrative organization at the university level does not fall within the province of this book. However, Fig. 3 is included as an example of a workable arrangement. The size of the university is a decisive factor in determining the number of subdivisions and the number and type of specifically designated positions.

Castetter, in a book devoted to the function of personnel in educational administration, defines an administrative function as a body of "homogenous organizational activities usually brought together as the administrative responsibilities of one person." [35] Subordinates may be assigned to aid the head in discharging the necessary functional activities. Castetter then portrays a general idea of administrative function in the model reproduced below (Fig. 4) which sketches relationships and functions in a formal organizational structure which has divided its administrative functions into five categories.[36]

---

[35] William B. Castetter, *The Personnel Function in Educational Administration* (New York: Macmillan, 1971): p. 8.

[36] *Ibid.*, pp. 8–10.

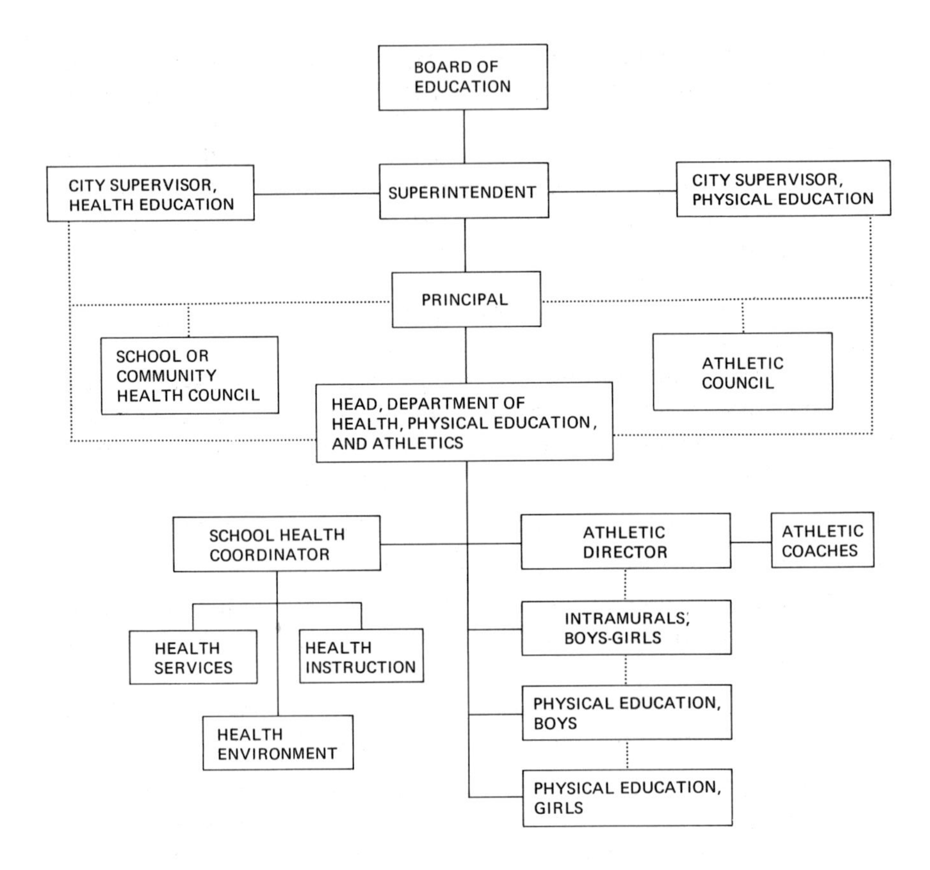

Fig. 2 Organization chart for health, physical education, and athletics in a large secondary school.

Figure 5 is an example of circular organization specifically designed for an administrative unit at the university level. However, it can quite easily be adapted to fit specific needs at any educational level. The advantages of the type of depicted outward flow of responsibility from general to specific are cited above.

It is an impossible task to point out all the ramifications and diversities in administrative plans. In every case the organizational chart is dictated by local conditions and therefore must be tailor-made to fit the situation at hand. No type of organizational chart is effective unless the involved personnel make it work. Therefore, it is mandatory to devote prime attention to the human element in any administrative scheme.

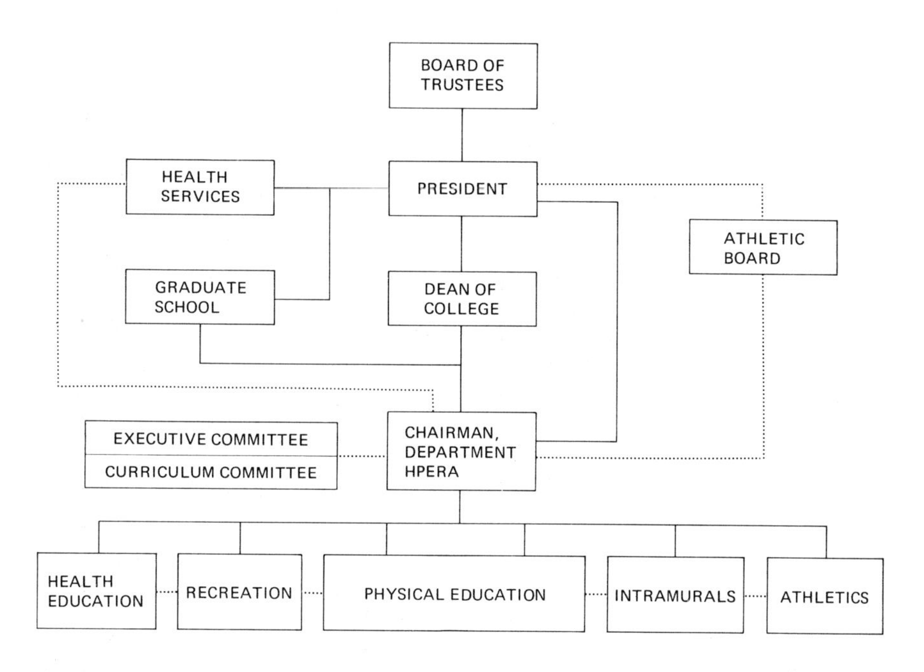

Fig. 3 Organization chart for health, physical education, and athletics at a university.

TYPES OF ADMINISTRATION

Types of administration in education, as in government, run along a continuum from dictatorship to anarchy. Sachs indicates that if this continuum were charted, democracy would fall somewhere along the midpoint but closer to anarchy than to authoritarianism. He goes on to say:

> [t]he authoritarian state is neat, in terms of power . . . whereas the very nature of argumentation and persuasion leads [the democratic process] away from neatness. In fact, the process is best described as fairly messy. In theory, democracy has beauty, and many ideals and ideal forms are ascribed to it. In this it resembles anarchistic theory, which proclaims that men, if properly educated, can become so "good" and just and righteous that they need no controls and no government—a magnificent ideal, indeed. But if in practice the democratic process is messy, the anarchistic is self-destructive. Despite numerous attempts, no modern anarchistic state has ever had

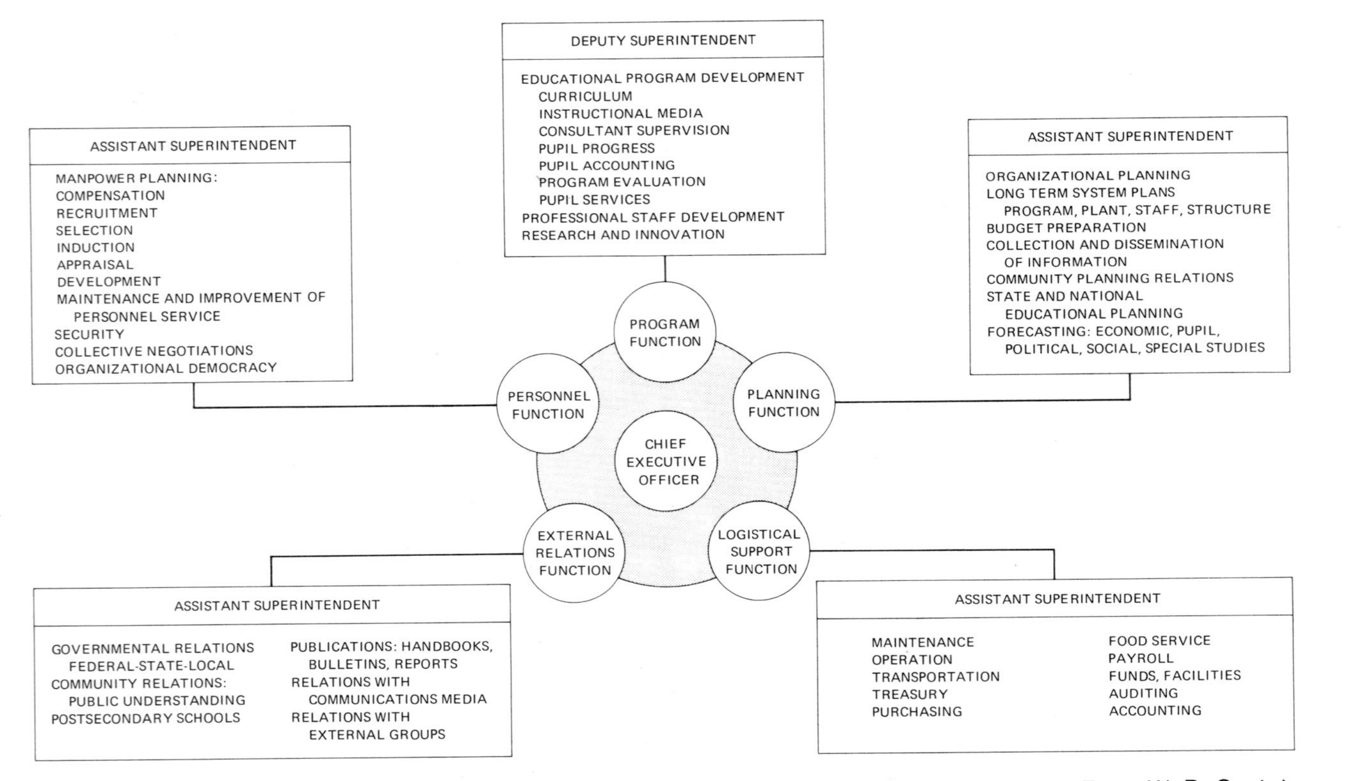

Fig. 4 Illustration of a formal organization structure showing relationships and functions. (From W. B. Castetter, *The Personnel Function in Educational Administration.* New York: Macmillan, Copyright © 1971, W. B. Castetter. Reprinted by permission of Macmillan Pub. Co.)

a long period of success, nor does a flourishing one exist as far as we know. Our great fear of anarchy is rather noteworthy in view of the fact that it is a universal failure.[37]

The administrator is the key to effective administration, and it is in the area of decision making that the administrator shows his or her true colors. The administrator may be truly a democratic leader or a political opportunist, may manipulate subordinates selfishly and ruthlessly or work with them for the good of all, may exhibit autocracy or apathy. Although, according to Strauss,[38] "it has become increasingly clear that no one form of [leadership] is universally appropriate for all personalities, cultures, and technologies," surely in the American political milieu if the administrator is not committed to the basic values of a free society, his or her effectiveness is greatly diminished, if not totally lost.

In general, the types of administrators, and thus of administration, can be classified as follows:

The Autocrat. Autocracy is considered to be the most basic form of leadership, and it is characterized by the use of powerful, authoritarian methods for obtaining desired results. Typically, the autocrat feels that he or she was chosen for an administrative position on the basis of being the best-qualified candidate, then deduces that she or he is necessarily the best qualified to make decisions and proceeds to do so! The autocrat makes all decisions, rules with an iron hand, enforces regulations without regard for circumstances, and generally ignores the human factor. However, this type of person may also act as a "benevolent despot"—one who, although making and enforcing all decisions, does so in a parental, protective manner which some teachers like. Typically, the benevolent despot is bound by tradition and therefore searches the past for truths to justify the present. Consequently, this effectively suppresses creativity and uniqueness among subordinates—the teachers.

The Laissez-faire Advocate. The person who avows this position does so in the belief that noninterference in the conduct of others will in the long run pay dividends. It can perhaps be said that more often than not, this type of administrator lacks self-con-

---

[37] Benjamin M. Sachs, *Educational Administration: A Behavioral Approach* (Boston: Houghton Mifflin Co., 1966): p. 59. Reprinted by permission.

[38] G. Strauss, "Organizational Behavior and Personnel Relations," in Industrial Relations Research Associates (ed.), *A Review of Industrial Relations Research* (Madison, Wisc.: The Association, 1970), p. 156.

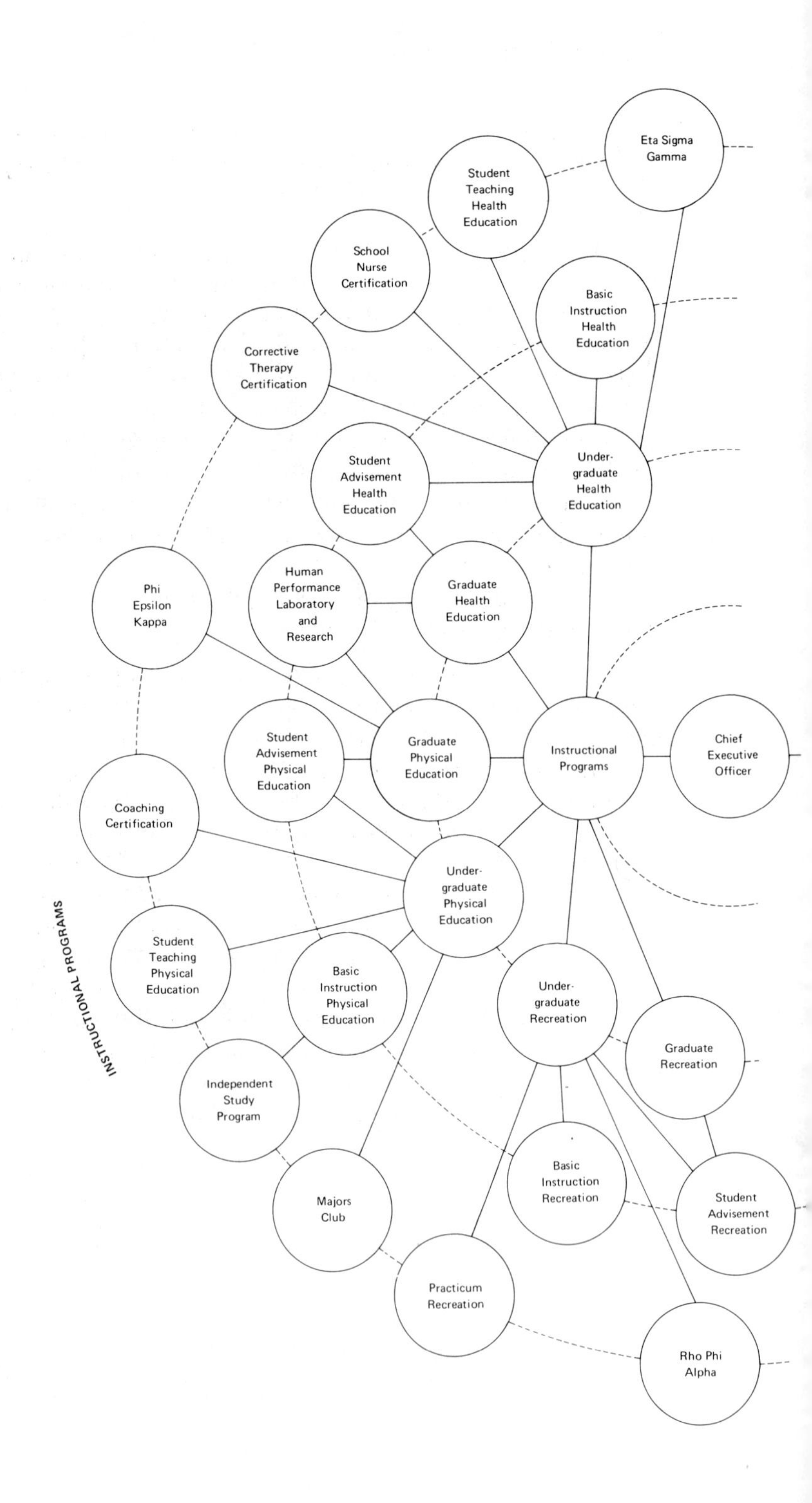

INSTRUCTIONAL PROGRAMS
Eta Sigma Gamma
Student Teaching Health Education
School Nurse Certification
Basic Instruction Health Education
Corrective Therapy Certification
Student Advisement Health Education
Under-graduate Health Education
Phi Epsilon Kappa
Human Performance Laboratory and Research
Graduate Health Education
Student Advisement Physical Education
Graduate Physical Education
Instructional Programs
Chief Executive Officer
Coaching Certification
Under-graduate Physical Education
Student Teaching Physical Education
Basic Instruction Physical Education
Under-graduate Recreation
Graduate Recreation
Independent Study Program
Basic Instruction Recreation
Majors Club
Student Advisement Recreation
Practicum Recreation
Rho Phi Alpha

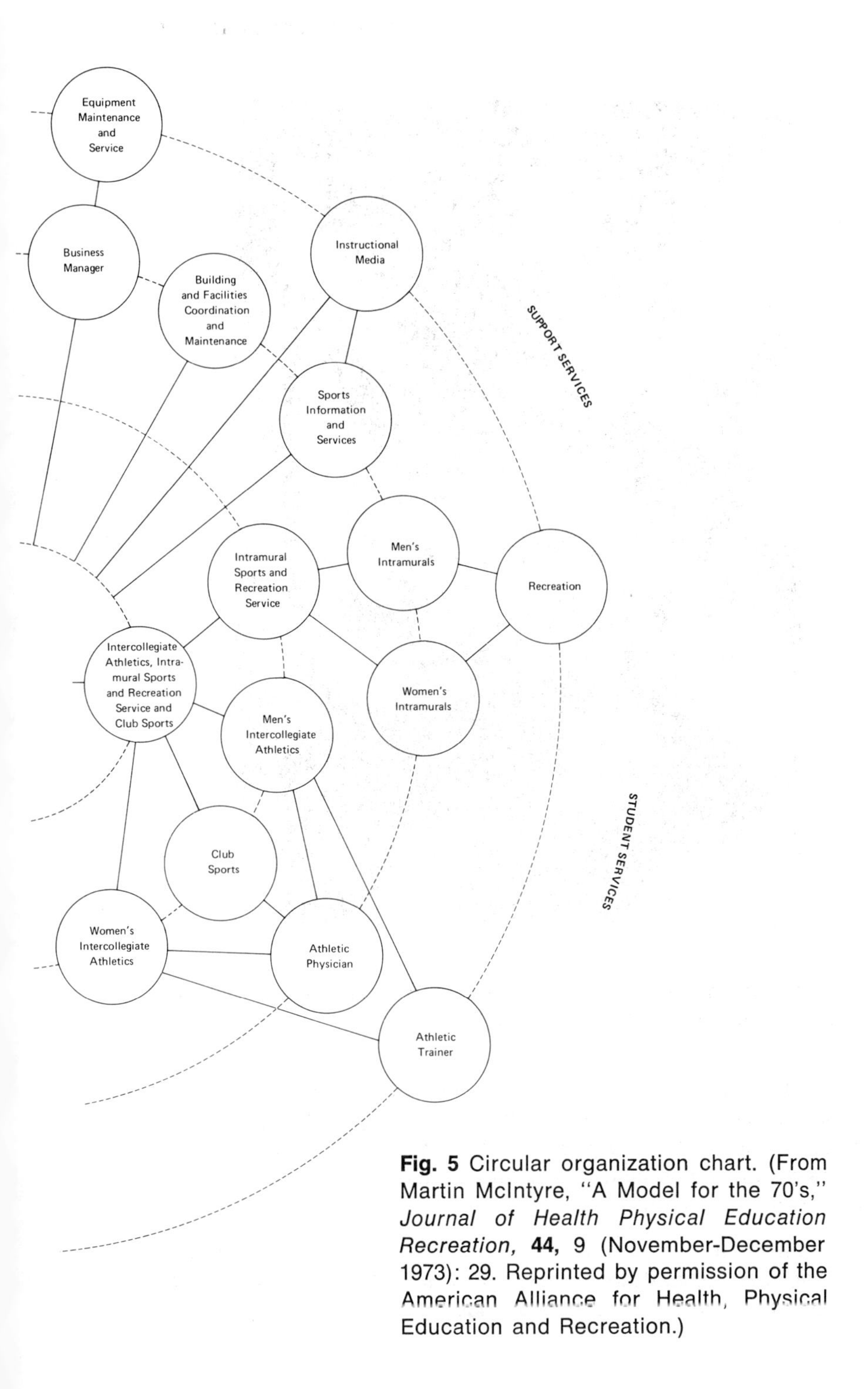

Fig. 5 Circular organization chart. (From Martin McIntyre, "A Model for the 70's," *Journal of Health Physical Education Recreation,* **44,** 9 (November-December 1973): 29. Reprinted by permission of the American Alliance for Health, Physical Education and Recreation.)

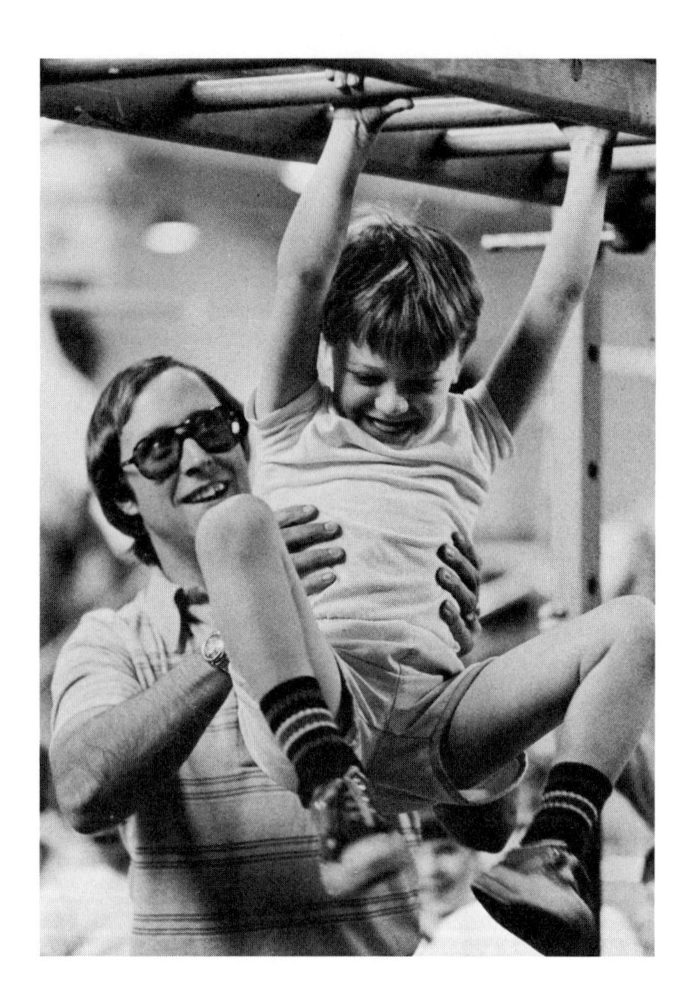

Fig. 6 Competent administration makes possible a joyful motor experience. (Courtesy Kent State University News Services.)

fidence. Often, too, an administrator of this type thinks that a hands-off policy is a democratic virtue. Perhaps the biggest danger in this type of administration is satisfaction with the status quo. Again, it can be said that some teachers prefer to teach in an atmosphere where no one "interferes."

The Anarchist. It is difficult at times to distinguish between anarchy and the laissez-faire position. Probably the basic difference rests in the anarchic theory of absence of rules and regulations along with the attendant belief that voluntary cooperative action will solve all issues. Unfortunately, too often everyone waits on everyone else to start the cooperative, voluntary ball rolling!

The Democrat. Democratic administration is characterized by attention to human relations and to a participative type of decision-making process. Nearly all administrative theory in this country naturally espouses democratic action as the most productive of good. Unfortunately, in spite of our heritage, many people do not really understand the implications of this concept. The myths surrounding it are many and varied. Griffith [39] says that "democracy is the most misunderstood term in educational administration" and tries to clarify that it does not mean, among other things, the abrogation of authority. Because of these common misunderstandings and because it is the authors' opinion that this is the most effective type of administration, Chapter 2 is devoted exclusively to a treatment of democratic administration.

Peter,[40] classifies managers (administrators) into only two groups: authoritative and participative. The authoritative manager makes independent decisions and issues orders based on them, influencing the behavior of subordinates on the basis of official position or financial pressure. The participative manager, on the other hand, shares directive power in a democratically constituted organization and also influences the behavior of others, but by consent.

Various studies have been conducted among groups operating under different types of administrative schemes to ascertain the effectiveness of the procedures used. In general, the results are similar to those cited by Luft.[41]

1. Autocratic and laissez-faire groups are not as original in their work or as effective as democratic groups.
2. There is more dependence and less individuality in autocratic groups.
3. Under the democratic leader, there is more friendliness and group spirit.

---

[39] Francis Griffith, "Six Mistaken Meanings of Democratic Administration," *Education Digest*, **32** (January 1967): 15.

[40] Laurence J. Peter, *The Peter Prescription* (New York: William Morrow & Co., 1973): p. 140.

[41] Joseph Luft, *Group Processes* (Palo Alto, Calif.: The National Press, 1963): p. 30.

4. Under autocratic leaders, there is more overt and hidden hostility, including aggression against scapegoats.

THE DECISION-MAKING PROCESS

Who is responsible for decisions? What time parameters govern decision making? Who is responsible for reviewing decisions? Is authority conferred on decision makers? Is such authority commensurate with the responsibility involved? All of these questions, in one form or another, are usually asked when staff members are involved in the decision-making process. Since this process is referred to throughout this book, it is desirable to explain how it might work under a democratic administration.

Obviously the most effective administrator is one who coordinates the efforts of the total group. Therefore, rather than making decisions alone, this person leads the group in a self-governing atmosphere in which the aim is consensus. If discussion is encouraged and a friendly climate prevails, all members should recognize that they have an opportunity *and a responsibility* to express their true feelings. If consensus cannot be achieved, compromises must be made until a mutually acceptable solution is found. Hence, even though some reservations may be retained, commitment to the group is felt, and all group members are willing to try a particular mode of action, with subsequent evaluation of it. Such a procedure is usually productive of high staff morale.

Any departmental problem can be used to show the process referred to in Fig. 7, the problem-solving process. For example, perhaps some female members of the staff have expressed concern about the fact that the coaches of the boys' varsity teams always get their choices of practice time in the various specialized facilities which must be shared by all. During a regularly scheduled staff meeting a spokesperson for the female coaches and the intramural supervisors explains why this practice appears to be rank discrimination against the majority of students and appeals for staff action.

As the rest of the group joins in the discussion it becomes apparent that there is a *need* to examine the problem in greater detail. A statement of the *definition* should include reference to each phase of the problem-solving process. Consequently, after attention is given to the necessity for objectivity, the definition of the problem, the first step in the problem-solving process, is stated as: "Shall all facilities be shared equally by all who have a legitimate claim for their use? If so, how shall the details for scheduling the

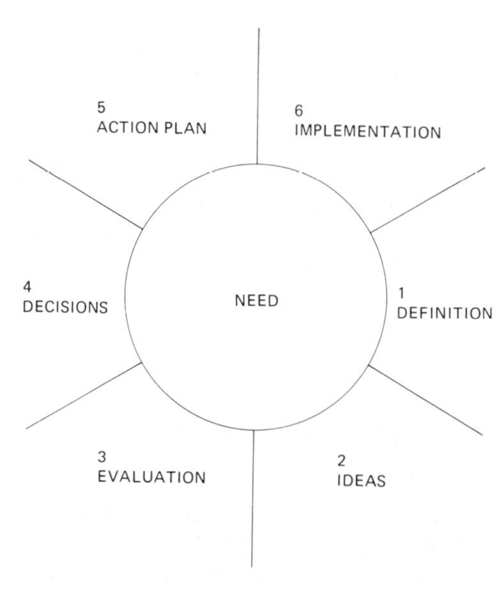
5
ACTION PLAN
6
IMPLEMENTATION
4
DECISIONS
NEED
1
DEFINITION
3
EVALUATION
2
IDEAS

Fig. 7 The problem-solving process. (Courtesy of Dr. Virginia Harvey, Professor, Counselor and Personnel Services Education, Kent State University.)

facilities be worked out? Who shall handle the necessary administrative details?"

The second step, the formulation of possible *ideas* for solving the problem, might be achieved through "buzz groups" which should include student representation and in which, hopefully, each member will "brainstorm" different ideas and suggestions. In the third phase, *evaluation*, a sifting process occurs wherein the pros and cons of the various suggestions are assessed in an attempt to clarify all positions.

The *decisions* of the process are concerned with the selection of ideas that have been evaluated. Attempts at consensus probably result in omitting some suggestions entirely, postponing others, and choosing still others on which to act. At this stage an *action plan* needs to be developed to which the total staff feels committed—a plan which explores all possible avenues leading to implementation. It would seem that relevant issues include the sharing of the least and the most desirable times for practice, transportation of students, and expenses for custodial care, electricity, and heat.

Divisions of responsibility can be assigned at this stage. For example, some members can contact other schools to learn how they have solved similar problems, and some can discuss with the principal the administrative ramifications of extended use of the facilities. The final stage, *implementation*, puts into play all implementation factors that were agreed upon, plus a continuous attempt at evaluation. If evaluation of the decision made is to be constructive, feedback must come from all concerned—students, staff, parents, and administrators—and there must be a willingness to readjust if it seems necessary. Feedback information can also be taxonomized; such procedures should help to ensure that needed adjustments are more adequate.[42]

ADMINISTRATIVE INTERRELATIONSHIPS

A quick reference to the formal organization charts (Figs. 1 through 5) reveals that many people and offices interrelate within the total administrative framework. However, the positions which are most often directly involved at the secondary school level are those of the superintendent, the building principal, and the department head, each of whom, in certain situations, is the "chief executive officer." What, then, are the usual functions of each of these offices, and how must the personnel in these positions interrelate to conduct an effective educational program?

The Superintendent

More than anyone else, the superintendent as chief executive officer is responsible to the board of education for the entire educational undertaking. In effect, the superintendent, as the liaison officer between the board of education, representing the public, and all the school personnel, must keep communication lines open and operable and must report on things ranging from the amount of money spent on custodial supplies to the effectiveness of individual teachers, from the request of teachers in a certain elementary school for a lounge where they can relax to a communication to teachers that some parents are complaining about the general unavailability of teachers for conferences concerning their children. The superintendent must take the ultimate blame when things go wrong and more often than not gets a major share of the credit when things go right.

---

[42] Jack M. Ott, Sheila Fletcher, and Donald G. Turner, "Taxonomy of Administrative Information Needs: An Aid to Educational Planning and Evaluation," *Educational Technology*, **8** (May 1973): 29–31.

In reporting an early attempt to delineate the leadership behavior of school superintendents, Halpin[43] describes two concepts of such behavior: (1) *initiating structure* (the definition of relationships between the administrator and the work group, together with the establishment of well-defined organizational patterns, procedural methods, and lines of communication), and (2) *consideration* (a prevailing atmosphere of friendliness and mutual trust and respect between the superintendent and members of the staff). As might be expected, the results of this study show that to be effective a leader must score well on both counts. Approximately 20 percent of Halpin's sample group approached this ideal. It is interesting to note that those who fell short tended to score better on "consideration" than on "initiating structure." Halpin theorizes that recent stress on human relationships has made superintendents more aware of this part of their job. Thus they may tend to overlook the importance of "initiating structure" or they may feel that attention to it is somehow undemocratic.

In a very large school system there may be one or more assistant superintendents. Their duties are usually designated, at least partially, by their titles, as in, for example, "Assistant Superintendent for Business," "Assistant Superintendent for Personnel," "Assistant Superintendent for Curriculum."

Regardless of the position, all educational matters must go through the superintendent to the board of education. Normally, it is considered to be one of the earmarks of the profession of education that individual teachers honor the channels as shown on the school's formal administrative chart. A teacher who feels he or she is being effectively blocked at a certain point on the chart can, in good conscience, announce intentions to request a hearing at the next higher level.

The Principal

The principal's first and most important task is the supervision of the teachers in the school. "Supervision" is another of the many words in administration which often carry an incorrect connotation. There is a big difference between being "snoopervised" by a principal who always visits a teacher unannounced, who scribbles notes on a scrap of paper during a few minutes visit, and who never communicates with the teacher regarding the visit made, and be-

---

[43] Andrew W. Halpin, *The Leadership Behavior of School Superintendents* (Chicago: University of Chicago Press, 1959): pp. 4–80.

ing "supervised" in a professional manner by a principal who usually, although not always, announces an intended visit, who stays for the entire period, and who then arranges for a conference with the teacher in order to evaluate the observed session in a friendly, constructive atmosphere.

Although the supervision of teachers is the principal's prime responsibility, the demands of routine work such as keeping a multitude of records have led to an abrogation of this more important responsibility in many instances. In such cases it seems clear that greater productivity at ultimately less expense will accrue from a separation of that part of administration which is concerned with the details that make instruction possible and that part which deals firsthand with the instructional cadre. (Refer again to Fig. 1.)

In the final analysis, the principal is responsible for developing a good school and therefore must be committed primarily to the community of teachers and students within the school. As Stanavage[44] says, "His [the principal's] concerns will be peculiarly and paramountly educational. The mechanical processes of organization and the minutiae of management will be delegated to office specialists, if and where the details cannot be handled by his own friendly computer." Hard-core reality forces us to conclude that friendly computers are incapable of dealing with today's brighter, better prepared, more aggressive teachers, not to mention brighter, more sophisticated students! Clearly, the handwriting on the wall indicates that the principal must become as skilled as possible in human relations and will be no less professional when participating as a member of the group rather than as the group's official leader and when assigning routine clerical work to office personnel. Effective principals possess certain qualities beyond the normal skills required for survival, including a low-key approach and a high boiling point.

The Department Head

This position is a little-understood one, but nearly everything that has been said about the superintendent and the principal qua administrators could be restated for the department head, who does not normally report directly to the board of education, but usually makes at least an annual written report for that body. The depart-

---

[44] John A. Stanavage, "Educational Leader: An Authentic Role," *Bulletin of the National Association of Secondary School Principals,* **51** (November 1967): 5. Reprinted by permission.

ment head is not involved with as many teacher visitations as the principal, but supervising them is still a prime function—especially in view of the concept of "specialized" teaching in physical education. He or she does not have as much record keeping to do as either the principal or the superintendent, but does devote a considerable amount of time to such tasks. What, then, are some of this person's duties, and in what ways, if any, are they unique to physical education?

The more important duties of the head of the physical education department are as follows:

1. To maintain an open, two-way line of communication between the department and the administration. This is perhaps even more necessary in physical education than in other departments because physical educators, by the very nature of their diverse duties, tend to be more in the public eye. Communication problems are symptoms of climatic dysfunction.
2. To keep the administration abreast of new developments and theories in physical education.
3. To interpret the field to the administration, the school board, the students, and the public.
4. To fit the department's objectives into the overall educational philosophy of the school—to be responsible for the development of objectives, syllabi, and courses of study.
5. To continuously evaluate and periodically revise the curriculum.
6. To budget for equipment and supplies.
7. To make plans for the purchase and care of equipment.
8. To formulate various necessary policies for the use of equipment and facilities. This is a great problem in physical education because of the attractiveness of the facilities.
9. To formulate the policies necessary for the conduct of the instructural program, including such things as the evaluation of students, the sharing of facilities, and the coeducational program.
10. To orient new teachers in the department.
11. To provide for in-service training such as visitations, demonstration lessons, and attendance at professional meetings.

12. To conduct research relative to the program.
13. To teach. It is the belief of the authors that everyone, including the administrator, should teach at least one class per semester. This will keep him or her aware of practical situations.
14. To make written evaluations of the teachers in the department. He or she must recommend merit increases, continued employment, and dismissals.
15. To schedule regular staff meetings and coordinate staff projects.
16. To plan for new facilities as needed.
17. To carry out the various duties connected only with interscholastic contests such as scheduling, writing of contracts, hiring of officials, and supervision of home contests. (This is covered in detail in Chapter 14.)
18. To establish a professional library, for both students and staff.
19. To make annual written reports.

If the department head is to perform all the listed functions well, even though many of them can be delegated to various members of the staff, he or she must have adequate time. Since there is no substitute for time, it is preferable to grant the head released time from instruction rather than to compensate him or her entirely by a differential in pay. How much released time is needed is difficult to determine, but generally the larger the department, the more released time is necessary, since the supervision of teachers and the motivation toward excellence remains the prime responsibility.

Clearly, leadership ability is the key quality that must be possessed by a department head. Concepts of leadership differ, and on occasion department heads cover up their deficiencies by defining "leadership" in a special way. Chapter 2 sheds more light on generally accepted tenets of democratic leadership.

DEFINITIONS

It may seem strange that a definition of the term "administration" was not given at the beginning of this chapter. However, after reading this far, the reader should have acquired some insight into the complexity of administration, and definitions will now be more meaningful.

Below are some of the more current definitions of "administration" found in articles and textbooks:

> ... administration is conceived as the guidance of cooperative human effort into clearly understood channels of responsible action for the purpose of achieving maximum effectiveness in program operation.[45]
>
> ... administration is mainly concerned with guiding human behavior in the service of some goal. Whatever the nature of the organization it is through human behavior that necessary tasks are accomplished. *The crux of administration is managing human behavior.*[46]
>
> Administration is the process of managing or conducting a program of activities. Broadly conceived, administration means constructive leadership which makes possible the teaching and learning process.[47]
>
> The essential task of management is to arrange organizational conditions and methods of operation so that people can achieve their own goals best by directing their own efforts toward organizational objectives.[48]
>
> Administration may be defined as the total of the processes through which appropriate human and material resources are made available and made effective for accomplishing the purposes of an enterprise.[49]

Note that a stress on leadership and the human factor is common to all those definitions. Although written many years ago, this last definition is a most cogent one. A definition can cover paragraphs, perhaps even pages, or, conversely, it can be stated as simply as: The function of administration is the process by which the job gets done! To be sure, this definition is much too simple unless all the ramifications of "the job" are considered.

CASE STUDY

Mr. George Simon had declared his intention to retire at the end of the current year. He had served as the Head of the Department of Physical

---

[45] Richard C. Havel and Emery W. Seymour, *Administration of Health, Physical Education and Recreation for Schools* (New York: The Ronald Press Co., 1961): p. 4. Reprinted by permission.

[46] Edward F. Voltmer and Arthur A. Esslinger, *The Organization and Administration of Physical Education,* 4th ed. (New York: Appleton-Century-Crofts, Educational Division, Meredith Corporation, 1967): p. 2. (Italics added.) Reprinted by permission.

[47] William L. Hughes and Esther French, *The Administration of Physical Education* (New York: A. S. Barnes and Co., 1954): p. 1. Reprinted by permission.

[48] Douglas M. McGregor, "The Human Side of Enterprise," in *Readings in Managerial Psychology,* ed. H. J. Leavitt and L. R. Pondy (Chicago: University of Chicago Press, 1964): p. 276. Reprinted by permission.

[49] American Association of School Administrators, *Staff Relations in School Administration* (Washington, D.C.: The Association, 1955): p. 17. Reprinted by permission.

Education for Boys for over 20 years, a position he retained when the departments for boys and girls merged. Although somewhat of an autocrat, he was not unapproachable. This, together with a deference to his age and experience, had allowed the staff, particularly the senior members, to work effectively under him.

The principal, a democratic administrator, relayed the notice of Mr. Simon's retirement to the staff and suggested that they consider selecting a new head from among the existing staff members.

There seemed to be two logical candidates for the position—one male, one female. The first, Mel Tipton, was a strong and domineering individual very much like Mr. Simon. Tipton had taught in the system for ten years and was highly regarded by the school administrators. The other candidate, Betty Jones, was a rather unassuming woman. Although she had less experience that Mr. Tipton, she had the ability to get people to work together.

At the next staff meeting, Mr. Simon informed everyone that he wanted to respect the wishes of the principal and was therefore open to suggestions as to how the group wished to proceed with the selection of the new department head.

1. What are the central issues in this case?
2. How should the staff proceed?
3. What guiding principles are involved?

SELECTED REFERENCES

Allen, Patricia. "An Investigation of Administrative Leadership and Group Interaction in Departments of Physical Education for Women of Selected Colleges and Universities." Ed.D. dissertation, University of Oregon, 1971.

Bolton, Dale L. *The Use of Simulation in Educational Administration.* Columbus, Ohio: Charles E. Merrill, 1971.

Button, H. Warren. "Doctrines of Administration," *Education Digest,* **32** (March 1967): 42–44.

Campbell, R. F., and R. T. Gregg (eds.). *Administrative Behavior in Education.* New York: Harper and Bros., 1957.

Castetter, William B. *The Personnel Function in Educational Administration.* New York: Macmillan, 1971.

Charters, W. W., et al. (eds.). *Perspectives on Educational Administration and the Behavioral Sciences.* Eugene, Oregon: University of Oregon, Center for the Advanced Study of Educational Administration, 1965.

Flower, George E. "Is Anybody in Charge Here?" *Education Canada* (September 1971): pp. 26–31.

Griffith, Francis. "Six Mistaken Meanings of Democratic Administration," *Education Digest,* **32** (January 1967): 15–17.

Halal, W. E. "Toward a General Theory of Leadership," *Human Relations,* **27** (April 1974): 401–416.

Hall, J. Tillman, et al. *Administration: Principles, Theory and Practice.* Pacific Palisades, California: Goodyear Publishing, 1973.

Halpin, Andrew W. *The Leadership Behavior of School Superintendents.* Chicago: University of Chicago Press, 1959.

———. *Theory and Research in Administration.* New York: Macmillan, 1966.

Hemphill, John K., Daniel E. Griffiths, and Norman Fredericksen. *Administrative Performance and Personality.* New York: Bureau of Publications, Teachers College, Columbia University, 1962.

Herman, Jerry. "A New Look at Organizing Administrative Functions," *The Clearing House,* **47** (January 1973): 273–276.

Johnson, James J. "Why Administrators Fail," *The Clearing House,* **48,** 1 (September 1973): 3–6.

Leavitt, H. J., and L. R. Pondy (eds.). *Readings in Managerial Psychology.* Chicago: University of Chicago Press, 1964.

Litchfield, Edward H. "Notes on a General Theory of Administration," *Administrative Science Quarterly,* **1** (June 1956): 3–29.

Luft, Joseph. *Group Processes.* Palo Alto, Calif.: The National Press, 1963.

McIntyre, Martin. "A Model for the 70's," *Journal of Health, Physical Education and Recreation,* **44,** 9 (November–December 1973): 28–30.

Manlove, Donald C., and Robert Buser. "The Department Head: Myths and Reality," *Bulletin of the National Association of Secondary School Principals,* **50** (November 1966): 38–41.

Mayhew, Lewis, and T. R. Glenn. "College and University Presidents: Roles in Transition," *Liberal Education,* **61** (October 1975): 299–308.

Ott, Jack M., Sheila Fletcher, and Donald G. Turner. "Taxonomy of Administrative Information Needs: An Aid to Educational Planning and Evaluation," *Educational Technology,* XIII (May 1973).

Penny, William John. "An Analysis of the Meanings Attached to Selected Concepts in Administrative Theory." Ph.D. dissertation, University of Illinois, 1968.

Peter, Laurence J. *The Peter Prescription.* New York: William Morrow, 1973.

Rockefeller, John D. *The Second American Revolution.* New York: Harper & Row, 1973.

Rubin, Louis J. (ed.). *Frontiers in School Leadership.* Chicago: Rand-McNally, 1970.

Sachs, Benjamin M. *Education Administration: A Behavioral Approach.* Boston: Houghton Mifflin, 1966.

Seidel, Beverly L. "The Use of the Group Process in the Administration of Departments of Physical Education in Selected Ohio Colleges and Universities." Ed.D dissertation, Case Western Reserve University, 1959.

Shami, Mohammed, *et al.,* "Dimensions of Accountability," *NASSP Bulletin,* **58** (September 1974): 1–12.

Spaeth, Marcia Jane. "An Analysis of Administrative Research in Physical Education and Athletics in Relation to a Research Paradigm." Ph.D. dissertation, University of Illinois, 1967.

Stanavage, John A. "Educational Leader: An Authentic Role," *Bulletin of the National Association of Secondary School Principals,* **51** (November 1967): 3–17.

Stewart, Beverly. "What Is Organizational Development and How Does It Apply to Schools?" *Education Canada,* **13** (June 1973): 19–21.

Voltmer, Edward F., and Arthur A. Esslinger. *The Organization and Administration of Physical Education* (4th ed.). New York: Appleton-Century-Crofts, 1967.

2

DEMOCRATIC ADMINISTRATION

STUDY STIMULATORS

1. Can a theory of systems analysis be made comparative with a theory of democracy?
2. Why is it imperative that responsibility be stressed in conjunction with the rights of individuals and groups?
3. What is a workable definition of the group process?
4. Why is not leadership exclusively a function of administration? What other personnel should play leadership roles?
5. What effect does a concept of accountability have on the educative process?
6. What is the teacher's role in the administrative hierarchy?
7. What are the "Elements of Democracy" as developed by the National Association for Physical Education of College Women? Do they seem to embrace the total concept of "democracy"?
8. In what way are the functions of a department head similar to those of a principal? How do they differ?
9. Should the leadership role be separated from the administrative role?

A leader is best
When people barely know that he exists,
Not so good when people acclaim him,
Worst when they despise him.
But of a good leader, who talks little
When his work is done, his aim fulfilled,
They will all say, "We did this ourselves." '

LAO-TSU, CHINESE PHILOSOPHER

INTRODUCTION

The processes of management, including systems analysis, as presented in Chapter 1, seem at least superficially to be incongruous with any value system that embraces a concept of democracy. Since the focus of this chapter is on democracy in administration, it is well to point out possible conflicts and how they can be, if not completely overcome, at least thwarted.

Whether administrative organization charts in education are depicted as vertical or circular, the reality of a hierarchy is inherent within them. Such reality seems incompatible with the basic values of democracy, such as human dignity, personal freedom, justice, and the opportunity for positive self-actualization, since a concept of hierarchy tends to embrace such values (or disvalues) as authority, power, control, and imposed discipline. Presently the latter values are given little status by much of American society. In fact, John D. Rockefeller III describes the revolution toward humanism as the Second American Revolution, and he believes that this revolution is one of "fulfillment," one that will ultimately "bring to fruition, in modern times, not only the letter but the spirit—the intent—of . . . the Declaration of Independence and the Constitution," the two great

IN CONGRESS, JULY 4, 1776.

The unanimous Declaration of the thirteen united States of America,

When in the Course of human events it becomes necessary for one people to dissolve the political bands which have connected them with another, and to assume among the powers of the earth, the separate and equal station to which the Laws of Nature and of Nature's God entitle them, a decent respect to the opinions of mankind requires that they should declare the causes which impel them to the separation. —— We hold these truths to be self-evident, that all men are created equal, that they are endowed by their Creator with certain unalienable Rights, that among these are Life, Liberty and the pursuit of Happiness. — That to secure these rights, Governments are instituted among Men, deriving their just powers from the consent of the governed, — That whenever any Form of Government becomes destructive of these ends, it is the Right of the People to alter or to abolish it, and to institute new Government, laying its foundation on such principles and organizing its powers in such form, as to them shall seem most likely to effect their Safety and Happiness. Prudence, indeed, will dictate that Governments long established should not be changed for light and transient causes; and accordingly all experience hath shewn, that mankind are more disposed to suffer, while evils are sufferable, than to right themselves by abolishing the forms to which they are accustomed. But when a long train of abuses and usurpations, pursuing invariably the same Object evinces a design to reduce them under absolute Despotism, it is their right, it is their duty, to throw off such Government, and to provide new Guards for their future security. — Such has been the patient sufferance of these Colonies; and such is now the necessity which constrains them to alter their former Systems of Government. The history of the present King of Great Britain is a history of repeated injuries and usurpations, all having in direct object the establishment of an absolute Tyranny over these States. To prove this, let Facts be submitted to a candid world. —— He has refused his Assent to Laws, the most wholesome and necessary for the public good. —— He has forbidden his Governors to pass Laws of immediate and pressing importance, unless suspended in their operation till his Assent should be obtained; and when so suspended, he has utterly neglected to attend to them. —— He has refused to pass other Laws for the accommodation of large districts of people, unless those people would relinquish the right of Representation in the Legislature, a right inestimable to them and formidable to tyrants only. —— He has called together legislative bodies at places unusual, uncomfortable, and distant from the depository of their public Records, for the sole purpose of fatiguing them into compliance with his measures. —— He has dissolved Representative Houses repeatedly, for opposing with manly firmness his invasions on the rights of the people. —— He has refused for a long time, after such dissolutions, to cause others to be elected; whereby the Legislative powers, incapable of Annihilation, have returned to the People at large for their exercise; the State remaining in the mean time exposed to all the dangers of invasion from without, and convulsions within. —— He has endeavoured to prevent the population of these States; for that purpose obstructing the Laws for Naturalization of Foreigners; refusing to pass others to encourage their migrations hither, and raising the conditions of new Appropriations of Lands. —— He has obstructed the Administration of Justice, by refusing his Assent to Laws for establishing Judiciary powers. —— He has made Judges dependent on his Will alone, for the tenure of their offices, and the amount and payment of their salaries. —— He has erected a multitude of New Offices, and sent hither swarms of Officers to harrass our people, and eat out their substance. —— He has kept among us, in times of peace, Standing Armies without the Consent of our legislatures. —— He has affected to render the Military independent of and superior to the Civil power. —— He has combined with others to subject us to a jurisdiction foreign to our constitution, and unacknowledged by our laws; giving his Assent to their Acts of pretended Legislation: — For Quartering large bodies of armed troops among us: — For protecting them, by a mock Trial, from punishment for any Murders which they should commit on the Inhabitants of these States: — For cutting off our Trade with all parts of the world: — For imposing Taxes on us without our Consent: — For depriving us in many cases, of the benefits of Trial by Jury: — For transporting us beyond Seas to be tried for pretended offences: — For abolishing the free System of English Laws in a neighbouring Province, establishing therein an Arbitrary government, and enlarging its Boundaries so as to render it at once an example and fit instrument for introducing the same absolute rule into these Colonies: — For taking away our Charters, abolishing our most valuable Laws, and altering fundamentally the Forms of our Governments: — For suspending our own Legislatures, and declaring themselves invested with power to legislate for us in all cases whatsoever. — He has abdicated Government here, by declaring us out of his Protection and waging War against us. —— He has plundered our seas, ravaged our Coasts, burnt our towns, and destroyed the lives of our people. —— He is at this time transporting large Armies of foreign Mercenaries to compleat the works of death, desolation and tyranny, already begun with circumstances of Cruelty & perfidy scarcely paralleled in the most barbarous ages, and totally unworthy the Head of a civilized nation. —— He has constrained our fellow Citizens taken Captive on the high Seas to bear Arms against their Country, to become the executioners of their friends and Brethren, or to fall themselves by their Hands. —— He has excited domestic insurrections amongst us, and has endeavoured to bring on the inhabitants of our frontiers, the merciless Indian Savages, whose known rule of warfare, is an undistinguished destruction of all ages, sexes and conditions. In every stage of these Oppressions We have Petitioned for Redress in the most humble terms: Our repeated Petitions have been answered only by repeated injury. A Prince, whose character is thus marked by every act which may define a Tyrant, is unfit to be the ruler of a free people. Nor have We been wanting in attentions to our British brethren. We have warned them from time to time of attempts by their legislature to extend an unwarrantable jurisdiction over us. We have reminded them of the circumstances of our emigration and settlement here. We have appealed to their native justice and magnanimity, and we have conjured them by the ties of our common kindred to disavow these usurpations, which, would inevitably interrupt our connections and correspondence. They too have been deaf to the voice of justice and of consanguinity. We must, therefore, acquiesce in the necessity, which denounces our Separation, and hold them, as we hold the rest of mankind, Enemies in War, in Peace Friends. ——

We, therefore, the Representatives of the united States of America, in General Congress, Assembled, appealing to the Supreme Judge of the world for the rectitude of our intentions, do, in the Name, and by Authority of the good People of these Colonies, solemnly publish and declare, That these United Colonies are, and of Right ought to be Free and Independent States; that they are Absolved from all Allegiance to the British Crown, and that all political connection between them and the State of Great Britain, is and ought to be totally dissolved; and that as Free and Independent States, they have full Power to levy War, conclude Peace, contract Alliances, establish Commerce, and to do all other Acts and Things which Independent States may of right do. —— And for the support of this Declaration, with a firm reliance on the protection of divine Providence, we mutually pledge to each other our Lives, our Fortunes and our sacred Honor.

John Hancock

Button Gwinnett, Lyman Hall, Geo Walton.

Wm Hooper, Joseph Hewes, John Penn

Edward Rutledge, Thos Heyward Junr, Thomas Lynch Junr, Arthur Middleton

Samuel Chase, Wm Paca, Thos Stone, Charles Carroll of Carrollton

George Wythe, Richard Henry Lee, Th Jefferson, Benja Harrison, Thos Nelson jr., Francis Lightfoot Lee, Carter Braxton

Robt Morris, Benjamin Rush, Benja Franklin, John Morton, Geo Clymer, Jas Smith, Geo Taylor, James Wilson, Geo Ross

Caesar Rodney, Geo Read, Tho M:Kean

Wm Floyd, Phil Livingston, Frans Lewis, Lewis Morris

Richd Stockton, Jno Witherspoon, Fras Hopkinson, John Hart, Abra Clark

Josiah Bartlett, Wm Whipple, Saml Adams, John Adams, Robt Treat Paine, Elbridge Gerry, Step Hopkins, William Ellery, Roger Sherman, Samel Huntington, Wm Williams, Oliver Wolcott, Matthew Thornton

Fig. 1 The Declaration of Independence, the foundation of democracy. (Courtesy the Kent State University Libraries.)

documents that are the bulwark of American democracy.[1] Inattention to democratic values in educational administration is at best hypocritical and at worst self-defeating if one wishes to administer effectively within society's accepted political framework.

On the other hand, it must be recognized that it is the prerogative of administration (management) to make decisions and to exert authority. As stated before, administration is responsilble for seeing that the job gets done. However, if administrators truly understand how deeply their decisions can affect the lives of those beneath them and if they understand the basic tenets of democratic leadership, they will tend to exercise their authority within the constraints of a humanistic philosophy lest their teachers fail to relate to the total educational endeavor.

According to Crockett,[2] the challenge is one of "enabling people to *live* democracy as well as to *theorize* democracy," one of making the democratic way of life more secure by making it more meaningful and thus more functional. Perhaps the following discussion on democratic administration, with its attention to how specific members of the hierarchy within education can operate democratically, will help meet this challenge.

THEORY OF DEMOCRACY

Democracy is the heritage of the American people. Since the government of the United States was founded upon this doctrine, it seems natural that the democratic ideology should permeate all phases of American life. The glib, everyday use of the words "democracy" and "democratic" among Americans seems to indicate that there is almost universal agreement on the general implications of these terms. However, history shows that no such agreement has ever existed, not even at the time of the formulation of the Constitution of the United States, the very document upon which America's democracy rests. In 1787, when the issues of the Constitution were being debated in Philadelphia, democracy had only a few, though eloquent, champions. Men like Benjamin Franklin and Thomas Jefferson spoke fluently on behalf of a democratic form of government, while Alexander Hamilton and others spoke

---

1 John D. Rockefeller III, *The Second American Revolution* (New York: Harper & Row, 1973: p. 11.

2 W. J. Crockett, "The Management Conflict with Democratic Values," *Business Horizons*, **16** October 1973): 13–19.

contemptuously of the "imprudence of democracy" because "the people seldom judge or determine right."[3] These authors of the Constitution did not radically disagree in philosophy, however, and after discussions and debates on all controversial issues, a compromise document on which there was fundamental agreement was drawn up. This pattern—discussion and debate followed by compromise—continues to be a basic method of democracy. "The Bill of Rights," the first ten amendments to the Constitution, was adopted at the initial session of the newly formed Congress in 1789. These amendments, based on the belief in individual freedom and worth, philosophically underlie the popular conception of democracy that has developed in America.

This philosophy also permeates American education. However, if, as Lewin[4] suggests, democracy must be learned anew by each generation, one can see that it is necessary constantly to teach democratic skills and methods. Basic to the practice of democracy is a clear understanding of its meaning, and since the processes of democracy must by nature be flexible, the task of the schools in educating for democracy becomes at once one of the most important issues of our day. Some people suggest that education has failed miserably in this respect in the past decade as evidenced, for example, by the fact that many students attack the teachers and vandalize the schools that have set them free. This is but another example that the concept of democracy is not well understood. The concept is not synonymous with the concept of freedom, if by freedom is meant the license to do "one's own thing" regardless of the results.

If education for democracy is accepted as one of America's basic needs, several congruent aspects are revealed. Not the least among these is the necessity for teachers to feel that they, too, are participating in a democratic climate. How incongruous it is that the students in American schools are instructed in democracy, often in a self-governing atmosphere, while their instructors are participating in a regulatory atmosphere which stifles virtually all freedom and creativity! Predictable backlash has caused some teachers to become extremely militant, demanding among other things a voice in every decision made; conversely, other teachers simply settle more deeply in a rut of mediocrity and complacency.

---

[3] Saul K. Padover, *The Living U.S. Constitution* (New York: The New American Library of World Literature, 1953): p. 18.

[4] Kurt Lewin, *Resolving Social Conflicts* (New York: Harper and Bros., 1948): p. 230.

Teaching involves much more than instruction; in fact, teachers have been known to say that at times instruction seems to be the least of their duties. This seems to dictate that the manner in which policies and procedures within the school system are established has an important bearing upon the spirit in which they are carried out. That the National Education Association views this facet of education as a continuing concern is readily apparent from the following two quotes, expressed some 20 years apart:

> Teachers . . . are most likely to work and think to the limits of their capacities when they have voices that count in deciding the purposes of their work, and when they feel that their efforts are indispensable parts of doing jobs which they have helped to plan.[5]

> When teachers are accepted as people of dignity and worth, as responsible people, as people who are trying in the only way they see to be adequate teachers, they tend to see themselves in more positive ways and to become more adequate in their relationships with students.[6]

As the nature and operation of democracy becomes more clearly defined and understood, the group process, an important aspect of democracy, becomes increasingly important. Although educators generally concede that teachers are using the group process more often and more effectively in the classroom, there is considerable doubt that the process is widely employed by administrators in relation to the teachers working under them. As was stated in Chapter 1, the task of administration is to get things done and not, as often seems the case, to nourish existing administrative policy and practice. Therefore, democratic administration is as desirable as democratic teaching if the school is to fulfill its responsibility to society.

In these days of teacher unrest, school personnel are quick to point out that administrators do too much talking about democracy for the amount and quality of effort they themselves put into the task. Democratic human relations cannot be advocated with integrity when schools and departments tend to be administered in an autocratic manner and staff members have little or no voice in problems which directly concern them.

---

[5] National Education Association, Educational Policies Committee, *Learning the Ways of Democracy* (Washington, D.C.: The Association, 1940): p. 375. Reprinted by permission.

[6] Association for Supervision and Curriculum Development, 1962 Yearbook, *Perceiving, Behaving, Becoming: A New Focus for Education* (Washington, D.C.: Association for Supervision and Curriculum Development, 1962): p. 74. Reprinted by permission.

ACCOUNTABILITY

New educational realities require action in terms of being accountable, flexible, and attuned to the times. However, if a system of accountability is to be effective, all groups related to the educational process must be reassured that analytic accountabilty is diagnostic, not judgmental, and that the total accountability program is for the benefit of all those engaged in the process of education.[7] In defense of administrators, it must be pointed out that their task is an increasingly difficult one. On one hand, the public cries for "accountability" in education; "accountability" seems to pertain primarily to financial matters, although some parents are demanding better, more productive teaching as well. Quantifying "the life of the mind"[8] is no simple task, and teachers generally believe that they should be held accountable only for those things that they can influence directly or indirectly. The implementation of "logical, systematic, and realistic accountability," then, must include (1) a clear statement of educational goals, (2) an identification of the types and measures of accountability to be used, (3) a delineation of responsibility of specific personnel, (4) a listing of those to whom education is accountable, (5) an identification of the levels of accountability, (6) the collection of pertinent data, and (7) a clear statement of how the results of accountability are to be used.[9] Note that cost as such is not even mentioned, although it is undoubtedly subsumed in one or more of the listed points. Even if it were possible to find a process that would guarantee better education by close attention to financial factors, the process would seem to be fraught with the danger of dehumanizing the educational undertaking to an even greater extent. Accountability, according to one author, leads to a robotlike individual whose human spirit is inextricably bound to a "dictatorial and closed system of education."[10]

Many teachers, internalizing a strong commitment to "academic freedom," have thus felt it imperative to leave the field of education; others, in spite of the agony involved, continue to strive for the ecstasy that accrues when it is realized that at least some students' lives have been affected positively.

---

[7] A. R. Olson, "The Hot Buttons in Accountability," *Planning and Change,* **7** (Summer 1976): 4–14.

[8] W. H. Danforth, "Management and Accountability in Higher Education," *A.A.U.P. Bulletin,* **59** (June 1973): 135–138.

[9] Mohammed Shami *et al.,* "Dimensions of Accountability," *NASSP Bulletin,* **58** (September 1974): 2.

[10] Gerald Teller, "What Are the Myths of Accountability?" *Educational Leadership,* **31** (February 1974): 455–456.

Teachers, too, cry for "accountability." They seem in some cases to distrust the ability of administrators; therefore, they feel a right to circumvent administrative decisions by any means possible. One educator, in addressing the question, "Is Anybody in Charge Here?" states that it makes little difference whether an administrator has the authority to make and enforce regulations if the persons over whom authority is to be exercised refuse to accept it. If they refuse to accept it, then to all intents and purposes, regardless of the legal aspects involved, such authority simply does not exist.[11] Situations such as this which show a mistrust of an administrator's ability have caused many of them to vacate their posts. Others, even though they recognize that they are no longer entirely trusted, continue to "strive with joy."

The remainder of this chapter is devoted to a brief description of the group process, an important procedure in democracy, and to specific examples of how this technique can be employed in educational leadership situations which affect the process of education.

GROUP PROCESS

Group process, or democratic process, refers to the manner in which individuals function in relation to one another when working toward a common goal.[12] The term, although a generic one which refers to many and often vague modes of operation rather than to a specific method, usually presupposes some knowledge of and skill in one of three widely utilized theories about groups:

1. *the field theory,* generally attributed to Kurt Lewin, which stresses the individual and his or her relation to the group.
2. *the interaction process analysis* of Robert Bales, which places more emphasis on groups in an observational scheme, and
3. *the system theory* of George Homans, which stresses a set of principles drawn from behavioral psychology organized around the concepts of activity, interaction, and sentiment.[13]

---

[11] George E. Flower, "Is Anybody in Charge Here?" *Education Canada,* **11** (September 1971): 26–31.

[12] Hilda Clute Kozman (ed.), *Group Process in Physical Education* (New York: Harper and Bros., 1951): p. 99.

[13] Clovis R. Shepherd, *Small Groups* (San Francisco: Chandler Publishing Co., 1964): pp. 21–46.

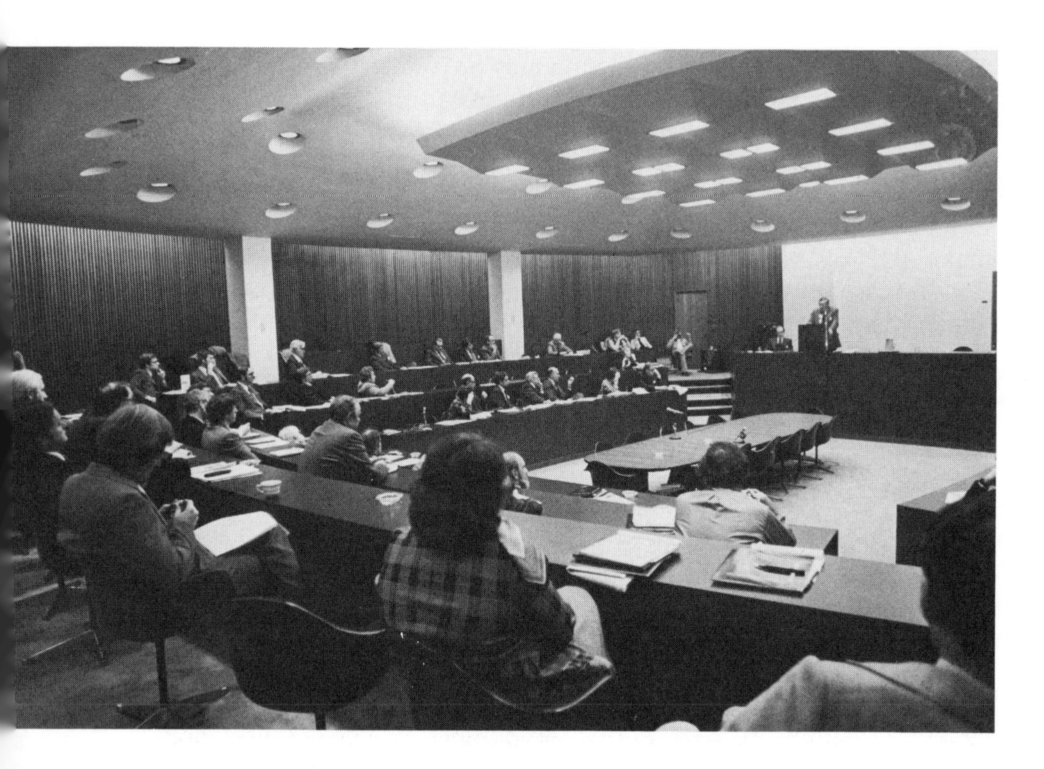

Fig. 2 Seating arrangements can facilitate the use of the group process. (Courtesy Kent State University Audio-Visual Services.)

According to Shepherd, each of these theories has merit in a specific situation, as the following quote shows.

> . . . Lewin's field theory seems to be most useful as a perspective with which to approach the analysis of a group. Bale's [*sic*] IPA seems to be the most useful as a scheme for the analysis of the behavior of members of a group, . . . and Homan's system theory seems to be most useful as a device to synthesize the findings of studies of small groups.[14]

Regardless of the basis of the belief in the worth of a particular theory, one of the outstanding characteristics of the group process is an emphasis upon cooperative social action. This implies that in any educational undertaking—whether it is the selection

---

[14] *Ibid.,* p. 36. Reprinted by permission.

of uniforms, the purchase of equipment, or a curricular decision—everyone participates to the best of his or her ability. This is based upon the belief that those who must abide by policies should participate in making them. Finally, underlying the entire process is the Jeffersonian tenet that people are basically moral, that informed people will come to agreement on fundamentals, and that intelligent, free inquiry will conquer wrong.

At this point it is well to indicate again that the administrative function is not relegated to a single level. One tends to think of the principal and superintendent as administrators which, of course, they are. However, as the modern school becomes more complex and more highly organized, there are many lower echelons of administration, such as department heads, deans of boys and girls, and guidance counselors. (See Fig. 1, Chapter 1.) Since the typical physical education teacher deals primarily with two of these administrators (the department head and the principal), most of the examples used in this chapter refer to these positions.

It is essential to recognize that leadership is not exclusively a function of administration. In a democracy, leadership is situationally centered and therefore leadership roles might be thrust upon teachers, parents, students, and custodians at various times. A cogent definition of educational leadership which implies this changing role, given by the Association for Supervision and Curriculum Development in its 1960 Yearbook, *Leadership for Improving Instruction,* is as follows: ". . . that action or behavior among individuals and groups to move toward educational goals that are increasingly mutually acceptable to them."[15] To prevent incorrect inferences from being made, it must be noted that democracy does not make leadership or administration easy. In fact, the opposite is more probably true. Nor does democracy demand that all people be leaders. However, democracy provides unparalleled opportunities for leadership to individuals whose natural or acquired talents qualify them for such positions. It provides opportunities for everyone, regardless of talent, to have a voice in the selection of leaders. And it demands that leaders operate within a framework of regulations which rest ultimately upon *the consent of the governed,* one of the basic beliefs of the founders of our Constitution. An acceptance of the concepts by the administrator may result in a value dilemma because although recognizing the role of the individual in

---

[15] Association for Supervision and Curriculum Development, 1960 Yearbook, *Leadership for Improving Instruction* (Washington, D.C.: Association for Supervision and Curriculum Development, 1960): p. 27.

the organizational structure, the administrator is at the same time aware of his or her own specialized knowledge and skill. Perhaps in the long run such inevitable value conflict may be healthy for the life of the organization.

Many theoreticians believe that the leadership role must be differentiated from the administrative role and even invested in different individuals. Some of them even suggest that leadership roles in an educational institution might better be borne by "human engineers" rather than scholar-teachers. At any rate, it seems imperative not only that the kinds of leadership which are needed to facilitate the educational process be more thoroughly researched and delineated, but that new and more tangible ways be found to apply present knowledge about leadership function and skills to the process of school administration.[16]

In order to develop specific examples of administrative or leadership tasks which are meaningful, it is perhaps imperative to supplement any somewhat nebulous definition of democracy with a more precise concept of the elements of democracy; this will then serve as a frame of reference for suggested practices.

No one definition of democracy is so generally accepted that it can function as a criterion for delineating examples of democratic practices, but this presentation will use the Elements of Democracy developed by the National Association for Physical Education of College Women[17] in 1948. These Elements, and a brief description of each of them, are given below.

Belief in the uniqueness and worth of each individual. The central value in a democracy is belief in the worth of the individual because he or she is an individual. This concept does not prescribe identical treatment for individuals who are of unequal ability, but it does advocate a policy of equal consideration for individuals whose needs may require different treatment.

Responsibility for one's own actions. In spite of the extreme worth of the individual, democracy does not imply unrestrained freedom of action. Nor does it restrict the freedom to be different. If freedom of difference in thought or action is intelligently directed so as not to restrict the rights of others, democracy encourages its

---

[16] Louis J. Rubin, *Frontiers in School Leadership* (Chicago: Rand McNally & Co., 1970): pp. 1–9.

[17] Professional Leadership Committee, National Association for Physical Education of College Women, *Practices of Promise in the Understanding and Use of the Democratic Process* (Boston: The Association, 1949): pp. 1–46.

maximum use. An awareness of what ultimate effect an individual's actions has on others is fundamental.

Belief and skill in cooperative action. Democracy values responsible cooperative action. Democracy, then, places a premium upon the group process. However, although the belief in cooperative action is easily embraced, the skill in cooperative action must be learned. This requires opportunities for practice. If such opportunities are frequent and under skilled leadership, learning is enhanced.

Awareness of democratic principles and of ways they are evidenced in one's actions. Democracy is an inclusive skill. It is possible for one to encompass many of the isolated skills underlying the first three Elements and yet not be effective in applying these skills in group action. Since democracy is based upon the right of the group to make its own decisions, skill in group action is imperative.

If, as suggested in Chapter 3, administrative policies ought to be written and distributed to all staff members, it would seem that a statement of administrative philosophy ought also to be written since such philosophy obviously undergirds all other policies and all administrative practices. Figure 3 is an example of a policy of this type which is presently in operation and which also expresses much of the philosophy presented in this chapter.

In the remainder of this chapter an attempt is made to show examples of specific practices under each of these Elements of Democracy which are functions of department heads and principals. Some of these duties were mentioned in Chapter 1, but here they are embellished within the framework of a specific mode of action. Finally, in order to show the role of the individual teacher in the democratic process, isolated examples of teacher responsibility are examined briefly. For the sake of emphasis, although it results in some repetition, each Element is discussed separately under each position.

The Principal

The roles of the principal in any given school situation are diverse. In addition to being responsible for the management of the building and other physical matters, and for maintaining good relations with the public, the principal is responsible for improving teach-

---

Kent State University

School of Health, Physical Education and Recreation

School Policy No. 19

Philosophy of Administration

The administrator is the key to effective administration since ultimate authority is legally invested in him. However, all administrative theory today recognizes the vital role of the individual to the overall administrative task. The competent administrator, the one who is truly a leader, as well as all the individuals working under him, must embrace the following tenets of democracy if the School of Health, Physical Education and Recreation is to function efficiently as well as humanely:

1. WE BELIEVE in the worth of each individual.
2. WE BELIEVE in the uniqueness of each person.
3. WE BELIEVE in decision making through cooperative action.
4. WE BELIEVE that all persons affected by a decision should have a role in the process of decision making, although not necessarily in the decision itself.
5. WE BELIEVE that all data pertinent to the decision-making process shall be available to those involved in making the decision.
6. WE BELIEVE that administrative authority functions through the consent of the governed.
7. WE BELIEVE that leadership is situationally centered.
8. WE BELIEVE that a function of administration is the implementation of policy.
9. WE BELIEVE that the administration is accountable to its faculty, its students, and, through its representatives in the University, to the State of Ohio.

THEREFORE, WE BELIEVE that all individuals and units within the School must ACT in a manner consistent with these beliefs and, likewise, all must assume the responsibility for their actions.

Fig. 3 Policy on administrative philosophy. (Reprinted by permission of Carl E. Erickson, Dean, School of Health, Physical Education and Recreation, Kent State University.)

ing-learning processes. He or she should always be cognizant of the primacy of this role, for in the long run it matters little whether the educational process is carried on in an architect's dream of a modern, efficient physical plant or in an old building which, though outmoded, is kept as clean and attractive as possible. The outmoded building may somewhat deter, but never obviate, effective teaching and learning.

Since the principal's primary role is to encourage good instruction and to evaluate and improve the curriculum, it is necessary for him or her to keep abreast of emerging trends and to try to incorporate them into the school. This task may be almost insurmountable unless department heads and others keep him or her informed of new theory in a particular field. Many physical educators have failed in this responsibility in the past. For example, how many principals are aware of the move toward a structured discipline of physical education revolving around human-movement phenomena, and away from the traditional approach to a teamsports-oriented curriculum incorrectly titled "gym,"[18] not to mention a conceptual, meaningful approach toward teaching such movement?[19]

Belief in the uniqueness and worth of each individual. The principal is responsible for a *planned* orientation of new teachers to the philosophy, goals, and policies of the particular school. Too often matters of this nature are not common knowledge, and a new teacher may unwittingly err, either by omission or commission.

The principal is the one person who can most foster a spirit of creativity among teachers by encouraging the use of experimental teaching methods and materials. He or she should not disapprove of an individual teacher's procedures until that teacher has had a sufficient period of time to prove or disprove their merit.

When faculty meetings are held, the atmosphere should be a permissive one which provides opportunities for one and all to express freely their opinions, needs, and problems without fear of reprisal. The faculty should feel free to formulate policies without administrative dominance. If conditions such as these exist, it is likely that there will be pleasant personal relationships among faculty members in spite of differences of opinions, since such a climate fosters mutual understanding and respect.

Instead of making all the decisions and informing the faculty

---

[18] Beverly L. Seidel and Matthew C. Resick, *Physical Education: An Overview*, 2d ed. Reading, Mass.: Addison-Wesley Co., 1978, pp. 1–10.

[19] Beverly L. Seidel, Fay R. Biles, Grace Figley, Bonnie Neuman, *Sports Skills: A Conceptual Approach to Meaningful Movement*. Dubuque: W. C. Brown Co., 1974.

of them in the form of administrative edicts, the democratic principal should appoint committees to solve problems and to formulate policies. The membership of such committees should be determined by interest and proficiency. Once appointed, the committees should be delegated authority along with responsibility. All decisions should be aired thoroughly before being put into effect.

Responsibility for one's own actions. It is rather obvious that this particular tenet has more application to an individual than to a position such as principal; however, there are some practices which are apropos. If faculty members are to feel a responsibility for their actions, they must be *encouraged* to act for the good of the school. Such actions are typified by continuous evaluation of curriculum, policies, and practices.

Belief and skill in cooperative action. Cooperative action such as planning sessions before the opening of the school year in which administrative functions are decentralized and shared is implied here.

A principal who encourages personal growth will do everything in his or her power to see that individual faculty members are allowed the time to attend professional meetings and are reimbursed for their expenses.

Not the least of the principal's obligations is to see that communication channels are open among faculty, administration, and students, and that such communication is conducted on an ethical basis.

Awareness of democratic principles and of ways they are evidenced in one's actions. The principal who is acutely aware of and sincerely believes in this tenet of democracy adopts an administrative philosophy aimed at releasing student and teacher powers rather than imposing rules and regulations. By the same token, the principal makes individual faculty members and students aware that decisions made by them carry attendant responsibilities.

The principal who encourages group action will make individuals feel a responsibility to contribute to discussions and decisions. Morale of the faculty will be high if such a climate is fostered.

The Department Head

It should be pointed out that many of the practices cited under "The Principal" could be reemphasized as functions of a department head. For example, just as the principal should orient new staff members to the philosophy and goals of the school, so should the department head orient all new staff members to matters which are unique to physical education, such as policies on uniforms, purchase of equipment, sharing of facilities, and grading. However, in order to avoid repetition, these are not mentioned. Also, it is apparent that many schools do not have department heads. (In this case it is hoped that the principal will see fit to delegate to some member of the physical education staff such responsibilities as familiarizing new staff members with departmental policies.) Nevertheless, this position is discussed because many schools do function under this type of administrative system and because the trend toward consolidation makes this position increasingly more plausible.

One of the most important duties of the department head is to keep informed of new developments in his or her field and to educate the principal and staff members about them. It stands to reason that staff members look to the department head for inspiration and assistance.

Belief in the uniqueness and worth of each individual. Perhaps one of the most significant contributions a department head can make along these lines is to encourage self-expression among individual staff members. If this is done, individual teaching methods and procedures may vary widely in spite of the fact that all are following the same course of study. Normally, one of the complaints most frequently voiced by teachers in large schools is that the prescribed course of study stifles initiative and creativity. It seems that this complaint could not be raised if the department head fulfilled his or her function. Along these same lines, surely the department head needs to guarantee that new teachers are observed and supervised to a certain extent. This observation does not have to be done by the department head; in fact, duties such as this should be delegated to some of the senior staff members on occasion. It should be pointed out, too, that in some cases such observation will also be conducted by a supervisor from the Board of Education. Regardless of how the operation is handled, the individual teacher should usually be informed of the upcoming visit and should subsequently receive the benefit of an evaluative session conducted in a constructive atmosphere. Not the least important part of this process is an awareness of the differences in individual capacities and therefore in expected accomplishments.

The department head needs to make possible periodic staff meetings in which problems are aired freely and differences of opinion are respected.

Now and then acute problems may arise which make it desirable to alter teaching schedules. The astute department head and an understanding staff will make such adjustment possible. Here empathy is more valuable than mere sympathy!

Responsibility for one's own actions. Through an understanding of the democratic process the department head fosters a climate which encourages staff members to attack departmental problems as a group, to suggest solutions, and to formulate policies. Occasionally a person may consider his or her work finished once a solution to a problem has been suggested. If so, it is the duty of the department head to make this staff member aware of his or her part in sharing the work and results accompanying the solution.

Unfortunately, the department head needs to emphasize to staff members that each of them is responsible for class management and group welfare and that the manner in which they fulfill assigned responsibilities reflects on them, the department, the school, and the profession.

Belief and skill in cooperative action. If cooperative action is desired, the department head must make such action possible. He or she can do this through regular staff meetings at which *all* staff members attend, where group and individual problems receive the benefit of staff attention. At such sessions, perhaps chaired by a different staff member each meeting, free expression of opinion is encouraged, an effort is made to draw any reticent individual into discussion, staff members refrain from using status such as seniority to influence decisions, and majority and minority groups are abetted in finding common grounds for constructive compromise.

Awareness of democratic principles and of ways they are evidenced in one's actions. In addition to the specific examples mentioned before, the following practices seem relevant. If the department head has indeed fostered a permissive atmosphere in which teachers are not bound by imposing regulations, the staff should be aware that their attendant responsibilities include such things as conducting classes in a democratic manner, contributing to group discussions and decisions, and reflecting departmental professional philosophy at all times. If certain staff members are not aware of this role, it is the department head's responsibility to so instruct them.

The Teacher and the Coach

The overall effectiveness of an instructional and athletic program will be little better than that of the weakest member of the staff. Principals and department heads are quick to point out that staff members often abrogate their leadership function and then project their ineffectiveness to the nominal leaders of the school. Democratic leadership practices do not end with the administration. Indeed, all the democratic administration in the world is of little avail if staff members do not show their conviction of the worth of the process by their actions.

Belief in the uniqueness and worth of each individual. Every staff member wants to be treated as an individual. He or she must recognize that all other staff members are individuals with ideas and opinions of their own. Each must be treated with integrity and each must be respected for what he or she is.

Responsibility for one's own actions. Unless each staff member feels an obligation to complete assigned work, the total function of the department and school will be disrupted.

A staff member should think through potential outcomes of staff action before voicing approval or disapproval. Once decisions are made, each member of the staff is expected to share in the work *and in the results* involved. It would be remiss not to mention that the latter point is one of the prime advantages of democratic action. All the people involved in making a decision must share in the responsibility for that decision. If results go awry, neither the principal nor any other single individual can be blamed. The group made the decision; the group must share in the consequences of the decision.

Belief and skill in cooperative action. A staff member who is allowed time and expenses to attend professional meetings has an obligation to be a conscientious, intelligent participant. Further, he or she should share impressions of the professional meetings with those from the staff who were unable to attend.

Just as the staff member desires open, professional lines of communication between self and the administration, so should the staff member keep open such avenues for communication with the students.

Members of the staff should feel a responsibility to voice fully their personal opinions regarding staff concerns; however, they should refrain from forcing their ideas on others.

Awareness of democratic principles and of ways they are evidenced in one's actions. Staff members who believe in this concept of democracy attempt to conduct their classes in a democratic manner, realizing that students learn democratic skills better through practice than through mere verbalization.

Each member of the staff must feel a responsibility not only to attend all staff and faculty meetings but also to voice opinions, make decisions, and accept the responsibilities which accompany the decisions.

SUMMARY

Democratic administration demands that all leaders justify themselves by being ever mindful of the rights, aspirations, and potentials of those being led. Leaders who are aware of this will delegate responsibility, authority, and various leadership functions to members of the group. In a democracy, final authority and responsibility rests with all individuals. Therefore, the members of a group need to relinquish to designated leaders only that degree of authority and responsibility which they themselves are incapable of handling. To quote Haiman:

> . . . leadership skills . . . are simply functions that need to be performed in any democratically operated group, and whoever can do them most conveniently and effectively should be turned to for leadership at that point. Every member of a democratic group should share leadership to the utmost of his ability. Hence, the man who is nominally *the* leader needs to fulfill only those responsibilities which the group itself, because of inability or inconvenience, cannot perform. The more mature the group, the less the man designated as leader will have to do.[20]

As was mentioned earlier in the chapter, education for democracy is generally accepted as one of America's basic needs. If this need is to be met as effectively as possible, leaders in education must constantly express by words and actions their faith in the democratic ideology, so that teachers will be inspired to accept their inimitable responsibility for the never-ending task of educating American children toward an acceptance of and belief in democratic values.

---

[20] Franklyn S. Haiman, *Group Leadership and Democratic Action* (Boston: Houghton Mifflin Co., 1951): p. 111. Reprinted by permission.

CASE STUDY

The physical education staff at Taylor High School consisted of two experienced teachers and three young relatively inexperienced instructors. They were completing a rather frustrating year in which they taught from a syllabus furnished by the principal. Since there was no appointed department head, the members of the department worked independently of each other.

The principal, a former physical education teacher, called periodic meetings of the group, but these meetings were generally merely reporting sessions. Little time was ever reserved for staff discussion.

The three younger instructors met informally once or twice and decided that they should seek some means of changing these conditions. They wished to become involved in the decisions that affected them and they truly felt that the curriculum could be improved. The two older and more experienced teachers listened to them but declared that they did not want to "rock the boat."

There was to be one more staff meeting before the end of the term. The three younger staff members met again to determine the best way to seek a change in the present procedure.

1. What are the issues in this case?
2. How should the three younger staff members seek involvement and change?
3. What principles of administration are involved in this case?

SELECTED REFERENCES

Association for Supervision and Curriculum Development 1960 Yearbook, *Leadership for Improving Instruction.* Washington, D.C.: Association for Supervision and Curriculum Development, 1960.

Association for Supervision and Curriculum Development, 1962 Yearbook. *Perceiving, Behaving, Becoming: A New Focus for Education.* Washington, D.C.: Association for Supervision and Curriculum Development, 1962.

Cohen, Michael D., and James G. March. *Leadership and Ambiguity.* New York: McGraw-Hill, 1974.

Coleman, Peter. "Leadership and Loyalty," *Education Canada,* **14** (September 1974): 29–37.

Crockett, William J. "The Management Conflict with Democratic Values," *Business Horizon,* **16** (October 1973): 13–19.

Danforth, W. H. "Management and Accountability in Higher Education." *A.A.U.P. Bulletin,* **59** (June 1973): 135–138.

Flower, George E. "Is Anybody in Charge Here?" *Education Canada* **11** (September 1971): 26–31.

Haiman, Franklyn S. *Group Leadership and Democratic Action.* Boston: Houghton Mifflin, 1951.

Kozman, Hilda Clute (ed.). *Group Process in Physical Education.* New York: Harper and Bros., 1951.

Lewin, Kurt. *Resolving Social Conflicts.* New York: Harper and Bros., 1948.

National Education Association, Educational Policies Committee. *Learning the Ways of Democracy.* Washington, D.C.: The Association, 1940.

Padover, Saul K. *The Living U.S. Constitution.* New York: The New American Library of World Literature, 1953.

Professional Leadership Committee, National Association for Physical Education for College Women. *Practices of Promise in the Understanding and Use of the Democratic Process.* Boston: The Association, 1949.

Rubin, Louis J. *Frontiers in School Leadership.* Chicago: Rand McNally, 1970.

Seidel, Beverly L., and Matthew C. Resick. *Physical Education: An Overview,* 2d ed. Reading, Mass.: Addison-Wesley, 1978.

Shepherd, Clovis R. *Small Groups.* San Francisco: Chandler Publishing, 1964.

Teller, Gerald. "What Are the Myths of Accountability?" *Educational Leadership,* **31** (February 1974): 455–456.

3

ORGANIZATIONAL POLICIES AND PROCEDURES

STUDY STIMULATORS

1. What is a workable definition of a policy?
2. What are the relationships among policies, principles, and rules?
3. What are the purposes of establishing administrative policies within a department of physical education?
4. What suggestions can be made in order to expedite the formulation of policies for a department?
5. What areas of administration should be covered by policies in order to increase the efficiency of a large department of physical education and athletics?
6. What factors determine the type of administration adopted by the faculty or administration of a department of physical education and athletics?
7. How do crisis situations affect decision-making and policy-making?

Since it is reason which shapes and regulates all other things, it ought not itself to be left in disorder.

EPICTETUS

All administration takes place within the structure of an organization, whether it be formal or informal. Even within the formal organization there are informal groups. Good administration is determined by the decision-making process, and therefore the organization of any unit, educational or not, should be constructed to enhance the process of decision-making. The military type of organization may not be the most feasible for an educational institution.

Since decisions are rarely independent of all other action, there is a need to give guidance or directions to the decisions being made by the members of an organization. Griffiths states:

> Practically every decision is one of a *sequence.* It is almost impossible to determine which decision on a certain state of affairs was the original decision. Furthermore, it is almost impossible to determine which decision of all those made is a unique one. Each decision made appears to tie into another decision reached previously. From this we note the sequential and interrelated nature of decision. This is a deviation from the dictionary or commonly accepted definition in that a decision rarely terminates or settles a controversy: it alters, changes its direction, or sometimes prolongs it.[1]

Most decisions are not made from policies and generalizations or principles. Most problems come unannounced and are consid-

---

[1] Daniel E. Griffiths, *Administrative Theory* (New York: Appleton-Century-Crofts, Educational Division, Meredith Corporation, 1959): p. 76. Reprinted by permission.

ered acute at the time they appear, even though sometimes they can be anticipated. As soon as one begins to formulate policies, one reverses this logical sequence of events. Hansen points this out in the following statement:

> Finally, decisions aren't really made in the way that most of us tend to think: they aren't made by reasoning from general principles of human values, educational goods, or great moral verities. They are made by going from a whole host of specifics to an ultimate generalization derived from these specifics. Whether we like it or not, decisions are made inductively, from specific to the general, rather than deductively from the generalizations to the specific. This is complicated, but it is important for as soon as we try to make decisions within a framework which insists that decisions must derive from a general principle rather than from the specific situation at hand, we are reversing the clear logic of the practical decision-making process.[2]

Special problems arise in times of a crisis; hence, many of the options normally considered in a decision are ignored. In times of crisis important values may be overlooked because the decision time is short, because of emotional tensions at the time of the crisis, or because of the threatening behavior of those involved (crowd control). Under these conditions there is not the usual careful weighing of evidence and the anticipating of consequences. Also under stress the decision maker has a tendency to use the consultative services of others to a lesser degree, and as a result may make more aggressively personal choices. Once practice is established under these circumstances, it is difficult to change when normal deliberations indicate that the decision made under stress was not the correct one.

For these and other reasons which are shown later in this chapter, it is almost mandatory that most organizations arrive at the point of policy formulation at the earliest possible time. Personnel within the organization must perform the functions assigned to them which entail the making of vital decisions. However, the implementation of a policy is the responsibility of the administrator under whose jurisdiction the policy was formulated.

---

[2] K. H. Hansen, "Design for Decision," *National Association Secondary School Principals Bulletin,* **51** (November 1967): 105. Reprinted by permission.

POLICIES DEFINED

Policy statements are found all the way from governmental agencies to plant management. There is, however, just as great a range of interpretations of the meaning of the word "policy" as there are types of organizations. A cursory examination of any dictionary would uncover such meanings as "shrewdly prudent procedure in any affairs," "prudence, practical wisdom or expediency," or "course dictated to prudence or expediency." Since policies are vital to the decision-making process as discussed earlier in this chapter, the following definition is proposed: *A policy is a statement of a prudent course of action adopted and pursued by an organization.* A policy is not to be confused with either a restricted rule or a broad concept or principle. It must have a degree of flexibility necessary for decision making within its framework and yet must set the guidelines which result in a degree of consistency of performance. Many of the statements found in policy bulletins are so restrictive that they demand enforcement rather than interpretation and application. Shea and Wieman illustrated the distinction when they used the following examples:

> Rule
>
> All students (in this institution) must maintain an overall academic average of 2.0 in order to be eligible to participate in extra-curricular student activities.
>
> Policy
>
> All students, including distinctive groups, should be required to demonstrate satisfactory levels of academic achievement to assure qualitative and quantitative progress toward a degree as determined by the faculty of an institution.
>
> Principle
>
> The establishment and maintenance of scholarly standards of performance for students in institutions of higher learning represents the chief means of providing assurance that the primary function and purpose of these institutions in relation to their role in the continuing development of the person, and in preparing a well-prepared, active, and contributing citizenry for this nation will be fulfilled.[3]

Thus it can be seen that rules and regulations, policies and principles, perform specific functions within the framework of the organization of any institution. Although principles influence poli-

---

[3] Edward J. Shea and Elton E. Wieman, *Administrative Policies for Intercollegiate Athletics* (Springfield, Ill.: Charles C Thomas, 1967): p. 55. Reprinted by permission.

cies, the remainder of this chapter will deal only with policies and their impact upon the administration of the physical education program.

THE PURPOSES OF ADMINISTRATIVE POLICIES

The formulation of a set of policies is a demanding and time-consuming process. The results of this work must prove the work of the operation. Some of the purposes of writing a set of policies are the following:

1. A set of policies reveals the ends or goals of the department. A review of a set of policies brings to light the philosophy of the department as expressed in operational terms.
2. A set of policies permits the staff to translate alternatives into action. This ensures some degree of expediency, since ground covered need not be crossed again in like problems.
3. A set of policies prevents inconsistency in solutions which might occur if problems were solved without regard to past performances.
4. A set of policies permits a degree of flexibility in the solution of local problems not possible under ironclad rules and regulations. This allows a group with divergent views to operate within the framework of the policies.
5. A set of policies performs the function of good public relations, since others are made aware of the bases of decisons which are not compatible with their own views.
6. A set of policies helps the staff realize that decisions which affect them adversely are not made on a personal basis.

SUGGESTIONS FOR THE FORMULATION OF POLICIES

Policy making is an arduous and time-consuming task which may involve a number of people. A number of ways this procedure can be expedited are listed below.

1. The staff should be involved in the planning and writing of departmental policies. Sharing the responsibility for formulating policies brings with it the responsibility for seeing that they are adhered to by the group.

2. Conflicts should be anticipated and policies set up to avoid them. For example, when a school has an extensive out-of-doors program, a rainy day schedule should be ready. Or when a heated rivalry comes to the crucial point, the staff should be prepared to offer protection to the fans, participants, and officials.
3. Talents on the staff should be utilized. Some staff members have the insight to see through to the heart of problems, while others are expert in writing proposals. Both types can contribute.
4. Policies should be written and distributed to all members of the staff and to superiors within the organization. It is preferable to keep one format and even one color of paper to attract the attention of the reader to the fact that this is a policy statement. A loose-leaf-type policy booklet permits easy revision.
5. Policies should not be made so restrictive that they become rules and regulations with no chance for deviation from them. The administrator cannot be placed in a straitjacket, but rather must be guaranteed some degree of flexibility.
6. Policies should be reviewed periodically. When the conditions warrant it, they must be revised. Small changes can be handled simply by making addenda.
7. All facets of administration cannot be covered by policies. As with all good things, policies can be overdone. Until there is evidence of need, policies should not be written.

AREAS NORMALLY COVERED BY POLICIES

In business or education policies may be few or many and in some cases likened to a large city telephone directory. In the area of physical education and athletics there are some areas which lend themselves to coverage by a series of departmental policies. Among these are the following:

Policies that govern relationships with outside agencies. If the city recreation department is a separate entity, are the facilities of the school available to it? Under what conditions? What is the relationship with the alumni concerning tickets, parking, and service? What is the role of the Boosters' Club? If services are needed, what is the relationship with the City Health Department?

Policies that govern relationships with other departments within the school. If the school has its own doctor and nurse, who determines whether an athlete is fit to play? Who determines whether a student is fit to take part in an activity? If the gymnasium is a multipurpose unit, what factors determine the right of the drama club to have play practice? What factors determine the right of the band to practice on the game field the day before a big performance? What is the procedure for obtaining proper custodial services for special events?

Policies that govern the line chart of responsibilities (chain of command). To whom can a staff member appeal for a review of a superior's decision when it seems unfair or discriminatory? To whom is a staff member responsible under changing circumstances?

Policies that govern the use of facilities within the department. What group has priority for the use of the gymnasium floor at different times of the year: intramural teams, girls' activities groups, or varsity teams? Is dancing allowed on the floor? When and under what conditions?

Policies concerning safety provisions. Are medical examinations required of all students? What procedures follow an accident or group calamity? Is insurance provided for all students? for athletes? In the case of an athletic injury, what types of medical services are available? What types or kinds of supervision are mandatory for dangerous activities?

Policies concerning budgeting and finance. Who is responsible for the budget allocations to the various activities? How is equipment borrowed, checked out, and returned? Who oversees the repair of equipment?

Policies concerning professional activities of staff. Are staff members given any compensation for the expense of attendance at conventions and clinics? How are substitute teachers obtained and who pays them? What is the procedure for arranging to have a staff member accompany students on an authorized field trip?

Policies concerning class administration. Under what conditions may a student be excluded from a physical education class? What procedure must be followed? What is the policy on dress for class? on showers? on tardiness? What is the policy on locks and lockers?

Policies must be made according to local circumstances. Some of the above may be used in certain schools and entirely unnecessary in others. The larger the administrative unit, the more necessary it becomes to formulate policies in any of the above areas. Figure 1 is a copy of a sample policy bulletin.

Department of Health, Physical Education
and Athletics

Policy Bulletin No. 1 October, 1978

Medical Care and Supervision

1. All students who participate in physical education classes must produce evidence of a physical examination.
2. Students injured in class will be given first aid treatment. Any further treatment is to be rendered by the family physician or medical center.
3. All students must have on file in this office a medical emergency card signed by the parents or guardian. (Cards are distributed to all students the first day of class.)
4. All costs or expenses incurred as a result of an accident are to be borne by the family.
5. School insurance is available to cover accidents and injuries of this nature. Parents may wish to purchase this insurance or they may wish to make their own arrangements.

George A. Lee, Head
Department of Health, Physical
Education and Athletics

Fig. 1 Sample of a policy bulletin.

CASE STUDY

Miller Senior High School is the only high school in a medium sized city. Up to the present, facilities have been adequate, but recently the department head has felt a pinch. It had been the practice to permit outside groups to use both the pool and the gymnasium for a nominal fee.

In recent weeks the requests were becoming more numerous and were coming from small groups such as a single scout troop. The requests were made far in advance so that, although the facility was free at the time, it was difficult to predict what school groups would want to use it. As a result Mr. Lee, the Department Head, found himself denying requests of students in his own school on the grounds that the facility, gymnasium or pool, was already booked for that date.

The students complained to the principal and also to their parents. Several of the parents called the school to express their unhappiness with the conduct of this phase of the school's administration.

1. What are the essential factors in this case?
2. What solutions are open to Mr. Lee?
3. How can this confusion be prevented in other facets of the organization?

SELECTED REFERENCES

Fuoss, Donald E., and Robert J. Troppmann. *Creative Management Techniques in Interscholastic Athletics.* New York: Wiley, 1977.

Griffiths, Daniel E. *Administrative Theory.* New York: Appleton-Century-Crofts, 1959.

Hall, J. Tillman, et al. *Administration: Principles, Theory and Practices with Applications to Physical Education.* Pacific Palisades, Calif.: Goodyear Publishing, 1973, Chap. 2.

Hansen, K. H. "Design for Decision," *National Association of Secondary School Principals,* **51** (November 1967): 105–113.

Havel, Richard C., and Emery W. Seymour. *Administration of Health, Physical Education, and Recreation for Schools.* New York: Ronald Press, 1961, Chap. 6.

Holsti, Ole R. "Crisis, Stress and Decision Making," *International Social Science Journal,* **23** (1) 1971.

Sells, James. "Need a Staff Policy Book?" *The Physical Educator,* **18** (May 1961): 61–62.

Shea, Edward J., and Elton E. Wieman. *Administrative Policies for Intercollegiate Athletics.* Springfield, Ill.: Charles C Thomas, 1967, Chap. 3.

Voltmer, Edward F., and Arthur A. Esslinger. *The Organization and Administration of Physical Education* (4th ed.). New York: Appleton-Century-Crofts, 1967, Chap. 3.

4

LEGAL RESPONSIBILITIES OF TEACHERS, SUPERVISORS, AND COACHES

STUDY STIMULATORS

1. What is negligence? What factors are necessary for proof of negligence?
2. How does civil law differ from criminal law?
3. Why are the individual teachers responsible for acts of negligence in most states?
4. What are the moral and legal implications of a teaching contract?
5. On what grounds may contracts be terminated?
6. What are the areas of potential danger in physical education?
7. How can a teacher or coach guard against lawsuits?

Every man is equally entitled to protection by law....

ANDREW JACKSON

Teachers, supervisors, and coaches are not expected to receive a legal education prior to assuming their responsibilities within the school. However, their future, their family's welfare, and even the school's welfare may be placed in jeopardy by a single preventable act. When this statement is combined with the facts on the hazardous areas in physical education, one can see that the situation has the potential to be explosive. Fortunately, the test for the behavior of physical education teachers is usually the behavior of a prudent physical education teacher, however nebulous this may sound. Then, too, the teacher is aided by (1) the lack of knowledge of the general population concerning its legal rights, (2) the legal precedence which has already been established in regard to the school, and (3) recent changes toward the legal responsibilities of school districts and away from those of the individual. These points will be expanded in other parts of this chapter.

This chapter is written to provide the teacher and prospective administrator with the information which will enable them to function more effectively within the legal framework of their environment. The authors hope that they can accomplish this by pointing out areas of potential negligence, by exposing certain legal fallacies, and by explaining a few simple legal principles on which the responsible teacher may base his or her behavior. The excuse "But I didn't know" is no more valid in the case of a school accident than in the breaking of a speed law. The principle of "unqualified action" is in force here. Stated simply, this principle means that one is ignorant in this area at one's own risk, whether the question at stake is a motor violation or a certified teacher's failure to perform a duty. The very fact that a person is certified by the state as a teacher in the area of physical education presupposes his or her awareness of the areas of potential danger to students from the environment or those conditions imposed on the teacher. Unlike the ostrich, the teacher must be alert to the possibilities of problems before they arise.

It is not the purpose of this chapter to threaten readers with imminent dangers within their profession or to have them refrain from teaching certain bona fide activities because there are hazards inherent in them. Generally, the courts have been exceedingly generous in their interpretations of the risks involved in physical education and have justified the position of the vigorous activity in schools, since the values outweigh the risks. The physical educator should not regard this teaching field in a lesser light.

Since most states still follow the concept of common law, in a legal sense the teacher bears the burden of carrying out the activities program. In essence she or he is the administrator and as such must be aware of the legal implications of his or her position.

THE HAZARDS IN PHYSICAL EDUCATION AND ATHLETICS

Since children are in the act of moving, the gymnasia and playing fields are the sites of more accidents than almost any area in the school setting. This is particularly true at the junior and senior high school levels as shown in the statistics in Tables 1 and 2. From a sampling of over 35,000 accidents under school jurisdiction it was determined that the majority of them occurred on the playfields, in physical education classes, during intramural activities, or during interscholastic sports. The accidents in the latter two categories occur most often at the junior and senior high school levels, as can be expected.

The courts are well aware of the danger potential inherent in these activities. However since it is assumed that no instructor or coach would willfully or wantonly cause injury to a student in his or her charge, all instructors and coaches must avoid negligence, in the legal sense, by being aware of the areas of potential injury or accident, as shown by the figures in these tables.

Table 1 Student Accident Rates for Boys by School Grade*

Location and Type	Totals	K	1–3	4–6	7–9	10–12	Days lost per injury
Shops and labs	.61	0	†	.03	1.01	1.95	.65
Buildings general	1.60	1.82	1.08	1.33	2.41	1.66	.89
Grounds unorganized activities	1.68	1.40	2.62	2.70	.73	.23	.99
Apparatus	.34	.67	.78	.36	.03	.01	1.39
Ball playing	.36	0	.26	.85	.23	.08	.86
Running	.45	.32	.68	.78	.20	.03	.92
Grounds miscellaneous	.43	.29	.47	.54	.44	.29	.97
Physical Education	3.19	.27	.66	2.05	5.92	5.98	1.14
Apparatus	.24	.09	.11	.20	.42	.34	1.24
Class games	.28	.10	.16	.31	.41	.30	.79
Baseball (hardball)	.04	0	.01	.04	.04	.07	.98
Softball	.20	0	.04	.26	.31	.29	1.10
Football	.15	0	.01	.04	.30	.38	1.74
Touch football	.31	0	.01	.12	.62	.71	1.36
Basketball	.53	.01	.01	.13	1.02	1.40	1.07
Hockey	.02	0	0	.02	.02	.05	1.01
Soccer	.15	0	.02	.15	.27	.20	1.10
Track and field events	.15	.01	.01	.09	.38	.21	1.73
Volleyball and similar games	.14	0	.02	.10	.21	.31	1.00
Other organized games	.43	.02	.13	.32	.80	.69	1.10
Swimming	.06	0	0	†	.09	.20	.94
Showers and dressing rooms	.09	.01	†	.02	.24	.16	1.02
Intramural sports	.22	0	†	.08	.41	.59	.84
Interscholastic sports	.87	0	†	.04	1.20	3.16	1.00
Special activities	.06	.05	.01	.06	.07	.12	1.47
To and from school (MV)	.19	.40	.22	.13	.20	.15	3.55
To and from school (not MV)	.26	.31	.34	.31	.24	.11	1.54
Total school jurisdiction	9.11	4.55	5.41	7.27	12.63	14.23	1.08

* *Accident Facts*, 1972 edition (Chicago: National Safety Council): p. 90. Tables are based on reports of more than 35,000 school jurisdiction accidents which occurred during the 1968–69 school year. The rates shown denote the number of accidents per 100,000 student days. Reprinted by permission.

† denotes less than 0.005.

Table 2 Student Accident Rates for Girls by School Grade*

Location and Type	Totals	K	1–3	4–6	7–9	10–12	Days lost per injury
Shops and labs	.09	.01	†	.01	.17	.22	.53
Buildings general	.98	.68	.66	.84	1.35	1.17	.99
Grounds unorganized activities	.94	.87	1.46	1.67	.24	.12	1.09
Apparatus	.26	.38	.56	.34	.03	.02	1.36
Ball playing	.13	0	.06	.41	.05	.01	.87
Running	.26	.19	.45	.42	.06	.04	1.11
Grounds miscellaneous	.24	.29	.25	.31	.16	.20	1.39
Physical Education	1.89	.14	.52	1.45	3.66	2.72	1.04
Apparatus	.30	.08	.14	.17	.57	.41	1.25
Class games	.21	.02	.12	.27	.30	.20	.90
Baseball (hardball)	.01	0	†	†	.02	†	.83
Softball	.12	0	.01	.13	.25	.12	.97
Football	†	0	0	0	.01	†	1.00
Touch football	.01	0	0	.01	.03	.03	2.06
Basketball	.21	0	†	.05	.47	.45	.75
Hockey	.02	0	0	†	.02	.07	.46
Soccer	.10	0	†	.09	.23	.12	.98
Track and field events	.09	0	.01	.09	.20	.09	1.32
Volleyball and similar games	.20	0	.03	.12	.42	.35	.70
Other organized games	.28	.01	.10	.30	.45	.34	1.18
Swimming	.05	0	†	.01	.10	.09	.66
Showers and dressing rooms	.05	0	†	.01	.13	.08	.99
Intramural sports	.04	0	.02	.04	.06	.04	2.66
Interscholastic sports	.04	.01	†	.05	.05	.10	2.28
Special activities	.05	0	.02	.06	.06	.11	1.52
To and from school (MV)	.14	.29	.13	.14	.14	.19	8.26
To and from school (not MV)	.17	.16	.19	.14	.14	.13	1.33
Total school jurisdiction	4.57	2.45	3.25	4.66	6.02	5.00	1.32

* *Accident Facts*, 1972 edition (Chicago: National Safety Council): p. 90. Tables are based on reports of more than 35,000 school jurisdiction accidents which occurred during the 1968–69 school year. The rates shown denote the number of accidents per 100,000 student days. Reprinted by permission.

† denotes less than 0.005.

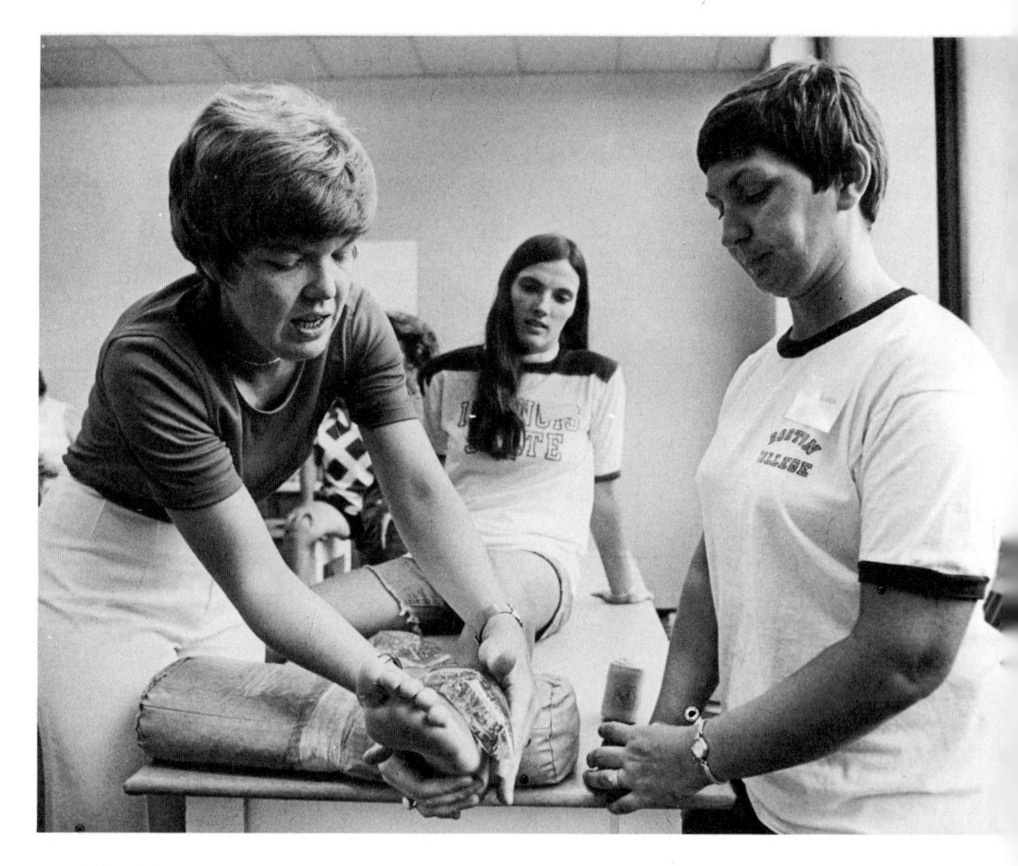

Fig. 1 Treatment by trained personnel. (Courtesy of Indiana University News Bureau.)

Negligent Action

Negligence, in the legal sense, is the *unintentional* failure to perform one's duties up to the standard expected of a prudent individual under similar circumstances. At times it would seem that the prudent individual is a figment of the imagination of the court and the twelve people who make up the jury. Ordinarily, teachers and coaches are judged by what action their peers would expect under similar circumstances. The fact that a teacher is certified by the state indicates a degree of expected behavior. Good intentions do not safeguard the wrong-doer against being subjected to a lawsuit, since negligence denotes an unintentional failure on the part of an individual.

SOURCES OF LEGAL RESPONSIBILITIES

The legal responsibilities of school personnel stem from a number of diverse sources and, at times, confuse both the experienced teacher and, especially, the neophyte. Sometimes even the legal profession must gain clarification from a higher tribunal. An examination of some of the principal sources of laws and regulations reveals the following.

The Federal Constitution and the State Constitution. The Constitution of the United States outlines legal responsibilities of individuals by what is implied and written in the Bill of Rights and what is purposely omitted. Specifically, the Fifth, Seventh, Ninth, and Tenth Amendments to the Constitution are significant in this respect. These are given below.

> *Amendment 5* No person shall be held to answer for a capital, or otherwise infamous crime, unless on a presentment of indictment of a Grand Jury, except in cases arising in the land or naval forces, or in the Militia, when in actual service in time of War or public danger; nor shall any person be subject for the same offence to be twice put in jeopardy of life or limb; nor shall be compelled in any criminal case to be witness against himself, nor be deprived of life, liberty, or property, without due process of law; nor shall private property be taken for public use, without just compensation.
>
> *Amendment 7.* In Suits at common law, where the value in controversy shall exceed twenty dollars, the right of trial by jury shall be preserved, and no fact tried by a jury, shall be otherwise re-examined in any Court of the United States, then according to the rules of the common law.
>
> *Amendment 9.* The enumeration in the Constitution, of certain rights, shall not be construed to deny or disparage others retained by the people.
>
> *Amendment 10.* The powers not delegated to the United States by the Constitution, nor prohibited by it to the States, are reserved to the States respectively, or to the people.

Common law. The concept of common law is inherited from our ancestors in Europe, especially England, as is much of our judicial system. The entire concept of common law is based on the former principle of sovereign immunity, whereby the king or queen could do no wrong. Although sovereign rule was rejected in this country, the rights of sovereigns were transferred to other governmental patterns and the agencies within these patterns. In essence, school districts and school boards are considered arms of the state government and as such are immune to legal action resulting from negligence unless this immunity is removed by statutory law. Most states are still considered basically common-law states with only slight changes in statutory law which may waive the immunity of boards, protect teachers or give them immunity, or permit the purchasing of insurance and other such deviations. The trend is definitely toward an increasing number of statutes which are replacing common law in the area of negligence within the school.

State statutes. Laws passed by state legislatures supersede common law as specified by that particular piece of legislation. This legislation may remove the entire concept of immunity or may give local boards permission to act independently on some phases of the negligence problem. Several examples of these variations are found in the examples of legislation given below.

1. The governing board of any school district is liable as such in the district's name for any judgment against the district on account of injury to person or property arising because of the negligence of the district, or its officers or employees.
2. Boards of education are authorized to purchase insurance for purposes of paying damages to person(s) injured in school.
3. Governmental immunity of the boards of education is waived to the extent of the insurance purchased.

Interpretation of the law. When the legislature of a state passes a law, the citizens of the state may question its meaning. At this point they may have just two means of recourse at their disposal. First, if they disagree with the legislation, they may make a test case and have the matter brought before the courts. Second, they ask the attorney general for a clarification or interpretation of the law. The opinions by the attorney general may still be challenged in the courts. In some cases, the interpretation of the attorney general remains in effect for decades until another overt action is initiated. A case in point is the opinion of the Attorney General of Ohio in 1933 on the question of whether tax monies could be used to buy athletic equipment. He stated:

> . . . I am of the opinion that the term physical education which the statutes of Ohio direct shall be included in the curriculum of the public schools of Ohio does not include what is commonly called 'interscholastic athletics', that is the playing of games in competition by picked teams representing the several schools. Interscholastic ath-

> letics is not a proper school activity within the scope of 'physical education' as the term is used in our statutes. That being the case, it is not a proper subject for which the Director of Education may, in his discretion, prescribe or approve as part of the courses in physical education and therefore it is not within the powers of a board of education to expend public funds for necessary 'apparatus' to enable the school teams to engage in such interscholastic athletics or to support or promote such activities in any respect.[1]

This ruling determined the course of expenditures of monies for athletic programs until the Attorney General was again asked for his opinion in August 1962. After studying the 1933 opinion, the 1948 opinion, and several court decisions from other states, he replied:

> Despite the full control and supervision of interscholastic sports, I concur with the 1933 opinion that the board of education cannot use public funds from general or special taxes to equip students participating in interscholastic football.[2]

At a later date the legislature passed a law permitting a limited use of monies for athletics by local boards. The reader can see the force of the interpretation of the law by duly constituted officers.

Precedence. As we saw in the previous section, the force of a precedent may influence the opinion of the attorney general. How a case was decided in a state many miles removed may have much weight upon a civil trial for negligence in a local court. Lawyers for both defendant and plaintiff call upon the courts to consider decisions in similar cases or cases involving similar legal principles.

City ordinances. The city is chartered by the state and hence has the power to pass such ordinances as are necessary to make the municipality a safe place in which to live, earn a living, and rear children. At times, the ordinances of a city may be in variance with the laws of the state. They can be more stringent but cannot be more lenient. For example, in the case of an "attractive nuisance" such as a swimming pool, the state may demand that the pool be surrounded by hedges, but the city ordinance may demand that it also be surrounded by a metal fence equipped with a lock. The teacher and the school are bound by the ordinances of the city within which the school is located.

---

1 *Auditor's Messenger* (Columbus, Ohio: Auditor of the State, State of Ohio, April 1964): p. 2.

2 *Ibid.*, p. 2.

School board rulings. The schools of the states are chartered by the state boards of education under systems of standards set up by the state boards. The individual school boards have the right to make rules and regulations concerning the standards for admission, dress, curriculum, and conduct of students within this framework. So long as these rules and regulations are reasonable, the board may punish the offender for infraction of these rules by commensurate punishment, which may include suspension or dismissal.

Civil Law versus Criminal Law

The reader will find it easier to distinguish between civil law and criminal law by thinking of the latter as concerning offenses against the state and of the former as involving offenses against an individual or a group of individuals. A person may be tried in both civil and criminal courts, and in fact a person found guilty of a criminal act may be more apt to be found guilty in a civil suit. This does not constitute what is known as "double jeopardy," or the retrial of an individual at the request of the state. Under this principle, a person found innocent of a crime may not be retried, even when additional evidence pointing to his or her guilt is uncovered.

Under civil law only a preponderance of evidence is needed for guilt (and the guilt may be partial or shared). All jurors need not be convinced of the defendant's guilt. On the other hand, under criminal law guilt must be established "beyond a reasonable doubt"; the guilt cannot be only partially established, and all jurors must agree on the guilt of the defendant.

The remainder of this chapter is concerned with the civil law as it affects the liability of individuals for negligence.

Factors Necessary for Proof of Negligence

Any person can sue another for negligence. If repeated suits become harassment, then the defendant may ask the court for an injunction against additional suits. Fortunately, negligence is difficult to prove and many individuals who wish to sue are discouraged by their lawyers when there are insufficient grounds for legal action. In a case of negligence, the following factors must be present.

1. The defendant must have a "duty" toward the plaintiff. In many states a person does not have a legal duty toward a stranger even though the stranger's life may hang in the balance. Since lawsuits have arisen from cases of improper aid, some states have passed

forms of "good samaritan" laws. These have been passed in order to encourage people to aid others in difficulty. In recent years the newspapers have carried stories of cries of help being unanswered in times of drownings, murder, rape, and accidents. In the state of Ohio, persons giving first aid outside the hospital or doctor's office cannot be sued unless they either get or expect remuneration for the help they give.

Teachers, supervisors, and administrative personnel have a duty toward the students entrusted into their care.

2. A "tort" or wrong must have been committed to the plaintiff, his or her property, or character. His or her physical or mental health may have been impaired; his or her books, clothing, watch, or vehicle may have been damaged; or his or her character may have been defamed.

3. The person having the duty must have "breached" that duty by an act of omission (nonfeasance) or an act of commission (misfeasance). In other words, a person with a duty cannot always avoid trouble by doing nothing at a time when a decision is to be made. That person who does nothing is often as liable as one who performs his or her function incorrectly.

4. The commission or omission of duty presented in (3) above was directly related to the injury itself by an unbroken chain of events. In other words, the act was the *proximate* cause of the injury. A series of events which are unbroken in their effect upon the other may lead to a tort or wrong to a person.

Teachers may fail to act in their capacities as teachers or they may act imprudently, but if no tort or harm results, then that teacher cannot be held for negligence, even though the act may have been an unwise one in the eyes of all concerned. Action against such teachers must be administrative rather than legal. All four factors mentioned above must be present in order for the case to be one of legal negligence.

Defenses Against Liability for Negligence

It is often stated, rather facetiously, that when one faces a lawsuit the best defense is a good lawyer. Although the statement contains more than a little truth, the lawyer too looks for defense in one of several factors. These are:

Assumption of risk. There are inherent dangers in most physical activities. Ordinarily, the benefits from physical activity outweigh the possible dangers. It is on this premise that physical education is justified as a subject within the schools. There is also danger involved in chemistry, home economics, and industrial arts, as well as driver education. At a sporting event, both spectators and players assume a normal risk. From the spectator's standpoint, a risk is assumed when a person goes to a baseball game and sits in the stands. A foul ball may fall on him or her or strike one after hitting another object. Although assuming the possibility of this danger, one does not assume the risk of being hit by a can of beer from the the stands above or of being hit by a bat thrown into the stands by an angry player. The risks that players face are numerous. The football player assumes the risk of a broken leg; the basketball player assumes the possibility of having a hand broken; and the wrestler assumes that a shoulder may be dislocated.

In any sport, when an accident occurs which is a result of normal occurrences in that sport, the players assume the responsibilities of these injuries.

Acts of God. There are some acts which cannot be foreseen by mere mortals. These are called pure accidents, or acts of God. Of course, God is often blamed for many misfortunes that are caused by humans. When an accident occurs which probably could have been foreseen, the person responsible for this act often blames God as a defense. If a sewer line running under a field were to collapse suddenly while students were on the field, the resultant injuries would probably be considered accidents. On the other hand, if a golf coach were to send the players out onto the course during a severe electrical storm and the lightning struck one of the players, the coach might be hard put to justify that action as one of a prudent individual.

Contributory negligence. Occasionally a person disregards advice and warning in performing an act. When an accident occurs under these circumstances, the person may have contributed to the accident by the negligent actions. Under these circumstances the person responsible is relieved of liability, in spite of a breach of duty by omission or commisssion of some phase of responsibility. In schools the children above the third grade are deemed to be responsible persons. Beyond this point each person is judged by how other members of his or her peer group would react under similar conditions. The ability to read, respond to directions, and to reason are factors which determine the nature of contributory negligence.

In several states comparative negligence is used to determine liability for a tort. The negligence of the injured is compared with the negligence of the person responsible for the student's welfare. A judgment is made on the basis of which negligence affected the course of action to a greater degree.

The lack of a proximate cause. As was indicated in the section on "proof of negligence," since an unbroken chain of events is necessary for proof of negligence, a break in the chain of events absolves the person for the damages beyond the break in this chain of events, even though the actions before this break were of an imprudent nature. An example of this situation is a case in which a student with a back injury was moved by a teacher without medical assistance. Although the student suffered no serious consequences at the time, he or she later reinjured the back at home and became paralyzed. The teacher would not be held responsible for the paralysis of the student.

Permission and Waiver Slips

Teachers and coaches at times work under the assumption that permission and/or waiver slips are a safeguard against a charge of negligence. Nothing could be further from the truth. Each of these factors should be treated separately, although they both may be combined in one notice to the parents or guardians.

A permission slip simply gives the school the right to permit a student to take part in an activity. It also serves to inform the parents that there are assumed possibilities of injury, no matter how remote.

A waiver slip, in contrast to a permission slip, requests that the parent disclaim any right to bring suit for damages suffered in the activity in question. The fallacy of this procedure lies in the fact that neither parents nor guardians may waive the rights of minors. Very recently a young man brought suit for an injury he suffered eight years earlier at a junior high school. He was within his rights since in his state the statute of limitation was two years after a minor reached the age of twenty-one. Problems arise for both the plaintiff and the defendant when the evidence is dependent upon the memories of all participants and witnesses. Although the length of time might seem unfair to the defendant, any changes in the law to rectify this condition might lead to the loss of other rights for minors. Some states have removed this right of minors to sue by changing the statute of limitations.

The waiver slip may well deter the minor from suing, since he or she may be unaware of his or her rights under the law. However, a more positive protection for the teacher is obtained by purchasing liability insurance. This functions much like the malpractice insurance carried by the members of the medical profession. Such a policy can be obtained as part of a home owner's policy or as part of a professional association membership. Most states have passed laws which permit the school boards to purchase liability insurance to cover transportation of students. Such insurance may protect the driver, the pupil, and the school board.

Another positive step the teacher can take is to record all accidents carefully with statements by witnesses and participants. An accident form should be available to facilitate the recording of all facts. Records of serious accidents should normally be kept beyond the time determined by the statute of limitations in the state in which the accident occurred.

Contracts

Coaches, teachers, and supervisors go through their professional lives signing contracts without being fully aware of the consequences of these signatures. There are a number of different types of contracts for which they are responsible. Among these are the standard teacher's contract, the supplemental contract for extracurricular duties, contracts with suppliers of materials, and contracts with other institutions. Most of these contracts have common elements.

Contracts are legally binding documents which involve consideration from both sides. (For the teacher it indicates the expectation of services for a specified sum of money.) These contracts are binding upon both parties for the length of time specified in the contract or until it is broken by mutual consent. Fulfillment can be enforced by law. Contracts are interpreted in the public interest as expressed in relevant statutes. Unless there is evidence to the contrary, the courts will sustain the spirit of the contract under the assumption that the parties involved had a legal purpose in mind when they signed the document.

Contracts begin with the offer and terminate with a fulfillment of the terms by both parties. An offer is legally binding unless it is terminated by the passage of a specified time, by a withdrawal before acceptance, by a rejection by one to whom it was offered, or by a counteroffer by the one to whom the original offer was made.

A contract is deemed to have been accepted when signed, prior to a withdrawal date, by a person of legal age and of sound mind. Prior to fulfillment a contract may be terminated for a number of reasons. Among these are: (1) either of the parties involved failed to perform without a legal excuse, (2) one of the participants made the contract while concealing pertinent information, and (3) the participants agreed mutually to terminate the contract.

Since public school contracts involve Boards of Education, there are several considerations which should be discussed. Boards of education cannot legally delegate their authority to any of school's administrative personnel. This includes the Superintendent of Schools, who nonetheless might well do all the preliminary negotiations with the person to be employed. Contracts with school personnel, in most states, can only be completed at the meetings of the Board which have been legally called. Any contract with a Board of Education implies adherence to the regulations of the Board and also to those regulations it may make during the tenure of the contract.

Although the teacher signs a contract annually, he or she may be on a continuing contract, or *tenure*—the right to hold a position indefinitely. Tenure is granted to a teacher with suitable experience and education who has proved his or her ability during a probationary period. Under these circumstances the teacher must be given a contract every year unless a drastic charge of immorality, inefficiency, or gross insubordination is proved at a hearing. Tenure, and the security it provides, may bring out better performance in the teacher, but in some instances the institution is saddled with a teacher whose incompetence was not discovered during the probationary period. At the college and university level, tenure is determined by the individual institutions and published in the faculty handbook. The probationary period varies according to professional rank.

The trend in many states now is to handle all coaching and intramural assignments with a supplemental contract. This permits the Board to pinpoint responsibilities such as Head Coach of Football and Assistant Coach in Basketball separately from the terms of the primary teaching contract.

Several years ago long-term contracts were in vogue in the college and professional coaching ranks. Many of these were broken, some under undesirable circumstances. There were instances where coaches wanted the security of the long-term contract without the responsibility of fulfilling the same. Buying up the contract of a professional coach at a set percentage of its tenure value has been practiced. Occasionally, when this could not be arranged, professional teams were paying the salaries of three managers simultaneously.

There are several other types of contracts associated with athletics, in addition to those of personnel, such as: (1) game contracts between institutions, (2) contracts with game officials, and (3) (in larger institutions) contracts dealing with concessions at athletic contests.

At times, moral considerations are strong enough to void a contract. A school system ordinarily will not stand in the path of professional advancement by one of its staff unless the educational process of that school system would be measurably impaired. The teacher and coach have a moral responsibility to fulfill the contract when such impairment might result. Neither the school nor the teacher can achieve much gain when a teacher is kept unwillingly or when a school system must retain a teacher beyond his or her point of effectiveness.

Areas of Potential Negligence and Liability

Since legal judgments are based on how a prudent person would act, by implication an individual is expected to be able to foresee the areas of potential danger and thus avoid the possibilities of injury to children. As was pointed out earlier in this chapter, as a subject in the school system, physical education has many areas of concern from the standpoint of student safety. In the following paragraphs these areas are explored so that the reader may become aware of some of these responsibilities. It is impossible to list all areas of concern, but typical examples will serve as guidelines to actions in similar activities and circumstances.

Poor selection of activities. A certificated teacher is assumed to possess the knowledge of both the nature of the activities in his or her field and the growth and development levels of the students under his or her care. The teacher is then obligated to select those activities within the range of experience of the students and which contribute to the students' development. The over-zealous teacher at times may select activities beyond the capabilities of some of the students in the class. If an accident occurs during such an activity, the teacher may be asked to defend that choice of activities either in an open meeting or in a court of law. In either case the teacher may be forced to support that position with evidence. The first source of such evidence might well be the syllabus or course of study developed by the teachers who teach in the school system. A second source may be the curricular guide normally accepted by the profession. Still another source is the testimony of curricular experts in the field.

Provisions for individual differences. Accidents in physical education are readily avoidable by a common-sense approach to teaching. No student should be forced or shamed into participating in an activity she or he feels is beyond personal capabilities, although such a student may be encouraged to extend those capabilities. Furthermore, activities of an extremely difficult nature should be reserved for the interest clubs rather than the normal physical education classes.

Provision of protective procedure. In activities in which protective equipment is mandated by the safety of the students, any deviations from the use of such equipment should be carefully avoided. Sports such as football, baseball, field hockey, and fencing are generally played with equipment which has been accepted as essential for the welfare of the participants. When drills or practices are conducted without this protection, the instructor must maintain much closer supervision than is normally necessary. Similarly, safety harnesses are sometimes necessary for such activities as tumbling, apparatus, and diving, and headgear should be worn in activities like wrestling to prevent injuries to the ears and head.

Accidents that could have been prevented if protective equipment had been used are difficult to explain or defend. Since the nonuse of these articles is just a matter of haste, laziness or unwillingness to put up with some discomfort, the defense of such action in a court of law is extremely difficult.

Hazardous conditions. Since physical activities have many inherent dangers to participants, a competent teacher should try to eliminate all hazards that can be foreseen. Whenever possible, all hazardous obstacles should be removed from the play areas. Among those found in the indoor play areas are sharp corners or edges on the walls or portable baskets, swinging doors which open onto the playing areas, and portable seats which extend into this space. In the outdoor play areas "chuck holes" due to washouts, ice formations in early spring and late fall, and light poles which are unpadded near the sidelines are the more common obstacles. In the latter case a few bales of straw wrapped around these posts would offer a great deal of protection.

The instructor or coach in any of these areas is responsible for reporting these conditions and either alleviating them or scheduling events so as to avoid such areas.

Use of faulty equipment. The responsibility for the maintenance of equipment in a usable and safe condition rests primarily with the teacher and coach. If after reporting (in writing) unsafe equipment, a teacher is told to continue the activity, the responsibility normally shifts to that teacher's superior. A daily inventory of all equipment might disclose such faulty equipment as frayed climbing ropes, faulty trampolines and diving boards, faulty swings and slides, and faulty gymnastic equipment, including mats. Whenever playground equipment is found to be hazardous, in addition to reporting this to the proper authorities, the teacher or coach should make the equipment inoperable. A comprehensive quarterly inventory should be made at which time a thorough inspection of all equipment is made and conditions recorded.

All safety equipment such as headgear and pads should also be carefully inspected. A faulty face guard may result in a fractured nose or a pierced eye. Sometimes something as innocuous as a repaired baseball bat may lead to a legal action if the repaired bat breaks and results in an accident to one of the participants. All high school and little league coaches have gone through the procedure of repairing bats at some stage of their careers. One lawsuit resulted from the use of baseball bats which did not have large enough knobs on the handles.

Inadequate supervision. School children are entitled to supervision throughout the school day both within the classroom and during free play. Most states simply demand that supervision be adequate for the surroundings. Thus a play area that is divided into segments by the design of the buildings may necessitate additional supervisory personnel. Supervision must also be maintained in the halls, the locker rooms, and the shower rooms. Since the physical education program includes outdoor space and indoor space, together with locker and shower areas, the task of supervision becomes complicated. Early dismissal of a portion of the class may result in a problem in the shower or locker areas. The law, although not clear, has been interpreted to mean that "area" supervision is sufficient, since the instructor cannot be everywhere at one time.

It is always assumed that the instructor has given directions as to expected behavior in the different areas under his jurisdiction.

Poor selection of play sites. Although the instructor may have to contend with inadequate space, the utilization of the area available becomes a potential problem. Thus, for example, the use of a common boundary between two adjoining basketball courts or of two overlapping outfields in softball have both been made issues in separate court cases. Yet many teachers are forced to use the limited space they have in this way to guarantee additional or greater participation.

Selecting a play area near a street becomes dangerous when students are forced to retrieve balls that have rolled into the street and in the face of oncoming traffic. Fields in this type of area should be surrounded by cyclone fence. The expense can never equal that of a maimed or killed child under these circumstances.

Field events need special consideration since there have been several recorded deaths from the shotput and discus throwing. These two activities should be practiced and performed where errant tosses will not result in injury to other participants or spectators.

Running cross-country meets across streets and highways should be avoided whenever possible unless police protection is available.

Attractive nuisances. Laws concerning attractive nuisances vary widely in the different states. Whereas an off-limits or no trespassing sign may be sufficient in one state, a locked cyclone fence may not be sufficient in another. The equipment in the gymnasium and the swimming pool are attractive to young people. Climbing ropes, swings, and trampolines are especially enticing and should be put away or made inoperable even when one hour elapses between usage, unless the gymnasium can be secure at all times. Doors to the swimming pool should have special locks and these should be closely scrutinized so that access becomes impossible at times other than when use is controlled.

Track equipment such as vaulting poles, javelins, and even hurdles should be removed and stored when not in use. In addition to the preventing of injuries, these procedures help keep the equipment in good condition.

In the gymnasium, if climbing pegs are used, the lower ones should be removed to prevent unsupervised use.

Transfer of confidential information. In general, educators in school systems of the same or higher order freely exchange information on the personal and academic development of the students. In one county in Ohio, the question of the legality of transferring information on personal behavior was raised. The issue was resolved by the transference of only that information which could be verified. This may serve as a guideline for those who wish to maintain the practice of exchanging this type of information with other school systems.

Improper organization. Occasionally activities are so organized that the students are in danger of being struck by other members of the class. For example, using a single mat for continuous tumbling may result in an accident. The use of lines in relays without proper intermittent space may cause children to be hurt needlessly.

Imposition of unreasonable squad rules. There have been literally hundreds of cases litigated which concerned the length and style of hair worn by athletes when these styles were in opposition to squad rules. Approximately half of these cases were found in favor of the athlete. Then, too, the number of court cases that dealt with drinking, dormitory behavior, and dress codes helped to overload the court calendar.

Unreasonable eligibility rules. Most of these types of cases are found at the college and university levels. At times, conference eligibility rules differ from those of the member institution. Whenever an athlete's eligibility or scholarship is threatened, there is always the possibility of a lawsuit. Most of these cases are settled by the answer to a basic question or premise: Is participation in athletics a privilege, or is it a right? If it is a right, all other students in the institution must be bound by the same restraints. The courts have not always agreed with this latter premise.

The rights of an individual to compete. Recently there have been a number of law suits filed to make varsity competitive opportunities accessible to girls or women on teams which were formerly open only to boys and men. Along the same line, the right of a legal adult to move to a new community and be eligible for interscholastic competition, regardless of the parents' residence, has caused concern in athletic administration.

Examples of lawsuits in the preceding paragraphs may be found in a fine compilation by Appenzeller entitled *Athletics and the Law,* as found in the references at the end of this chapter.

Proprietary Function versus Governmental Function of Schools

Earlier in this chapter the governmental function of schools was explained. As the sovereign arms of the state, schools cannot be sued unless such provisions are made by statutes. Thus in their governmental capacities, schools, represented by the boards of education, can be sued only through the passing of special provisions. However, at times the boards of education function as the proprietor of a building or buildings which are bought, sold, leased, or rented. The protection that the school board enjoys in its governmental role does not apply in its dealings in business or when it is making a profit from an activity. When the school board rents a facility to an agency, it is serving in its proprietary function, and as such, may be liable for any torts committed. In many cases, this is extended to include those events for which the school charges admission. Among these activities are plays, exhibitions, and athletic contests.

Respondeat Superior and Supervisor's Responsibility

Respondeat Superior is the responsibility of one person for the acts of employees or subordinates. Under common law as it developed in England, the master was responsible for the acts of all servants. Since the ultimate master in the public schools is the state, the common law mentioned above was in conflict with the common law which proclaimed that the state could do no wrong. Therefore, in common law the principle of Respondeat Superior was not enforceable. To permit the passing of responsibility to a higher authority (for example, the school district), the states passed legislation that permits the waiving of immunity in either specific selected torts or in all cases of negligence. Most states waive immunity only for accidents which involve school transportation.

As a general rule, supervisory personnel, since they serve only in an advisory capacity, are not included in the direct line of responsibility for negligence that applies to the teachers within a school system. For instance, when a teacher is working in a hazardous system, relief of responsibility can be received only by written permission from the department head or principal.

Wanton and Willful, or the "Cheap Shot"

This chapter was devoted mainly to the acts of negligence or unintentional failure to perform one's duties. Recently there has been a rash of incidents in both professional and amateur sports which may be described as wanton and willful acts. Professional sports have tried to deal with these problems by a series of severe fines and suspensions. Amateur sports have the option of suspension, but lack the regulatory agency to levy fines.

Recently the Illinois Appellate Court handed down a verdict (*Nabozny* v. *Barnhill*) which may serve as a precedent and have far-reaching influence for future cases dealing with injuries inflicted beyond the scope of fair play. The basis of the ruling was that: (1) players involved are trained and coached by knowledgeable personnel; (2) a recognized set of safety rules governs the conduct of competition; and (3) these safety rules are designed primarily to protect the players from serious injury. A reckless disregard for these rules cannot be excused. A player is liable for injury in a tort action if his or her conduct is such that it is deliberate, willful, or with reckless disregard for the safety of the other players.

Perhaps a few lawsuits settled in favor of the plaintiff would reduce the number of incidents of bat-throwing, the use of the beanball, and "blind siding" after the whistle has blown.

General Conclusions

Although the field of physical education is among the most hazardous of all teaching areas, there needs to be very little restriction on the quality of the programs planned and executed for the students. The courts are well aware of the inherent risks in physical activities and thus acknowledge the fact that the values exceed the risk expectancy. It is assumed that programs are based on knowledge of the needs of children and are executed by well-trained and prudent instructors. As a result, very few suits are concluded with adverse results to the instructor. This chapter was written to alert the administrator and instructor to their rights and responsibilities under the law.

CASE STUDY

Rope climbing was the activity of the day in Mr. George's twelfth grade class. As Tommy Smith returned to his squad after a climb, he remarked to Mr. George that the rope looked frayed at the upper attachment. Mr. George thanked him and walked over to the rope, looked up, gave the area a cursory examination, and then proceeded to his office.

The next day the class met at the same hour, and after several other activities, they proceeded to work on rope climbing. At the midpoint of this activity, Charlie Long, a 200-pound senior took his turn and just as he neared the top, the rope gave way and Charlie crashed to the floor. The floor was covered with a single mat. Charlie hit the floor with a thud and lay in a twisted position.

Mr. George gave Charlie first aid treatment and summoned medical assistance. Charlie was taken to the hospital where it was discovered that he had received a spinal injury and would not have the use of his legs in the immediate future, if ever. Within a month, Mr. George was informed that he was being sued for negligence.

1. What are the essential issues in this case?
2. What are the possible outcomes and legal bases of these?
3. What legal principles are found in this case?

SELECTED REFERENCES

Accident Facts, 1972 edition. Chicago: National Safety Council, 1972.

Appenzeller, H. *Athletics and the Law.* Charlottesville, Va.: The Michie Company, 1975.

Auditor's Messenger, Columbus, Ohio: Auditor of the State, State of Ohio, April 1964.

Chambless, Jim R., and Connie J. Mangin. "Legal Liability and the Physical Educator," *Journal of Health Physical Education Recreation,* **4** (April 1973): 42–43.

Grieve, Andrew. "State Legal Requirements for Physical Education," *Journal of Health Physical Education Recreation,* **42** (April 1971): 19–23.

Hofeld, Albert F. "Athletes—Their Rights and Correlative Duties," *The Trial Lawyer's Guide,* Vol. 19. Chicago: Callaghan & Company, 1975, pp. 383–406.

Johnson, T. Page. "The Courts and Eligibility Rules: Is a New Attitude Emerging?" *Journal of Health Physical Education Recreation,* **44** (February 1973): 34–36.

Leibee, Howard C. *Liability for Accidents in Physical Education, Athletics, and Recreation.* Ann Arbor, Mich.: Ann Arbor Publishers, 1952.

Muniz, Arthur J. "The Teacher, Pupil Injury and Legal Liability," *Journal of Health Physical Education Recreation,* **33** (September 1962): 28.

National Education Association Research Division. *Who is Liable for Pupil Injuries?* Washington, D.C.: National Commission on Safety Education, National Education Association, 1963.

Nolte, M. C. *Duties and Liabilities of School Administrators.* West Nyack, N.Y.: Parker, 1973.

Rice, Sidney W. "A Suit for the Teacher," *Journal of Health Physical Education Recreation,* **32** (November 1961): 24–25.

Shroyer, George F. "Legal Implications of Requiring Pupils to Enroll in Physical Education," *Journal of Health Physical Education Recreation,* **35** (May 1964): 51–52.

———. "Personal Liabilities of Secondary School Physical Educators," *The Physical Educator,* **21** (May 1964): 55–56.

5

PERSONNEL ADMINISTRATION

STUDY STIMULATORS

1. What is the principal purpose of personnel programs?
2. What avenues might a prospective teacher follow in seeking employment?
3. What functions does the department head perform in personnel management?
4. Communication is essential for good organizational behavior. What are some considerations for proper communication within an organizational unit?
5. Personnel benefits often determine staff morale. What areas must be considered under this topic?
6. How can personnel grievances be dealt with in an academic setting?

If men are to be precluded from offering their sentiments on a matter, which may involve the most serious and alarming consequences that can invite the consideration of mankind, reason is of no use to us. . . .

GEORGE WASHINGTON

The resolution of problems dealing with personnel is one of the greatest challenges the administrator has to face. It is the administrator's duty to attempt to keep staff members working at their individual optimum capacities and in harmony with other staff members. This is a difficult task requiring constant sensitivity and a thorough knowledge of human relations.

Over the years society has developed an educational system that prepares individuals to assume professional and staff positions in major social institutions including education, industry, business, government, and hospitals. All these institutions have developed personnel programs designed to create the most favorable conditions possible for employees. The objective of personnel programs is to aid the individual employee to develop maximum effectiveness in his or her work.

Departments of physical education and athletics are staffed by individuals with academic degrees and expertise in specialized activities. As in every department in an educational institution, the administrator of the department of physical education and athletics has a duty to administer the most effective personnel program possible.

This chapter deals with (1) recruitment and selection of teachers, (2) personnel management, and (3) personnel benefits.

RECRUITMENT AND SELECTION OF TEACHERS

Since the success of any department in a school depends on the quality of the staff, great care should be exercised in selecting staff members by personnel directors of school districts.

Recruitment and selection of teachers requires that the person searching for a teaching position and representatives of the school district be brought together. This is made possible in three principal ways:

1. *College and University Placement Bureaus.* Most colleges and universities have placement bureaus. Their function is to assist students in obtaining positions in many areas of endeavor, including teaching. When students reach their senior year they should contact their university placement bureau to obtain and complete the necessary application forms. A copy of a student's transcript is usually required. The placement bureau staff maintains contact with representatives of school districts that are searching for teachers and invites them to the campus to interview prospective candidates, or school districts request permission to send representatives to the campus to screen candidates. University placement bureaus advertise in school newspapers, on bulletin boards, on campus radio and television stations, and by other means, the schedule of school district representatives who will visit the campus and the kinds of teachers they are seeking. Students may then sign up for an interview at a specific time with a particular representative.

2. *School District Personnel Departments.* Central administration offices in most school districts maintain personnel departments. The number of persons assigned to the personnel department depends upon the size of the school district. One of the functions of the personnel department is to recruit and select teachers for new positions or as replacements for teachers who have resigned. In a small school district recruitment and selection of teachers may be a function of the superintendent or assistant superintendent of schools. In the larger school systems a director of personnel and staff will be responsible for recruitment and selection of teachers.

The Department of Health, Education and Welfare now requires that teachers be employed in individual school districts in direct ethnic ratio to the numbers of students, for example, Anglo, Mexican-American, and black.

3. *Private Teachers' Agencies.* Private teachers' agencies are located in many of the major metropolitan areas of the United States. Their function is to assist public school systems, colleges, and universities, which are searching for faculty, to locate qualified persons and to provide a placement service for individuals who seek teaching or administrative positions in education.

A teacher who registers with private teachers' agencies pays a nominal fee. In addition, the teacher must agree to pay the agency a percentage (usually five percent) of his or her first year's salary if the agency obtains a position for the individual.

Regardless of whether the person applies for a position through the university placement bureau, a school district personnel department, or private teachers' agency, there are certain general procedures followed by the applicant. These procedures include the completion of application forms, submission of an official university transcript, recommendations from professors and other individuals familiar with the professional and personal qualifications of the applicant, and a personal interview.

PERSONNEL MANAGEMENT

To conduct an effective physical education program, a competent staff must be assembled. The size of the staff obviously depends on the number of students to be served and the magnitude of the physical education and athletic programs. The staff includes a department head, a given number of instructors and/or athletic coaches, and support personnel (secretaries, locker room supervisors, and maintenance persons).

As the key person on the staff, the administrative head's principal job is to provide leadership, to mold all staff members into a coordinated group working effectively to achieve the departmental goals (see Chaps. 1, 2). In addition, the department head is responsible for the general organization, administration, and supervision of the total program. The department head's duties include:

1. interpreting and implementing the policies of the institution;
2. interpreting and implementing the specific policies of the physical education department;
3. recommending changes in policies when the need arises;
4. representing the department in policy matters both inside and outside the department;

5. making emergency decisions;
6. providing continuous evaluation and appraisal of the department to ensure that adequate standards are being met;
7. establishing sound standards for the financial operation of the department;
8. attempting to keep all areas of the department in proportion and balance;
9. assigning staff members to their respective duties;
10. recommending the appointment and promotion of staff members.

In addition, the department head must be concerned with communication, e.g., keeping all staff members informed of the changes that affect them. The department head must maintain good relations with the principal and other school district administrators, must delegate responsibility and authority, and, finally, should have an advisory council of senior staff members to advise him or her on important departmental matters.

Qualifications of the department head include the desire to be an administrator and knowledge of administrative skills, integrity, intelligence, good human-relations skills, excellent health, professional knowledge, decision-making ability, and the desire to accept responsibility.

Staff members of the physical education department should possess the same qualifications as other teachers in the school systems; for example, the bachelor's or master's degree (in physical education) and state teacher certification. Besides being skilled in teaching and coaching a wide variety of sports activities, the staff person should be capable and comfortable in at least one or two activities. The staff member is expected to get along well with other members of the staff and to fit into the general operation of the department and the school.

Orientation

Most school systems provide an orientation program for new teachers. The object is to help these faculty members become acquainted with the operation of the school system as rapidly as possible. The program includes meetings to discuss such diverse topics as policies, rules and regulations, and the benefits provided by the school system, plus other pertinent information.

In-service Education

Progressive school systems include in-service education for teachers as part of their personnel program to improve the teaching-learning process and to help teachers update their knowledge. In practice, in-service education is conducted in specific disciplines by appropriate departments. For example, the department of physical education might conduct workshops for physical education teachers in new techniques of teaching swimming, golf, tennis, first aid, or any other physical education activity. In athletics, workshops may be conducted in new concepts and methods in any one of the varsity sports offered in the school district athletic program.

Code of Ethics

All professions have developed codes of ethics as guides for the conduct of the members of that profession. The profession of education is no exception as shown by codes of ethics developed by organizations such as the National Education Association and the American Association of University Professors. Some years ago a committee of the American Alliance for Health, Physical Education and Recreation prepared a code of ethics for the guidance of teachers of physical education. It is an excellent statement and still applicable today. Following is the preamble and code of ethics:

> *Preamble:* Believing that the strength of our American democracy and its influence upon the course of events everywhere in the world lies in the physical, mental and moral strength of its individual citizens; believing that the schools of America possess the greatest potential for the development of these strengths in our young citizens; believing that the teachers of physical education have a unique opportunity, as well as a responsibility to contribute greatly to the achievement of this potentiality; believing that all teachers of physical education should approach this great responsibility in a spirit of true professional devotion, the American Association for Health, Physical Education, and Recreation proposes for the guidance of its members the following:
>
> PRINCIPLES OF ETHICS
>
> 1. Inasmuch as teachers of physical education are members of the teaching profession, the American Association for Health, Physical Education, and Recreation endorses without reservation the Code of Ethics for Teachers, adopted by the National Education Association.
>
> 2. The aim of physical education is the optimum development of the individual. To this end teachers of physical education should conduct

programs and provide opportunities for experiences which will promote the physical development of youth and contribute to social, emotional, and mental growth.

3. In a democratic society every child has a right to the time of the teacher, to the use of the facilities, and a part in the planned activities. Physical education teachers should resist the temptation to devote an undue amount of time and attention to the activities of students of superior ability to the neglect of the less proficient.

4. The professional relations of a teacher with pupils require that all information of a personal nature shall be held in strict confidence.

5. While a physical education teacher should maintain a friendly interest in the progress of pupils, familiarity should be avoided as inimical to effective teaching and professional dignity.

6. The teacher's personal life should exemplify the highest ethical principles and should motivate children to the practice of good living and wholesome activities.

7. To promote effective teaching, the teacher of physical education should maintain relations with associates which are based on mutual integrity, understanding, and respect.

8. The physical education teacher should cooperate fully and unselfishly in all school endeavors which are within the sphere of education. He should be an integral part of the school faculty, expecting neither privileges nor rewards that are not available to other members of the faculty.

9. It is an obligation of the teacher of physical education to understand and make use of proper administrative channels in approaching the problems encountered in education and in schools.

10. It is the duty of the physical education teacher to strive for progress in personal education and to promote emerging practices and programs in physical education. The teacher should also endeavor to achieve status in the profession of education.

11. Professional ethics imply that altruistic purpose outweighs personal gain. The teacher, therefore, should avoid using personal glory achieved through winning teams for the purpose of self-promotion.

12. It is considered unethical to endorse physical education equipment, materials and other commercial products for personal gain or to support anything of a pseudo-educational nature. Nor should a teacher profit personally through the purchase of materials for physical education by the school.

13. It is the responsibility of the teacher of physical education to acquire a real understanding of children and youth in order that he may contribute to their growth and development. To achieve this under

standing, it is essential that an earnest effort be made to foster and strengthen good school-home-community relationships.

14. It is the duty of every teacher of physical education to become acquainted with and to participate in the affairs of the community, particularly those concerned with making the community a better place in which to live. The teacher should take an active interest in the work of the various child- and youth-serving agencies, participating as a citizen, and as a leader of children, youth and adults.

15. Inasmuch as physical education will progress through strong local, state, and national organizations, the teacher of physical education is obligated to membership and active participation in the proceedings of professional organizations, both in general education and in the specialized field of physical education.

16. Institutions preparing teachers of physical education have an ethical responsibility to the profession, to the public and nation for the admission, education, and retention of desirable candidates for teaching. To meet this obligation, curriculum offerings must be in harmony with the highest standards of professional education.

17. Teachers of physical education should render professional service by recruiting qualified men and women for future teachers of America. The physical education teacher also has a professional obligation to assist in the learning, practice and understanding of student teachers in the field.[1]

Staff Morale

The morale of the staff of the department of health and physical education is the responsibility of the department head. However, it is also essential that all staff members cooperate to create the best morale possible (see Chap. 2).

The basis for good staff morale is good administration. This implies excellent leadership by the department head, a well-conceived plan for the progress of the department with a clearly stated aim and well-developed objectives. In addition, it implies excellence in curriculum, finance, facilities and equipment.

If good staff morale is to be attained, the department head must have concern for the staff and their welfare and must create an atmosphere of trust, honesty, and openness in the department, for example, through the delegation of responsibility and authority. The staff must realize the department head is interested in their

---

[1] Committee on Professional Ethics, "Suggested Code of Ethics for Teachers of Physical Education," *Journal of Health Physical Education Recreation* (June, 1950): pp. 323–324, 366. (Reprinted by permission of the American Association for Health, Physical Education, and Recreation.)

professional growth and that they will receive recognition for a job well done.

An aid to staff morale is the realization by staff members that they are a part of a recognized quality program. Within the department there must be a reliable communication system and adequate staff meetings to keep the staff well informed. Policy making must be shared by all members of the staff affected by the policy.

Other factors that provide for positive staff morale are: equitable work loads, both teaching and additional duties; satisfactory working conditions, which include adequate facilities, equipment, and reasonable class size; a salary which provides a decent standard of living; opportunities for promotion; and personnel benefits which provide for adequate welfare of individual staff members. Job descriptions also aid in staff morale. If staff members understand their exact duties and the parameters are established, doubts are eliminated.

The goal of personnel management is to obtain the best level of performance possible from each individual over a long period of time. The department head establishes the level of performance for the staff—sets the tone for the staff. If a department head who is dedicated to the work, on the job and available, who gets things done, and is constantly working to improve the department is likely to receive optimum performance from the staff. The department head's job performance tends to be emulated by the staff. Personnel management functions best when the department head has obtained the confidence of the staff by his or her honesty, sincerity, ability, and day-to-day actions. When the department members believe they are given every opportunity to grow professionally and when they are rewarded for good work (both on and beyond normal assignments), staff members will produce to the best of their ability.

Differentiated Staffing

One of the major problems of school administrators is how to make most effective use of teaching personnel. One of the new plans to capitalize on teacher strengths and individual differences is differentiated staffing.

Differentiated staffing has been described in *Nation's Schools:*

> There is no precise definition, but it implies a restructuring and redeployment of teaching personnel in a way that makes optimum use of their talents, interests, and commitments, and affords them greater autonomy in determining their own professional development. A fully differentiated staff includes classroom teachers at various respon-

sibility levels and pay—assigned on the basis of training, competence, educational goals and difficulty of task—subject specialists, special service personnel, administrative and/or curriculum development personnel (who may also teach a percentage of their time) and a greater number of subprofessionals and nonprofessionals, such as teaching interns and teacher aides.[2]

A public secondary school using the differentiated staffing concept for the physical education department might be organized as follows: instead of the traditional five instructors of equal status, there is one directing teacher and four staff teachers plus several paraprofessionals and aides. The staff teachers in the differentiated staffing plan may be at various levels ranging from a beginning level for new teachers with limited duties confined mainly to instruction under supervision (teachers at this level are on a probationary basis) through experienced teachers that teach with little or no supervision, and directing teachers who, in addition to teaching, may be involved in curriculum development, in-service training and serving as team teaching leaders, to the directing teacher who directs the physical education instructional program and is responsible for in-service training, research, long-range planning, and the administrative elements.

Another aspect of the differentiated staffing plan is the use of paraprofessionals and aides. Paraprofessionals usually have accumulated some college credits and knowledge of a specific field, in this case physical education. The paraprofessional may assist the staff teachers with both group and individual instruction, as well as the many peripheral duties involved in conducting classes. Aides are individuals with limited educational background but some technical or clerical abilities that can be of great value to a physical education department.

The concept of differentiated staffing has much merit and should be given consideration as a means of improving staff effectiveness.

ORGANIZATIONAL BEHAVIOR

Managing People Effectively

To obtain the goal of personnel management, which is the maximum level of performance possible for each individual in the department, the administrator must have an understanding of the fundamentals

---

[2] "Differentiated Staffing," *Nation's Schools*, **85** (June 1970): 43. Reprinted by permission.

of effective management of people. Following is information to aid administrators in this important task.

Human interaction. Physical educators, like all educators, primarily work in institutional settings—public schools, colleges, universities, the YMCA, YWCA, children's clubs, hospitals, and the armed forces. This means that each individual interacts with other individuals and groups in the physical education department, in the institution, and in many cases with persons outside the institution.

Human interaction is a complex process not totally understood; however, the physical education administrator must make every effort to understand human behavior and the dynamics of relationships between individuals and between individuals and groups in and out of the department, if the department is to be managed effectively.

The role of the individual in the institutional setting. Individuals who choose to work in an institutional setting must understand the roles they are expected to play in the specific institutions in which they work. In addition to competence in the tasks assigned, the person is expected to be cooperative with colleagues, by loyal to the chairperson and the institution, and to subscribe to the code of ethics of the profession.

Group dynamics. Group dynamics is the process by which people interact face to face in small groups. Richards and Cuffee indicate that groups vary considerably with respect to the degree and nature of the interaction between members, with the result that three types of groups emerge—interacting, coacting, and counteracting.[3]

Fiedler defines the interacting group as one requiring the close coordination of several members in the performance of the primary task. The ability of one member to perform his or her job may depend on the fact that another member has first completed his or her share of the task.[4]

Richards and Cuffee state that the major characteristic of interacting groups is the interdependence of its members. Basketball teams, tank crews, and small production units in organizations are examples. The leader's job is one of directing, channeling, guiding, and coordinating each group member's group.[5]

---

[3] Steven A. Richards and James V. Cuffee, "Behavioral Correlates of Leadership Effectiveness in Interacting and Counteracting Groups," *Journal of Applied Psychology,* **56,** 5 (October 1972): 377–381.

[4] F. E. Fiedler, *A Theory of Leadership Effectiveness* (New York: McGraw-Hill, 1967).

[5] Richards and Cuffee, *op. cit.*

The counteracting group, according to Fiedler, occurs when individuals are working together for the purpose of negotiating and reconciling conflicting opinions and purposes. These groups are typically engaged in bargaining and negotiating processes, with some of these members representing a point of view and the other members an opposing, or at least a divergent, point of view. Each individual member, to a greater or lesser extent, works at achieving his or her own party's ends at the expense of another's. The leader's task in counteracting groups is to facilitate communications and mutual understanding among group leaders in an effort to establish a climate conducive to the development of solutions that will resolve the conflict; in short, the leader acts as a moderator or conciliator.[6]

A third type of interaction between members of a group is coacting. Fiedler indicates that coacting members may perform their respective individual tasks independently of other members of the group. The faculty of a university is a good example of a coacting group, since each instructor can, and often does, conduct teaching, research, or writing activities with little dependence on other members of the faculty. Law firms and medical clinics are also typical coacting groups. Coacting groups need coordination only in the achievement of group goals and in those instances when the goals of an individual member may be in conflict with those of another member.[7]

Thus it is obvious that people interact in small groups, in the three types discussed, in refinements of each of these types, and in a variety of other ways, but they will interact.

Leadership. Much has been written in recent years about leadership. Leadership has been analyzed and dissected, yet there are some aspects that are not completely understood. Some authors write of the factor X in leadership, which indicates that there are intangibles in leadership that still defy interpretation.

Although some leadership traits are innate, others can be learned through formal education or experience. Essential leadership traits include intelligence, integrity, courage, dedication, humility, knowledge, confidence, clarity, a sense of timing, concern, common sense, and character.

Although knowledge of leadership traits is important if one is to understand leadership, Keith Davis believes that leadership is shown more by the way a person acts than by one's traits.[8] Davis

---

6 Fiedler, *op. cit.*, p. 20.

7 *Ibid.*

8 Keith Davis, *Human Behavior at Work*, 5th ed. (New York: McGraw-Hill, 1977).

states that as society has learned more about leadership, it has become increasingly evident that strong leadership is a result of effective role behavior. Thus leadership depends on acts, not on traits. Traits influence acts, but so do followers, goals, and the environment in which the acts occur. It follows that organizational leadership is role behavior that unites and stimulates followers toward particular objectives in particular environments. All four elements—leader, follower, goals, and environment—are variables that affect one another in determining suitable role behavior; at this point, it is apparent that leadership is a situational and contingency relationship.[9]

Scholars of the leadership process have analyzed styles of leadership and have described the various methods leaders use in interacting with the groups they lead. Although the terminology differs, in essence the leadership styles are: autocratic, democratic, and free-rein. The autocratic leader makes all the decisions for the group, and power is centralized in the leader. The democratic leader, by contrast, consults with the members of the group, encouraging their suggestions and ideas, which are then considered in the leader's decisions that affect the group. The free-rein leader is willing to delegate authority to members of the group. The group solves its own problems and establishes its own goals. Instructions from the free-rein leader are given in general terms; the members of the group then develop the specific details to complete assigned tasks. The free-rein leader acts as a coordinator of the activities of the group with a minimum of direction.

Although leaders will use all three styles—autocratic, democratic, and free-rein—in the conduct of the affairs of their organizations, their leadership is characterized by one predominant style. Some authorities on leadership suggest that adaptive leadership is best. That is, the leader adapts his or her leadership style to the situation and can be flexible in meeting the needs of the group.

Reddin has developed a model of effective leadership styles, as follows:

> 1. *Executive.* This style gives a great deal of concern to both task . . . and people. . . . A manager using this style is a good motivator, sets high standards, recognizes individual differences, and utilizes team management.
>
> 2. *Developer.* This style gives maximum concern to people . . . and minimum concern to the task. . . . A manager using the style has implicit trust in people and is mainly concerned with developing them as individuals.

---

[9] *Ibid.*, p. 109.

> 3. *Benevolent autocrat.* This style gives maximum concern to the task . . . and minimum concern to people. . . . A manager using this style knows exactly what he or she wants and how to get it without resentment.
>
> 4. *Bureaucratic.* This style gives minimum concern to both task . . . and people. . . . A manager using this style is mainly interested in the rules and wants to maintain and control the situations by their use, but is seen as conscientious.[10]

It is obvious that there are a variety of leadership styles and that each person who leads a group will adopt a leadership style that is compatible with his or her personality and will best meet the needs and solve the problems of the group he or she leads.

Power. Power is an important concept in administering the affairs of groups of people. There are two kinds of power—formal and informal. Formal power is the power vested in the office, the authority granted to the individual by virtue of position held. Informal power is achieved by how the leader relates to the group; it is based on the leader's personality and character. It is important to note that formal power is necessary for informal power to exist. Best administration occurs when formal power is supplemented by the informal power earned by the leader's personal leadership and the respect and cooperation he or she has earned.

Authority. One of the fundamental concepts of leadership is authority. In an institutional setting authority is directing the actions of those persons in the organization for the purpose of attaining the objectives and goals of the organization. Those in leadership positions are granted the right by the institution they serve to make decisions affecting other members of the organization. The effectiveness of authority depends on whether or not those persons affected by the decisions made by leaders accept the decisions. Just as there is formal and informal power in an organization, so too there is positional and personal authority. Positional authority is the authority the leader has by virtue of his or her position in the institution; personal authority is authority obtained through the leader's personality, respect, and character.

An important principle of administration is that when a member of the institution is given a responsibility, she or he is also given the authority to carry out the responsibility. When this principle is

---

[10] William J. Reddin, "Managing Organizational Change," *Personnel Journal* (July 1969): 503. Quoted with permission of *Personnel Journal* copyright 1969.

violated, frustration and confusion occur, resulting in poor administration.

It is essential that leaders in institutions understand that their authority is never final; even the top administrator in the organization is subject to higher authority (the board of directors or the board of education).

Influence. A leader's influence with the group is an important ingredient of success. Leaders build positive influence over a period of time, primarily by close personal contact with the group and with individual members of the group, during which time trust and confidence in the leader are developed. The group builds a sense of responsibility to the leader, and group teamwork emerges. Under these circumstances, the leader is in an excellent position to exert influence on the group.

Decision making. Making decisions is one of the most important and difficult functions of leadership. A commonly accepted definition of decision making is choosing between two or more alternatives. The decision-making process follows a series of logical steps: (1) define the problem, (2) analyze the available information, (3) develop alternative courses of action, (4) select one course of action deemed best by the decision maker or makers, and (5) implement the decision (the procedures used to put the decision into action). If this method of decision making is used, the chances are very good that the correct decision will be made. It should be noted, however, that many decisions made in an institutional setting are not clear-cut; there is often a gray area that prevents a precise decision. When this circumstance occurs, the decision maker must still make the decision based on the steps outlined above.

Control. Hicks and Gullett define control as follows: "Controlling is one process by which management sees if what did happen was what was supposed to happen. If not, necessary adjustments are made." [11]

The complexity of today's organizations—governmental agencies, industry, churches, schools, and others—requires controls by managers, to ensure that the organization is operating effectively in achieving institutional goals. In spite of negative feelings about control, most individuals welcome control in their lives to provide stability and order. This includes the time spent "on the job."

---

[11] Herbert G. Hicks and C. Ray Gullet, *The Management of Organizations*, 3rd ed. (New York: McGraw-Hill, 1976), p. 497.

One of the principal functions of administrators is to establish the necessary controls to provide equilibrium in the organization. According to Luthans, there are three basic elements inherent in the definition of control: "First, control sets the standards and objectives which serve as the guide for performance. Second, control measures and evaluates inputs and performance according to the standards and objectives. Third, control takes corrective action in the form of a control decision." [12]

Controls occur at all levels of public school education. Controls are established by teachers, department heads, principals, superintendents, and boards of education. All of these people are necessary for an effective school system. Once standards and objectives are established for school-system operations, techniques are developed to measure and evaluate human performance and the various functions in the operation of the school system. These techniques range from personal observation to budgets, accounting procedures, and audits. If the evaluation indicates that corrective action is necessary, administrative decisions can be made to better control and improve the situation.

Motivation. A persistent problem of persons in managerial positions is how to motivate the members of the organization to produce at their maximum capacity. Administrators exert much energy and time in attempting to produce the proper ingredients for motivation. Motivation is a complex phenomenon, as it is individual in nature. Events that motivate one individual do not necessarily motivate others.

Some years ago, A. H. Maslow developed levels of need priorities. From the lowest order to the highest order, they are: (1) basic physiological needs, (2) safety and security, (3) belonging and social needs, (4) esteem and status, and (5) self-actualization.[13] Of most concern to leaders are needs at levels 3, 4, and 5; however, it must be understood that these needs are based on the fulfillment of needs at the first two levels. The concerned administrator will make efforts to provide an environment that will fulfill the members' needs for belonging, social needs, needs for esteem and status, and finally, for self-actualization, when the individual reaches his or her maximum potential. The fulfillment of the five levels of needs should provide the individual with motivation to perform his or her duties in the organization in a highly acceptable fashion.

---

[12] Fred Luthans, *Organizational Behavior,* 2d ed. (New York: McGraw-Hill, 1977), p. 229.

[13] A. H. Maslow, "A Theory of Human Motivation," *Psychological Review,* **50** (1943): 370–396.

Another aspect of motivation that should be understood is intrinsic and extrinsic motivators. Intrinsic motivators come from within the individual; a person who derives direct satisfaction from performing the tasks involved in his or her occupation will be highly motivated to perform at an optimum level. Extrinsic motivation, on the other hand, is external to the individual and occurs in many forms, e.g., the organization's fringe benefits, a bonus offered for sales, or an athletic award for members of athletic teams. Although both types of motivation are important, it is obvious that intrinsic motivation is the more significant.

Communication. Communication is the process of exchanging information. The success of any organization is based on the effectiveness of its communication system. Most problems that occur in an institution are the result of a lack of communication. Vardaman and Halterman discuss the comprehensive nature of communication in today's organizations.

> By communication we mean the flow of material, information, perception and understandings between various parts and members of an organization . . . all the methods, means, and media of communication (communication technology), all the channels, networks, and systems of communication (organization structure), all the person-to-person interchange (interpersonal communication). . . . It includes all aspects of communication: up, down, lateral; speaking, writing, listening, reading; methods, media, modes, channels, networks, flow; interpersonal, intraorganizational, interorganizational.[14]

Effective organizations develop formal plans of communication which include such items as organizational goals, principles, policies, procedures, schedules, and job descriptions. The formal plan of communication for the organization is supplemented by an informal plan developed by the members of the organization. The informal communication plan is spontaneous and based on personal relationships. This plan attempts to fill the communication gaps not provided by the formal communication system and to control individual behavior by group pressure. If the organization has a rigid, impersonal formal plan of communication, the informal plan will often be in conflict with the formal plan.

The improvement of communication skills is a challenge to everyone, especially for persons involved in institutional affairs. Improvement of communication skills is summed up in excellent statement of rules, its Ten Commandments of Good Communication:

---

[14] George T. Vardaman and Carol C. Halterman, *Managerial Control through Communication* (New York: Wiley, 1968), pp. 3–4. Reprinted by permission.

1. *Seek to clarify your ideas before communicating.* The more systematically we analyze the problem or idea to be communicated, the clearer it becomes that this is the first step toward effective communication. Many communications fail because of inadequate planning. Good planning must consider the goals and attitudes of those who will receive the communications and those who will be affected by it.

2. *Examine the true purpose of each communication.* Before you communicate, ask yourself what you really want to accomplish with your message—obtain information, initiate action, change another person's attitude? Identify your most important goal and then adapt your language, tone, and total approach to serve that specific objective. Don't try to accomplish too much with each communication. The sharper the focus of your message, the greater its chances of success.

3. *Consider the total physical and human setting whenever you communicate.* Meaning and intent are conveyed by more than words alone. Many other factors influence the overall impact of a communication, and the manager must be sensitive to the total setting in which he or she communicates. Consider, for example, your sense of timing—i.e., the circumstances under which you make an announcement or render a decision; the physical setting—whether you communicate in private, for example, or otherwise; the social climate that pervades work relationships within the company or a department and sets the tone of its communications; customs and past practice—the degree to which your communication conforms to or departs from, the expectations of your audience. Be constantly aware of the total setting in which you communicate. Like all living things, communication must be capable of adapting to its environment.

4. *Consult with others, where appropriate, in planning communications.* Frequently it is desirable or necessary to seek the participation of others in planning a communication or developing the facts on which to base it. Such consultation often helps to lend additional insight and objectivity to your message. Moreover, those who have helped you plan your communication will give it their support.

5. *Be mindful, while you communicate, of the overtones as well as the basic content of your message.* Your tone of voice, your expression, your apparent receptiveness to the responses of others —all have tremendous impact on those you wish to reach. Frequently overlooked, these subtleties of communication often affect

a listener's reaction to a message even more than its basic content. Similarly, your choice of language—particularly your awareness of the fine shades of meaning and emotion in the words you use—predetermines in large part the reactions of your listeners.

6. *Take the opportunity, when it arises, to convey something of help or value to the receiver.* Consideration of the other person's interests and needs—the habit of trying to look at things from his or her point of view—will frequently point up opportunities to convey something of immediate benefit or long-range value to that person. People on the job are most responsive to the manager whose messages take their own interests into account.

7. *Follow up your communication.* Our best efforts at communication may be wasted and we may never know whether we have succeeded in expressing our true meaning and intent if we do not follow up to see how well we have put our message across. This you can do by asking questions, by encouraging the receiver to express his or her reactions, by follow-up contacts, by subsequent review of performance. Make certain that every important communication has a "feed-back" so that complete understanding and appropriate action result.

8. *Communicate for tomorrow as well as today.* Although communications may be aimed primarily at meeting the demands of an immediate situation, they must be planned with the past in mind if they are to maintain consistency in the receiver's view; but, most important of all, they must be consistent with long-range interests and goals. For example, it is not easy to communicate frankly on such matters as poor performance or the shortcomings of a loyal subordinate—but postponing disagreeable communications makes them more difficult in the long run and is actually unfair to your subordinates and your department.

9. *Be sure your actions support your communications.* In the final analysis, the most persuasive kind of communication is not what you say, but what you do. When a person's actions or attitudes contradict his or her words, we tend to discount what was said. For every manager, this means that good supervisory practices—such as clear assignment of responsibility and authority, fair rewards for effort, and sound policy enforcement—serve to communicate more than all the gifts of oratory.

10. *Last, but by no means least: Seek not only to be understood, but to understand—be a good listener.* When we start talking, we often cease to listen—in that larger sense of being attuned to the

other person's unspoken reactions and attitudes. Even more serious is the fact that we are all guilty, at times, of inattentiveness when others are attempting to communicate to us. Listening is one of the most important, most difficult—and most neglected—skills in communication. It demands that we concentrate not only on the explicit meanings another person is expressing, but on the implicit meanings, unspoken words, and overtones that may be far more significant. Thus we must learn to listen with the inner person.[15]

Rewards. Inherent in the management of people in an organization is the development of a system of rewards for services rendered. The basic reward is the economic reward, the salary or wages received. The money reward is important to the individual not only because of the goods and services it purchases, but also as a status symbol. The salary received indicates to the person the regard with which he or she is held by the employer.

Rewards are classified as extrinsic and intrinsic. The extrinsic rewards are primarily money. The intrinsic rewards are the satisfactions the individual receives from the work. For many people, including most individuals in the field of education, personal satisfaction for a job well done is a very powerful motivator.

Organizational managers should strive to provide their personnel with a combination of extrinsic and intrinsic rewards. It should be noted that individual concepts of rewards differ. People place different values on financial income and job satisfaction; salary is the most important reward for some persons and of lesser importance to others. By the same token, job satisfaction is of prime importance in the reward system for some and of little importance to others.

Business firms as well as systems of public and higher education provide fringe benefits as part of their reward program. In many instances fringe benefits rank high in the value system of members of organizations and are regarded as evidence of recognition and status.

Conflict. Conflict is a complex phenomenon, especially for those individuals who work in organizational settings. Basically, there is conflict within individuals, between indivduals, and between individuals and the organization. Conflict within individuals is characterized by frustration resulting from inability to realize personal goals which may be impeded by personal inadequacies, real or

---

[15] *Ten Commandments of Good Communication,* New York: American Management Association, 1955). Reprinted by permission of the publisher. © 1955 by American Management Association, Inc. All rights reserved.

imagined. Conflict between individuals is common in organizations, in part because of different points of view, lack of communication, or personality conflicts. Conflict between individuals and the organization may be due to institutional rules and regulations that are so rigid that the individual is denied the opportunity for individual and personal growth.

Students of the problem of conflict generally agree that conflict in organizations is inevitable, but that it should be kept to a minimum. This is one of the many challenges for institutional leaders.

Seniority. Seniority, or length of service to an organization, is a very important concept in industry as well as, though perhaps to a lesser degree, in education.

In industry, especially where labor unions are involved, salary raises and job security are based on seniority rather than performance. In many public school systems and some colleges and universities, a scale system for salary raises is used rather than rewarding faculty for merit. When the scale system for salary raises is used, those instructors with longest service to the college, university, or public school system, receive the largest salaries.

Although most educators would prefer to be judged on their performance, many, especially public school teachers, opt for the seniority concept of salary raises. One of the principal reasons for selecting the seniority concept is that it is often very difficult to evaluate teacher performance. Also, there is frequently a lack of trust in the ability of administrators to truly judge teaching ability. Many public school administrators prefer the seniority system because it is simpler to administer and there is less chance for misunderstandings and conflicts of opinion. One possible solution is a combination of seniority and performance.

A negative aspect of seniority is that in many cases, after the individual has spent a number of years on the job in the industry, business, or school system and built up seniority, it is difficult to leave for another position and lose the seniority. The individual is frequently "locked in" to the organization.

Equal Employment Opportunity—Affirmative Action

No discussion of personnel administration would be complete without reference to the federal laws pertaining to equal employment opportunity and affirmative action. The original equal employment opportunity act was Title VII of the Civil Rights Act of 1964. Educational institutions, at both the public school and the college and university levels, in their role as employer, are under the jurisdiction of Title VII of the Civil Rights Act of 1964. George P. Sape, Associate Counsel for the U.S. Senate Labor Subcommittee, writes as follows: "Title VII is the major federal statute designed to provide all persons an equal opportunity for meaningful employment, regardless of race, religion, color, sex, or national origin. It is this law which represents the federal effort to eliminate past patterns of discrimination in employment on the basis of the above-noted categories, and to insure that all future employment programs will allow free and open access to employment for all qualified applicants."[16]

According to Sape, the basic and fundamental concept of Title VII is found in section 703, which outlines discrimination in employment and makes it an unlawful employment practice when it is shown that a particular practice (or practices) discriminates against one of the protected classes enumerated in Title VII because it:

1. results in a failure or refusal to hire any individual because of such person's race, religion, color, sex, or national origin;
2. results in the discharge of any individual because of such person's race, color, religion, sex, or national origin;
3. differentiates between individuals with respect to compensation, terms, conditions, or privileges of employment because of such person's race, color, religion, sex, or national origin;
4. limits, segregates, or classifies employees or applicants for employment in any way which would deprive or tend to deprive any individual of employment opportunities, or otherwise adversely affect such person's employment status, because of such person's race, color, religion, sex, or national origin.[17]

Other federal government programs pertaining to equal employment opportunity include the following:

1. *Section 503 of the Rehabilitation Act of 1973.* This act requires government contractors and subcontractors to take affirmitive action to employ and advance in employment qualified handicapped individuals.[18] Section 504 of the Rehabilitation Act is designated to eliminate discrimination on the basis of handicap in any program or activity receiving federal financial assistance. Section 504 applies to all public school districts, colleges, and universities that receive federal financial assistance.[19]

---

[16] George P. Sape, *Federal Regulations and Employment Practices of Colleges and Universities,* Washington, D.C.: National Association of College and University Business Officers, 1974, p. 2.

[17] *Ibid.,* p. 7.

[18] *Ibid.,* P. SUPP-HAPP, p. 29.

[19] *Ibid.,* P. SUPP-HAP, p. 4.

2. *Title VI of the Civil Rights Act of 1964.* The purpose of this act states that no person in the United States shall, on the ground of race, color, or national origin, be excluded from participation in, be denied the benefits of, or be otherwise subjected to discrimination under any program or activity receiving federal financial assistance from the Department of Health, Education and Welfare.[20]

3. *Title IX.* Title IX of the Education Amendments of 1972, Public Law 92–318, passed by Congress on June 23, 1972, is designed to eliminate discrimination on the basis of sex in any education program or activity receiving federal financial assistance.[21]

4. *Age Discrimination in Employment Act of 1967.* This law covers the age group 40 to 65 and declares illegal any discriminatory actions on the basis of age in the critical areas of hiring, job retention, compensation, and employee benefits systems. Any employer of 25 or more workers is subject to the law.[22]

Affirmative action. Since January 13, 1973, all educational institutions (both public and private) with one or more federal contract(s) of $50,000 or more and 50 or more employees have been required to maintain a written affirmative action plan. Although the requirement to maintain a written affirmative action plan does not apply unless an institution has a federal contract of $50,000 or more, federal contracts during any 12-month period that have an aggregate total value exceeding $10,000 subject an institution to compliance with the executive orders and Office of Federal Contract Compliance Programs of the Department of Labor issued thereunder.[23]

The basic authority requiring affirmative action is Executive Order 11246, as amended by Executive Order 11375. These orders require each federal contracting agency to include in every contract entered into by that agency, provisions which obligate the individual contractor, in part, as follows:

> The Contractor will not discriminate against any employee or applicant for employment because of race, color, religion, sex or national origin. The Contractor will take affirmative action to insure that applicants are employed, and that employees are treated during

---

[20] *Ibid.*

[21] *Federal Register*, p. 38, 17979, July 5, 1973 and Supplement—Sex-12, August 28, 1975. (For further discussion of Title IX, see Chapter 15.)

[22] *Federal Regulations and Employment Practices of Colleges and Universities, op. cit.*, p. 4.

[23] *Ibid.*, P.AFA 2.

employment without regard to their race, color, religion, sex, or national origin. Such action shall include, but not be limited to the following: employment, upgrading, demotion, or transfer; recruitment or recruitment advertising; lay-off or termination; rates of pay or other forms of compensation; and selection for training, including apprenticeship.[24]

PERSONNEL BENEFITS

Modern personnel programs in public school systems provide a variety of benefits for teachers, staff, and administrators. The purposes of the personnel benefits program include: (1) to help the school system recruit and hold better personnel, (2) to help maintain good staff morale, and (3) to help the school employees obtain benefits they cannot usually attain for themselves by salary increases. Personnel benefits vary from school district to school district. Following is a discussion of the usual benefits available to school personnel.

Medical Examinations

Most public school systems require all prospective employees to obtain a medical examination. The examination should be given by a physician in the employment of the board of education, and the examination should be paid for by the board. Those school-system applicants who are poor health risks, especially teachers, should not be employed by the school district.

Persons who are employed by the school system should be required by the board of education to have periodic medical examinations at least every three or four years. These examinations should be performed by physicians approved by the board and paid for by the board. These periodic examinations are necessary to ensure that school employees maintain good health during their period of employment.

Health Insurance

Group health insurance. Most school districts make a group health insurance plan available to their employees. Hospitalization, surgical benefits, and medical care are provided either singly or in combination. Basic health insurance plans are in reality a prepaid installment method of paying medical expenses. They do not offer adequate protection against major medical expense. Therefore,

---

[24] *Ibid.*, P.AFA 2.

teachers and other school district employees should consider a supplementary major medical policy.

Group disability insurance. Group disability insurance is income insurance. It guarantees the employee a monthly income, usually 65 to 75 percent of monthly basic earnings, if the person becomes so disabled by injury or sickness that she or he can no longer work for a living. Some disability plans protect the employee for only a few months, while other plans, called group long-term disability insurance plans, protect the individual as long as he or she is "totally disabled." Income payments usually stop when the person recovers, dies, or reaches age 65.

Group Life Insurance

Group life insurance provides protection for a number of individuals as a group under a single policy. The intent is to provide low-cost insurance during a person's working years. Group life insurance is supplemental insurance; it is not intended to meet all of a person's life insurance needs.

Advantages of group life insurance include greater protection for dependents per dollar cost than any other benefit and coverage for many persons who might not qualify for individual life insurance, due to inability to meet physical requirements. However, there are disadvantages, the principal one being that it is term insurance, which provides protection for a contracted period, usually one year, after which the policy must be renewed. The policy does not have cash, loan, or paid-up values, and it may be cancelled when the teacher terminates his or her employment or retires.

Workmen's Compensation

Workmen's compensation is generally defined as damages recoverable from an employer by an employee in case of an accident. Many states now provide workmen's compensation for public school employees. The coverage and benefits available to employees vary considerably from state to state. School employees should become familiar with the workmen's compensation program in the state in which they are employed. In general the coverage includes medical expenses for specific injuries, partial disability, total disability, death benefits, and burial expenses. Weekly financial benefits paid to the employee usually range from 60 to 70 percent of the employee's salary, not to exceed a maximum weekly amount and a maximum number of weeks.

Leaves of Absence

Teachers may be absent from their assigned duties for a variety of reasons. To ensure uniformity of administration and fairness to all, school districts must establish policies to cover the various kinds of leaves of absence available to teachers. The most common types of leave are: sick leave, maternity, emergency, convention and conference, professional study and travel, and sabbatical.

Sick leave. In most school districts teachers are granted sick leave at full salary for a specified number of days. This makes it possible for the teacher to be absent from the job while recovering from an illness. Usually there is a provision for accumulation of unused leave from year to year to a maximum number of days. The amount of sick leave usually increases with length of service to the school system. Policies vary from school system to school system; a common allowance is one day of sick leave for each month of employment. Other school systems grant ten days of sick leave annually. Accumulated sick leave for a teacher is not usually transferred from one school district to another. There is always the possibility that sick leave may be abused by some individuals and used for purposes for which it was not intended. However, abuses are the exception rather than the rule, for teachers are expected to provide verification of the illness by a physician.

Maternity leave. Maternity leave assures the teacher a job in the school system when she is ready to return to active duty; maternity leave is usually leave without pay. It is usual practice to require that the teacher, prior to returning to work, submit a physician's certification that the teacher is in satisfactory physical condition to resume her duties.

Emergency leave. School systems usually have provisions for emergency leave. Emergency leave may be for a variety of reasons including death of a relative, medical and dental appointments, appointments with a lawyer or the courts, or required attendance at a religious service; it is usually of short duration and with pay.

Convention and conference leave. Administrators in most school systems recognize the value of teachers attending conventions and conferences in their disciplines. Generally permission to attend such meetings must be granted by the teacher's principal. Limitations in terms of time away from the teaching post are common. In most cases the teacher's pay is not docked. Some school systems provide all or some part of travel and per diem expenses.

Professional study and travel leave. In most school systems teachers may be granted a leave of absence to work toward an advanced degree. Teachers may also be granted permission to be absent from their teaching assignment to travel, provided the travel will benefit the individual in his or her teaching duties. School districts usually do not pay teachers who are granted professional study or travel leave.

Sabbatical leave. A sabbatical leave is granted to a teacher for an extended period of time, usually one or two semesters, with full or partial salary. Sabbatical leaves are granted after a given period of years (usually six) service to the school system. With the economic pressures on public school education, sabbatical leaves are not common in public schools. However, some school systems do make sabbatical leaves available to faculty members.

Sabbatical pay varies greatly among school districts; however, the usual pattern is full pay for a semester or half pay for a school year.

Sabbatical leaves are justified by the values accrued to both the school district and the teacher. Teachers are usually expected to engage in activities that will enhance their professional competence. Peripheral values include rehabilitation of the faculty member and freedom from routine and vocational pressure.

Tenure

Tenure is defined as a means of guaranteeing teachers security during satisfactory performance of duties. Prior to being granted tenure, it is common practice for the teacher to serve in a probationary status. The probation period is designed to enable the teacher to prove his or her worth to school officials and for school authorities to evaluate the teaching ability of the individual before offering tenure. The probationary period is usually three years, but the time may vary in different states and school districts. Tenure, which is guaranteed in some states, is a privilege granted by the individual school systems to teachers, not an obligation.

Reasons for tenure include security of employment, academic freedom, protection against dismissal, prevention of permanent employment to incompetent persons, and maintenance of staff stability. While many states have a tenure law, some do not. In lieu of tenure, some states are adopting the "continuing contract" which provides that a teacher's contract is automatically renewed for the next school year unless the teacher is notified by a specified date that the contract will not be renewed.

Retirement

All 50 states now have a retirement plan for public school teachers. The principal objective is to provide the teachers, after retirement from teaching, economic independence and the opportunity to live their remaining years in dignity and security. Retirement plans are a means by which school employees are required to save a portion of their income for their retirement years. Retirement plans are designed to provide teachers with a sense of security during their active careers, which, in turn, should result in more effective teacher performance.

It is necessary for our public education systems to provide effective retirement plans; most employees in governmental agencies, in business, and in industry are offered retirement plans. If public education is to compete for competent personnel, retirement plans must be provided. Another advantage of retirement programs is that school districts are able to retire professional school personnel, who reach retirement age, in an orderly fashion with the knowledge that these persons will have economic security.

State governments establish official administrative units for the state teachers retirement programs. Policy for the program administration is made by a board of directors. The usual practice is to appoint an executive director to administer the program. Effective management is essential since thousands of school personnel and millions of dollars are involved in each state teachers retirement program.

Membership in state retirement plans varies; the plan may include only teachers, or teachers and administrators, or all school personnel. Contribution plans also differ; the most common are (1) a joint contribution plan for which the cost is shared by the members and the school district and/or the state, (2) a plan for which the state or school district pays the total cost, or (3) a plan for which the members pay the costs.

In some states all new teachers, by law, must become members of the teacher retirement system. In states where teachers pay the entire plan's cost, or share the cost with the state and/or school district, the usual practice is to support the teacher's membership with a salary deduction. In most cases this ranges from five to eight percent. These contributions may be withdrawn when a teacher leaves the state school system; some states include the accrued interest.

The age at which a teacher becomes eligible for retirement and its available benefits is of utmost importance. Laws vary from state to state; retirement eligibility and benefits in the state of Texas follow:

1. *Normal-age retirement:* A member may receive full formula benefits at:
   a) age 65 with 10–19 years of service, or
   b) age 60 with 20 or more years of service, or
   c) age 59 or earlier with 36 or more years service, as shown in Table 2.
2. *Early-age retirement:* A member may receive a reduced annuity at:
   a) age 55 with 10–19 years of creditable service, as shown in Table 1, or

Table 1

Years of Service	Age at Date of Retirement 55	56	57	58	59	60	61	62	63	64	65
	Percentages										
10–19	47	51	55	59	63	67	73	80	87	93	100

Table 2

Years of Service	Age at Date of Retirement 55	56	57	58	59	60
	Percentages					
20–24	70	76	82	88	94	100
25–29	75	80	82	88	94	100
30	80	82	84	88	94	100
31	82	84	86	88	94	100
32	84	86	88	90	94	100
33	86	88	90	92	94	100
34	88	90	92	94	96	100
35	90	92	94	96	98	100
36	92	94	96	98	100	100
37	94	96	98	100	100	100
38	96	98	100	100	100	100
39	98	100	100	100	100	100
40 or more	100	100	100	100	100	100

b) age 55 with 20 or more years of creditable service, as shown in Table 2, or

c) any age with 30 or more years of creditable service, as shown in Table 2.[25]

The following example of how maximum retirement benefits are calculated is from the Teacher Retirement System of Texas.[26]

1. $\dfrac{\$11{,}398}{\text{5-year average salary}}$

(Average your highest five annual salaries earned on or about Sept. 1 through Aug. 31 of each year. Annual compensation cannot exceed $25,000).

2. $\dfrac{32}{\text{Total years of creditable service}} \times 2\% = \dfrac{64\%}{\text{Total }\%}$

3. $\dfrac{.64}{\text{Total }\%} \times \dfrac{\$11.398}{\text{Average salary}} = \dfrac{\$7294.72}{\text{Annual annuity}}$

4. $\dfrac{\$7294.72}{\text{Annual annuity}} \div 12 = \dfrac{\$607.89}{\text{Monthly standard annuity}}$

Another feature of teacher retirement plans is options in lieu of maximum benefits. For example, the Teacher Retirement System of Texas provides the opportunity to select one of four optional retirement plans in lieu of the standard annuity in order to provide income for someone following the member's death. The examples below are based on the retirement formula above and a 60-year-old member with a beneficiary age 61.

Standard annuity—Maximum benefits (see example above): $607.89 per month throughout the member's life with these payments ceasing upon death.

Option 1—100% joint life annuity: $528.01 per month throughout the member's life and upon the member's death, the same payments will continue throughout the life of the surviving beneficiary who was named at the time of retirement.

Option 2—50% joint life annuity: $565.16 per month throughout the member's life and upon the member's death, one-half of this payment

---

[25] Teacher Retirement System of Texas, *The ABC's of Teacher Retirement System in Texas* (Austin, Texas: The Teacher Retirement System, 1977): pp. 4–5. Reprinted with permission.

[26] *Ibid.*, p. 7.

($282.58) will continue throughout the life of the surviving beneficiary who was named at the time of retirement.

Option 3—60 monthly payments guaranteed: $602.97 per month throughout the member's life. If the member dies before 60 monthly payments have been made, payments will be made to the beneficiary until remainder of the 60 payments have been made. A total of $36,178 is guaranteed payable in this example.

Option 4—120 monthly payments guaranteed: $589.35 per month throughout the life of the member. If the member dies before 120 payments have been made, payments will be made to the bneficiary until remainder of the 120 payments have been made. A total of $70,722 is guaranteed payable in this example.

In the examples above, actuarial factors were 86.86% for Option 1, 92.97% for Option 2, 99.19% for Option 3, and 96.95% for Option 4.[27]

Many states make it possible to purchase credit for out-of-state teaching, although this option usually has limitations placed on the amount of credit that the teacher can claim. For example, a member of the Texas Teacher Retirement System, to obtain credit for each year of out-of-state service, must pay 12 percent of his or her annual salary rate for the first year of Texas service which is both after the out-of-state service and after September 1, 1956. This service can be purchased one year at a time.

Before any benefit can be computed using out-of-state service credit, the member must render at least ten years of creditable service in Texas.

Members may purchase one year of Texas service for each year of out-of-state service up to a maximum of ten years. A fee of five percent per year is added to the cost of obtaining out-of-state service, calculated from the date the member becomes eligible for the purchase.

Because of diverse retirement laws, it has been difficult for a teacher to transfer teaching service from one state to another except by purchase of years of service. This impedes mobility of teachers. Quite often teachers are reluctant to move to a better opportunity in another state after accruing some years of service in a state because retirement years will be lost. Reciprocity in teacher retirement programs between states is needed in the teaching profession.

Two other features of most teacher retirement programs are disability benefits and workmen's compensation. To be eligible for disability benefits the school employee must be a member of

---

[27] *Ibid.*, p. 17.

the state teacher retirement program for a given period of time, usually ten years. To be eligible for workmen's compensation, the individual must be injured while on duty.

Another means for public school employees to provide for their retirement years is through social security. In some states public school employees have social security in addition to state teachers retirement, while in other states social security is not available. In still other states there are local options by individual school districts.

It is recommended that teachers investigate the state teachers retirement plan in the state in which they teach.

Miscellaneous Benefits

In addition to the personnel benefits previously discussed in this chapter, there are other benefits available to public school employees. The number and kind of personnel benefits available vary from school district to school district. Some additional personnel benefits are:

Additional salary for additional duties. Most school systems now provide teachers with additional salary for additional duties. The most common additional duties include coaching athletic teams, directing musical groups, coaching debate teams, and directing school plays and drama groups.

Credit union. Many large school districts provide a credit union for the benefit of school employees. A credit union is a form of mutual investment corporation. The principal benefits to teachers and other school district employees are loans at lower interest rates than available at commercial banks, group purchase plans, and insurance protection plans. Most credit unions provide members the opportunity to purchase shares in the union. Interest on the shares is paid at a rate comparable to commercial banks.

Consultative services. Personnel departments in large school districts provide a consultative service for employees in a number of important areas which include job-related problems, financial problems, legal problems, social problems, health problems, and retirement problems.

Insurance for drivers of motor vehicles. Physical education instructors, athletic coaches, band directors, debate coaches, and other teachers frequently are required to drive motor vehicles owned by the school district, or their own private automobiles, to transport students to contests or meets. Some school districts provide the necessary insurance to protect teachers during the performance of their duties.

Visitation days. Teachers in many school districts are permitted a given number of days, usually two or three, to make visits to other schools, both within and outside the school district, to witness new or innovative programs that may enhance their effectiveness as teachers.

Parking. Free parking space is a benefit provided by most schools for teachers, administrators and other school personnel. For teachers who live beyond walking distance to their schools, assured parking space is an important convenience and time saver.

Free admission to athletic, cultural and theatrical activities. A benefit provided to teachers by many school districts is free admission to athletic contests, cultural and theatrical activities sponsored by the school in which the teacher is employed. Since schools desire that teachers attend as many school-sponsored activities as possible, both the teacher and the school benefit by this policy.

Grievances

For a wide variety of reasons teachers and other school personnel have real or imagined grievances which must be resolved as rapidly and effectively as possible. It is always best when these grievances can be solved at the lowest possible level, that is, by the person's immediate superior. However, when grievances cannot be solved at this level, other procedures are necessary. In the past, grievance procedures have not always been available to school personnel, and the problems may not have been solved to the person's satisfaction, resulting in dissatisfied and less effective individuals.

Public school personnel departments should develop effective grievance procedures with the involvement of teachers and other school staff personnel. The aim is to minimize grievances. But when grievances do occur, a systematic plan is needed to attempt to solve the problem. Procedures, in writing, must be established in the form of a series of appeals to the next highest administrative echelon. A grievance should originate with the grievant's immediate supervisor. In the case of a staff member the order of rank is department head, principal, superintendent and board of education.

One of the principal advantages of establishing grievance procedures is the psychological effect on school district employees. The knowledge that machinery is available to hear grievances can be a factor in establishing better staff morale.

CASE STUDY

Staff morale at Wilson High School was at a low ebb due to a number of factors, one of which was a mandated reduction in staff due to a drop in enrollment at the school. There were two untenured teachers in the Department of Physical Education. A committee of interested teachers was to meet with Martin Wise, the Department Head. Of the two untenured faculty the first, Pete Michaels, had two specialized teaching skills, aquatics and gymnastics. The second teacher, Mary May, was a good teacher, and a generalist. Mr. Wise was well aware of the Affirmative Action program; but, because of the coaching assignments, his staff was heavily weighted with men teachers. However, much of the physical education program in Wilson High School was coeducational.

1. What are some of the overriding issues in this case?
2. Which of these two teachers should be retained? What rationale can be used for the dismissal of the other?
3. Are there any policies or principles which evolve from the above case?

SELECTED REFERENCES

Anderson, R. H. "Organizing and Staffing the School," *National Society for the Study of Education Yearbook*, **72** (Winter 1973): pt. 2, 221–242.

Barrilleaux, L. E. "Accountability Through Performance Objectives," *Bulletin of the National Association of Secondary School Principals*, **56** (May 1972): 103–110.

Bernabei, R. "Differentiated Staffing: Where To Now?" *Man/Society/Technology,* **32** (April 1973): 265–268.

Brighton, Howard. *Utilizing Teacher Aides in Differentiated Staffing.* Midland, Mich.: Pendell Publishing, 1972.

Browder, Lesley, Jr. *Emerging Patterns of Administrative Accountability.* Berkeley, Calif.: McCutchan Publishing, 1971.

Bucher, Charles A., *Administration of Health and Physical Education Programs, Including Athletics* (5th rev. ed.). St. Louis, Mo.: C. V. Mosby, 1971.

———. *Administrative Dimensions of Health and Physical Education Programs, Including Athletics.* St. Louis, Mo.: C. V. Mosby, 1971.

Butefish, W. L. "Now for a Short Course in How to Keep Good Teachers," *American School Board Journal,* **159** (September 1972): 35.

Castetter, W. B. *Personnel Function in Educational Administration.* Riverside, N.J.: Macmillan, 1971.

Colvin, W., and E. Roundy. "Instrument for the Student Evaluation of Teaching Effectiveness in Physical Education Activity Courses," *Research Quarterly* (May 1976): 296–298.

Cooper, James M. *Differentiated Staffing: New Staff Utilization Patterns for Public Schools.* Philadelphia: W. B. Saunders, 1971.

Daughtrey, Greyson, and John B. Woods. *Physical Education and Intramural Programs: Organization and Administration.* Philadelphia: W. B. Saunders, 1976.

———. *Physical Education Programs: Organization and Administration.* Philadelphia: W. B. Saunders, 1971.

Davies, G. H. "Single Physical Education Departments and Equality for Women," *Journal of Health Physical Education Recreation,* **44** (April 1973): 62–63.

Day, James F. *Teacher Retirement in the United States.* N. Quincy, Mass.: Christopher Publishing House, 1971.

Day, W., and D. Hamer. "Trends in Ascertaining Physical Education Faculty Workloads," *Journal of Health Physical Education Recreation,* **44** (April 1973): 63.

Dunn, K., and R. Dunn. *Practical Approaches to Individualizing Instruction: Contracts and Other Effective Teaching Strategies.* Englewood Cliffs, N.J.: Prentice-Hall, 1972.

English, Fenwick, and Donald K. Sharpes. *Strategies for Differentiated Staffing.* Berkeley, Calif.: McCutchan Publishing, 1972.

Field, David A. "Accountability for the Physical Educator," *Journal of Health Physical Education Recreation,* **44** (February 1973): 37–38.

Fiorino, A. John. *Differentiated Staffing: A Flexible Instructional Organization.* New York: Harper & Row, 1972.

Frost, Reuben B., and Stanley J. Marshall. *Administration of Physical Education and Athletics: Concepts and Practices.* Dubuque, Iowa: W. C. Brown, 1974.

Greene, Jay E. *School Personnel Administration.* Radnor, Pa.: Chilton Book, 1971.

Ingram, A. "Teacher of Physical Education Should Have These Attributes," *Physical Educator,* **34** (March 1977): 34.

Irwin, J. R. "Can Large Schools Be Humanized Through School Organizations?" *Bulletin of the National Association of Secondary School Principals,* **57** (May 1973): 143–145.

Johnson, M. L. *Functional Administration in Physical and Health Education.* Boston: Houghton Mifflin, 1977.

Kleinman, S. "Men vs. the Women in Physical Education: A Study in Non-Communication," *Physical Educator,* **27** (May 1970): 77.

Lawton, S. B. "Socio-Economic Environment and Promotional Opportunities," *California Journal of Educational Research,* **24** (September 1973): 152–164.

Lefkowitz, L. J. "Paraprofessionals: An Administration/School Board Conspiracy?" with reply by E. B. Michael, *Phi Delta Kappan,* **54** (April 1973): 546–549.

Lewis, James, Jr. *Differentiating the Teaching Staff.* W. Nyack, N.Y.: Parker Publishing, 1971.

Lutz, Frank W., et al. *Grievances and Their Resolution.* Danville, Ill.: Interstate, 1967.

Mansergh, Gerald G. (ed.). *Dynamics of Management by Objectives for School Administrators.* Danville, Ill.: Interstate, 1971.

Miller, Van, et al. *The Public Administration of American School Systems.* Riverside, N.J.: Macmillan, 1972.

Morland, R. "From Coach to Principal," *Journal of Health Physical Education Recreation,* **45** (June 1974): 38–40.

Norred, R. "Relating to Administrators," *Journal of Health Physical Education Recreation,* **45** (June 1974): 24–25.

Oberdorfer, J. "Balance of Interests: Community Control and Personnel Practices," *Urban Review,* **5** (September 1971): 11–19 and **5** (November 1971): 26–34.

Ridini, L. M. "Paraprofessional in Physical Education," *Physical Educator,* **27** (October 1970): 114–117.

Rubin, Louis J. *Improving In-Service Education: Proposals and Procedures for Change.* Rockleigh, N.J.: Allyn & Bacon, 1971.

Ryan, Kevin (ed.). *Don't Smile Until Christmas: Accounts of the First Year of Teaching.* Chicago: University of Chicago Press, 1972.

Schmid, W. William, et al. *Retirement Systems of the American Teacher.* New York: Fleet Press, 1970.

Seidel, Beverly. "Are Administrators Responsible for Teacher Unrest?" *Physical Educator,* **27** (March 1970): 22–24.

Thomas, D. "Don't Let the New Accountability Make More Problems Than It Solves," *American School Board Journal,* **160** (January 1973): 59.

Weber, Clarence A. *Leadership in Personnel Management in Public Schools.* Edited by William E. Amos. St. Louis, Mo.: Warren H. Green, 1970.

Whaling, T. "Managing the School System: A Performance Improvement Approach; Management Action Program (MAP)," *Bulletin of the National Association of Secondary School Principals,* **56** (November 1972): 32–39.

Yanke, P. "Organizing the Staff," *Athletic Journal,* **55** (March 1975): 3.

6

RELATIONSHIP OF PHYSICAL EDUCATION WITH HEALTH EDUCATION

STUDY STIMULATORS

1. How did physical education become aligned with health education as a combined field?
2. What different school functions are considered under the aegis of school health education?
3. What specific activities make up the content of a good health services program?
4. How does the way the school is organized affect the health of students?
5. What are the possible effects of the trend to separate the certification of physical education teachers from health teachers in the small school? the large school?

All great changes are irksome to the human mind, especially those which are attended with.... uncertain effects.

JOHN ADAMS

Although this textbook is written for those involved in the administration of physical education and athletics, this chapter deals with the relationship of physical education and athletics with health education. Even though the trend in certification is to separate these two fields of study, "health and physical education" have been used together for so many years that it is difficult to identify them as separate and distinct disciplines. Most states still certify teachers in "health and physical education." Even though the departments of health and the departments of physical education may be separated in larger teacher education institutions, they remain united in the smaller ones. What is more important is that their products, the teachers and administrators, still function in a united department at the middle school and the secondary school levels. The administrator continues to wear several hats.

One of the purposes of this chapter is to enable the student to understand the many ramifications of school health education and how it is arranged administratively. No attempt is made to discuss the many facets of the broad spectrum of allied health sciences, including community health. The interested student may continue this track by individual investigation of a number of available sources.

Much of the material from the remainder of this chapter has

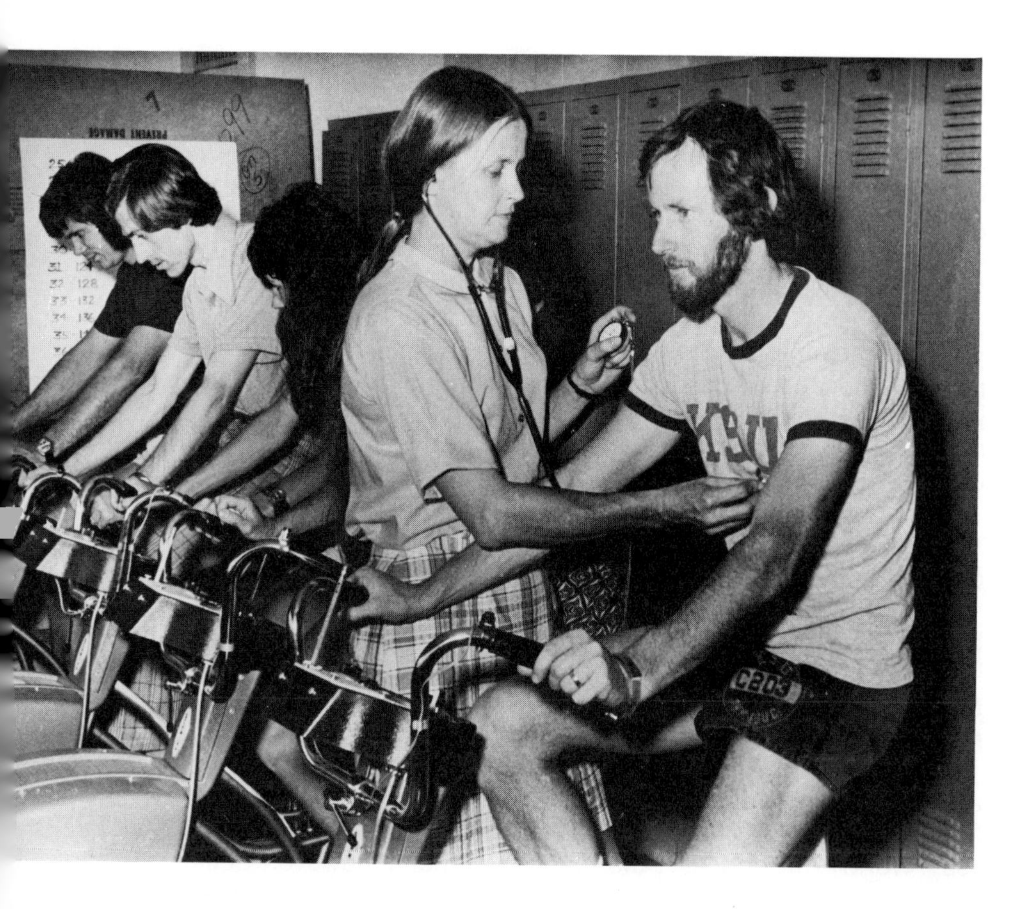

Fig. 1 Health educators and physical educators work toward a common objective—the health of the individual. (Courtesy Kent State University Audio-Visual Services.)

been taken directly from the text by Seidel and Resick entitled *Physical Education: An Overview,* since the objective in both books is to show the relationships, both past and present, between the two cognate fields of physical education and health education.

A SHORT HISTORY OF HEALTH EDUCATION

Although health and the effects on it of the environment figured in writings in Colonial America, the subject was not dealt with as a separate entity in the schools of that period. William A. Alcott (1798–1859) is considered the father of school health education because he wrote on the school environment and necessary health services. Even in his day, however, health was linked to physical education, as the writings of Horace Mann indicate. As a result of Alcott's efforts, Massachusetts became the first state to require by law the teaching of health (1850). Harvard College had initiated a course in hygiene by 1818.

During the latter stages of the nineteenth century, the "marriage" of health and physical education became almost complete, probably because: (1) heads of departments of physical education were mostly medical doctors, (2) the objectives had much in common, and (3) the curricular needs of both were met, to a great extent, in common courses.

This union continued well into the twentieth century, although Thomas Wood and others were disturbed by the lack of attention devoted to health education. There were organizations promoting health education, including some within the federal government, but health continued to play a secondary role in departments of health and physical education and in professional associations. Meanwhile, health *services* were fully accepted and played a major role in the school.

Until after World War I, no teacher training institution offered a major in health education. The first major program was established in Teachers College, Columbia University, in the year 1920–1921. World War II became the real turning point, however. Because of the exploding knowledge in health education and the pressures from health-allied organizations, a number of institutions began offering separate degrees in health education, including master's and doctor's degrees.

A trend noted in the early 1970s is to distinguish the fields of health education and physical education through separate certification requirements. The day of the joint major at either the undergraduate or the graduate level has come to an end. Although the two fields still have some common objectives, they will no longer have common facilities or personnel. The discipline of health education has come of age. The effects of the separation on either of the two related fields is a matter of conjecture at this time. In an age of exploding knowledge and specialization, one can hope that both will benefit, but with growing difficulties in the tax support of public schools, both may suffer.

DEFINITION AND PURPOSES OF SCHOOL HEALTH EDUCATION

Health is that quality of life which permits an individual to function optimally within the environment. Health has physical, mental, and social implications, which differ in individuals and groups. The necessary level of social and mental health of a student living in a residence hall may have little relevance for a hermit. In a similar sense, the level of physical health and fitness for a bank president is not the same as for a steelworker.

The broad programs that deal with efforts to control those conditions having an impact on the prevention of diseases, improvement of the condition of the body for everyday living, and the extension of the life span are known as "public health." These programs are concerned with the conservation and improvement of human resources from the cradle to the grave. School health is the action taken by a school to protect the health of students and other school personnel and to enhance the educative process.

Although health education is ordinarily a joint venture of school and community, this chapter will be concerned with school health education primarily and will refer to community health only when such reference is applicable. In maintaining this approach, we recognize nevertheless that the responsibilities for school health education may rest solely with the local health department or jointly with the schools and the local health department. For either organizational pattern, the purposes of the health education program should be the same.

1. To disseminate information to the students concerning health and those factors which have an impact on it. The information may range from the structure of the body to the use of community agencies for the solution of health problems.

2. To initiate a positive health attitude in the students. For example, the students may have adequate knowledge about the problems of smoking or weight control, but a change in attitude may be necessary before they will use that knowledge.

3. To influence the students to change their behavior now or in the future. In the final analysis, the test of health education is not what people know about the subject, but what they do about it.

It is often assumed that if a person acquires knowledge in a certain area, a change in attitude and behavior in that area will naturally follow. Most of us are examples of the fallacy of this assumption. Indeed, the order may be reversed. A child may respond to a teacher's or parent's "brush your teeth" or "wash your hands" long before he or she understands dental caries or the germ theory of disease. Then, too, a student with excellent knowledge may be faced with a personal problem that causes an attitudinal change in him or her.

In order to achieve the three purposes cited above, health educators organize the health experiences of students into three categories: health instruction, school health services, and the school environment. All three make important contributions to the students' knowledge of health. They will be more fully discussed in the following sections of this chapter. The diagram in Fig. 2 shows how the three areas of health education can be arranged for administration in a joint school and community health department.[1] A chart showing the relationships with physical education is shown in Chap. 1, Fig. 2.

HEALTH INSTRUCTION

Even though health, historically, was not a course in the academic sense of the word, some of what is considered health education was always taught in correlation with other subjects, as part of an integrated unit or project, or incidentally, during the great "teaching moments" which take place as a result of such happenings as tornadoes, hurricanes, earthquakes, or space landings. Under such circumstances, however, the great abundance of exploding health knowledge remained untaught, and serious gaps in health knowledge of students existed. Even with extensive planning, the teaching of health through a series of integrated projects or in correlation with subjects such as biology, physics, and social studies has been found wanting.

Every school needs a concentrated series of courses in health to deal with problems that confront students of different age and grade levels. Although some of these problems (such as acne) are of interest to only one grade or age level, many of the others cross many grade-level lines. The problem of drug abuse, for example, is beginning in the elementary schools and continuing throughout adult life.

The biggest problems confronting the schools are the selection of materials to be taught and the proper introduction and grade

---

[1] Cyrus Mayshark and Leslie W. Irwin, *Health Education in Secondary Schools,* 3rd ed. (St. Louis: C. V. Mosby, 1972): p. 33.

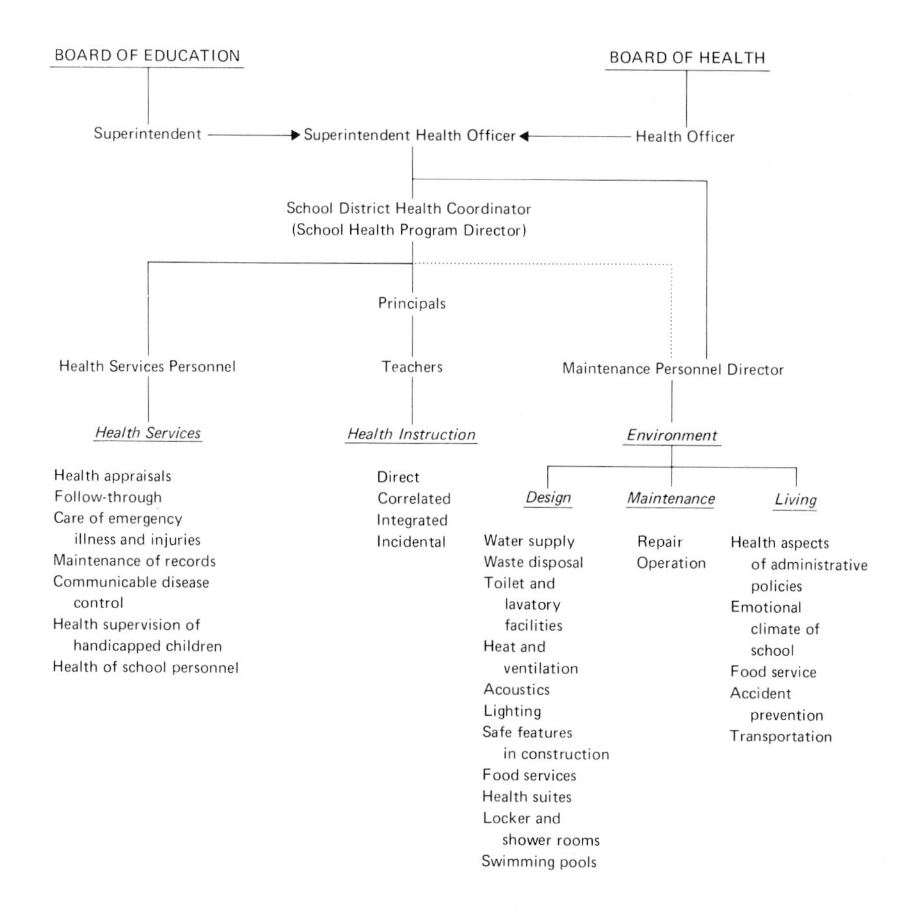

Figure 2

placement of such materials. Subjects which formerly were reserved for discussion at the upper secondary grades or college are now topics for study at the junior high school level, and rightly so. Among them are the following.

Human sexuality. Study begins in the early elementary grades with information about sex-role differences and continues throughout life. Early maturation and dating make the inclusion of proper materials at the junior high school level mandatory. The acceptance of pregnant girls in the total high school program and changes in the obscenity laws create a climate that underscores the need to continue the study of human sexuality.

Drug use and abuse. Problems relating to drugs are no longer confined to the very few in the lower echelons of society or to the adult age group. Since cases of drug addiction are being discovered in children not yet in their teens, instruction on the dangers involved in drug use must begin at the elementary level before the students are subjected to the pressures of peers to adopt a life style that includes the use of drugs. Use of and traffic in glue sniffing, marijuana, LSD, and heroin have legal as well as social implications.

Environmental problems. The pollution of the air we breathe and the water we drink has become a national emergency because it not only threatens our health but also constitutes aesthetic loss and diminishes recreation opportunities. The pollution of the nation's usable water may result in a severe water shortage in several decades unless the trend is reversed.

Radiation, in addition to polluting the air and water, accumulates in plants and animals, sometimes causing genetic changes in those forms of life. The effects of low-grade radiation are still virtually unknown. The dramatic effects of the "bomb" with its concussions, burns, and cancer-causing qualities are well established.

Pesticides, which were once proclaimed as saviors of humanity, are now suspected of causing a number of illnesses. Governmental agencies are urging caution and restraint in the use of most pesticides, and they have banned some entirely.

The use of food additives and substitutes has created hazards to the health of the user. Such additives and substitutes have been used to make food cheaper, more attractive, less fattening, and more appetizing. Some have been found to contribute to unhealthful conditions, especially as agents that may play a causative part in cancer, and they are now under study.

Mental health. The promotion of good mental health and the avoidance of mental illness are dealt with at all grade levels in order to emphasize the preventive rather than the curative aspects of this growing problem. The labor shortage attributable to mental health is among the nation's most critical, and it will not be easily solved. For this reason, early detection of minor problems and an emphasis on positive mental health are of crucial importance.

Social and ethical problems. The legal and ethical problems involved in organ transplants and in the control of the exploding population, for example, pose meaningful questions for both high school and college students. The very definitions of life and death are now being revised.

The topics suggested above, together with more traditional topics, such as rest, exercise, weight control, and consumer education, can make the contents of a relevant curriculum in health education from kindergarten through college vital and exciting. If such a course of study is to have meaning for the student, it must be taught from a psychological or problematical approach rather than from the exclusively physiological, or systems, approach that has been customary in the past. The development of concepts concerning health is more important than the accumulation of knowledge that rapidly becomes outdated.

SCHOOL HEALTH SERVICES

In addition to what students are taught about health in the formal classroom, many of their experiences in and about the school add to their knowledge and attitudes about health. Since participation in health services is often very personal, a good program may be the principal tool in reaching a student. Although few public schools today can fully qualify, a good health service program should contain the following aspects.

Periodic physical examinations. Some states require an annual examination of all students attending elementary and secondary schools, but most do not. Where there is no such requirement, a periodic physical should be given four times during a student's schooling: (1) on first entering school, (2) during elementary school, (3) during junior high school, and (4) during senior high school.

At one time physical examinations were conducted on school premises, but at present the usual practice is for the family physician to examine the child and send the results to the school. The change to the physician's examining room should ensure a more thorough examination than could be provided in the school. Equipment is available for any special testing that may be necessary, and complete records are kept on the child's growth and development. Different arrangements, however, must be made for children of needy families.

Special examinations. There are times other than the periods specified in the preceding paragraph when students will need to be seen by a physician. Athletes in contact sports and other vigorous activities, for example, should have examinations before being allowed to participate in athletics. The heart, lungs, teeth, and tonsils should be examined, and the student should be checked for hernia.

A special examination should also be given to students after a prolonged absence from school because of illness to ensure their readiness to participate in physical education classes or athletics.

Examination follow-up program. One of the valid criticisms leveled at schools in the past has been the failure to use information gained from physical examinations. In the desire to adhere to the principle of "privileged communication," the results of examinations were "locked away" and seldom referred to. The school should make use of these records in any way that will benefit the student. A physical examination loses part of its value if there is no attempt to correct those deviations from the norm which are correctable. Parents or guardians must be informed about the health status of their children. If the parents cannot afford to have corrections made because of their financial status, referral to an agency that takes care of such matters is in order.

Vaccination and inoculation program. Although most states have compulsory vaccination and inoculation programs against communicable diseases as a school entrance requirement, schools in the states that do not must formulate their own requirements. The principal communicable diseases are virtually nonexistent in the United States, but they still abound in many parts of the world, and any relaxation of our program could lead to an epidemic. The immunization program in schools is occasionally objected to on the grounds of religious beliefs. Even when exceptions are made in such cases, the communicable diseases can be kept at a non-epidemic level in the student population unless unusual circumstances prevail. Among the diseases for which immunization should be required for school attendance are smallpox, diphtheria, whooping cough, poliomyelitis, tetanus, and measles. Standard immunizations for these diseases, with the possible exception of that for poliomyelitis, do not guarantee lifetime immunity and do require booster shots at specified intervals.

A system of health referrals and health consultations. Every school system should have a definite policy of dealing with students with health problems, including exclusion from class and exclusion from school. Minor illnesses may be handled by health service personnel, but recurrent or prolonged problems should be referred to the home or a community agency for solution. Exclusion from school sometimes involves legal problems, since the responsibility rests with the school that the student can reach home and that someone willl be there when he or she arrives. The school's excluding officer must be sure that these conditions are met before releasing an ill student. All teachers should recognize symptoms in health and behavior that might be significant and refer students exhibiting such symptoms to the health service or counselor. Sight and hearing problems, especially, often develop between the periodic health examinations.

First aid and safety provisions. Most states have laws requiring each school building to provide a rest and recovery room for students. The room should contain cots, toilets, and lavatories. Since it is not feasible to have a doctor or even a nurse on duty at all times in each building, someone trained and certified in first aid should be readily available. Ideally, all teachers should be certified in first aid procedures.

A plan should be established for handling any type of emergency. The school should require each parent or guardian to complete a form containing pertinent information, including the name of the person to be notified in the event of an emergency. It should list the parent's name and phone number, family physician and phone number, and an alternative person to be notified when a parent cannot be reached, a person who has the legal right to make a decision regarding the child who is sick or injured. A form of this type is shown in Fig. 3. Such a form should be readily accessible and near a telephone.

The information it contains must be kept current to be effective. Athletic coaches and intramural directors who stay after school with large numbers of students should have easy access to this information, or they should have their squad members complete similar forms for their own use.

System of screening tests and observations. Since there may be three or four years between physical examinations, the school system should develop a series of screening procedures. Simple height and weight charts can bring to light deviations from the norm that occur between examinations and that can be investigated before they become serious. When combined with information on body typing, data on height and weight become extremely valuable.

Vision should be tested each year in the elementary grades. Either the Snellen or the Massachusetts Vision Test can be used. The latter is superior, though a little more costly, since it isolates conditions of farsightedness as well as nearsightedness. The classroom teacher can administer these tests with a minimum of training.

EMERGENCY INFORMATION

1. Student: Last name ____ First ____ Middle initial ____

Parents or guardians: Last name ____ Father ____ Mother ____

Address ____ Phone ____

Parent's emergency number (employer): ____ Phone ____

2. Family physician: Last name ____ First ____

Address ____ Phone ____

3. Other physician ____

4. In case of emergency, what hospital should be used? ____

5. Name of relative or friend who is approved to make decisions in case you cannot be reached. ____ Phone ____

6. In case none of the above can be reached, may we have permission to make a decision?

Yes ____ No ____

____
Signature

Figure 3

Hearing testing, in which audiometric devices are used, is much more sophisticated than vision testing and requires longer training periods for the tester. Ordinarily, the school speech and hearing therapist does this type of testing.

Health supervision of school personnel. Where state laws do not require that food handlers have medical examinations, the school board should do so. Since teachers, especially in the elementary schools, have very close contact with students, it should be mandatory that they be free of communicable disease. If nothing else, an annual certification of freedom from tuberculosis should be required. The trend in some states is toward annual examination of all teachers, paid for by the board of education. Some school boards will not release the first salary check until this condition is met. This type of plan is usually a local option of the board of education. The state of Maine, for one, requires that all teachers have an annual physical examination.

THE SCHOOL ENVIRONMENT

The location of the physical plant, the relationship of students to teachers, and the nature of the organization for instruction all have an impact on the health of the student. It is essential that the student be provided a most healthful school environment to enhance the learning process. A discussion on the effect of the environment on the student's health and the learning process follows.

The physical environment. A healthful school environment begins with the location of the school itself. It is difficult to change an established location, and therefore the initial selection of a school site affects students for decades. Is it near railroads, factories, or a main highway? Must most of the students cross the main part of the city to reach it? Is it located in the direction of the future growth of the city?

The disadvantages of old buildings located near noisy factories can be decreased by the use of tree screens between the noise and the school, by careful installation of acoustical tile, and by careful selection of courses to be taught on the noisy and quiet sides of the building.

The school environment also includes the color of the paint on the walls, lighting, humidity and heat, the condition of restrooms, and the adequacy of food services. Laboratories and workshops should be properly vented, and playfields, walks, and building approaches should be properly cared for.

Although most of these problems rest with the administration, an alert student body and teaching corps will ensure the maintenance of a healthful school environment. Because of their special expertise, health teachers and administrators have additional responsibility in these areas.

School organization and health. The manner in which the school day is organized and administered may have at least as much effect on the student as the physical makeup of the school. Among the factors to be considered are the following.

1. *Length of the school day.* It is estimated that the secondary school student now spends more than 1100 hours a year in school. There are advocates of a longer school day, but with the addi-

tional time spent on co-curricular work, most of the student's day is in fact spent in school. The school day is—and should be—gradually lengthened from kindergarten through senior high school, directly in proportion to the decrease in fatigue and the increase in attention span as the student grows older.

2. *Length of class period.* Similar to the problem of school day length is that of class period length. Fatigue and attention span must be considered, and shorter periods in the lower elementary grades permit frequent change in the types of activity. Such change is essential for a proper learning climate at that age level. Periods of 20–30 minutes are common at this level; periods of 40–45 are more usual in the junior and senior high school. At the college level the practice of dog-legging (double period on some days) is necessary to make efficient use of existing space when weekly meetings are variable.

3. *Homework policy.* Some schools have had to initiate a policy of limiting homework assignments to protect the students from demands for unreasonable amounts of work by teachers who seem unaware of the requirements of other disciplines. The school may curtail homework by establishing a time limit per assignment or by restricting homework for each subject to specified days of the week. For instance, English, language, and mathematics teachers may be permitted to give homework on Monday, Wednesday, and Friday, whereas the science, humanities, and social studies teachers are restricted to Tuesday and Thursday.

4. *Curtailment of outside activities.* Often a student gets involved in too many extra- or co-curricular activties, either by choice or because forced to by peer or parental pressure to participate. Some schools have restricted students to two or three extracurricular activities. Even though the activities sponsored by the school can be controlled, however, the student may still be subjected to a number of nonschool activities and lessons. The cumulative effect of school work, extracurricular activities, and private lessons may be detrimental to the student. When a student's mental and physical health are endangered by such excesses and pressures, the parents must be notified by the health or counseling services.

5. *Rewards for attendance.* A program of honoring students with perfect attendance records, though understandable in purpose, may actually perform a disservice to the teachers and student body. Some elementary school children come to school with communicable diseases in order to keep their records intact. The attendance

certificate becomes of greater significance than their own health or the health of others they come in contact with. The practice of making awards for perfect attendance is fortunately dying out.

6. *Sick-leave program for teachers.* A similar threat to general health may stem from the school's sick-leave policy for teachers. If the teachers must pay for their own substitutes after a maximum number of absences, some will come to school with such communicable diseases as influenza, thus exposing students and other members of the faculty. On the other hand, a program which allows the accumulation of sick days for future use may result in a similar response: the teacher may "save" them for a protracted illness.

7. *Time placement of difficult subjects.* In the self-contained classroom of the elementary school, teachers can arrange their courses to meet the needs of the students. Teachers can plan to teach more difficult subjects during that part of the day when the students are most rested and relaxed, or can alternate them with recreational types of classes, such as art, music, or physical education. Unfortunately, however, at most large secondary schools, not every student can have a desirable schedule. All subjects are taught during most hours of the school day, and the student must take them when they fit into the schedule and not when she or he is most fit to take them.

The Teacher and Student Health. The interpersonal relationships between the teacher and the students within the classroom have an impact on the health of the students. Among the considerations which contribute to student health are the following.

1. *The make-up program following absence.* Frequently the procedures followed in having the student make up missed work are in direct contradiction to the practices of good health. Following an illness that necessitated absence from school, the student is often inundated with make-up work to complete while he or she is still recovering. In other words, immediately on returning to school, he or she is expected to produce more than the healthy student.

2. *Seating arrangements.* Because it is practical (administratively) to follow some ascending or descending alphabetical order in seating students, a teacher may inadvertently place students with sight or hearing problems in positions that may retard their progress in class. Taking attendance, collecting written work, and grading may be facilitated by this arrangement, but students may suffer for it. A proper health service identifies the students with handicaps tactfully and without the knowledge of the other students.

3. *Fear of the teacher or subject matter.* In a class where there is actual fear of physical harm for either poor performance or failure to perform at all, the student may suffer impairment of health. If the teacher uses the technique of ridicule or embarrassment, the student may have a similar reaction. When exchanges between teachers and students occur in an atmosphere of mutual respect, stress and tensions are held to a minimum. Leniency in course requirements is not in any sense necessary to achieve this ideal, however. Students may learn to enjoy a difficult subject if they are encouraged whenever they show improvement and progress. Criticism of a student's actions may be offered in the interests of improvement, and creative self-expression is not stifled in a rush to conformity.

4. *Free expression.* Although the demand for student silence in a classroom may impair the learning process, the opposite may also be true. Young children forced to work in the bedlam that surrounds the overpermissive teacher may experience complete mental and physical fatigue at the end of the day. Studies have shown that excessive noise causes physical fatigue among factory workers, and one can reasonably assume the same effect on students.

5. *Overemphasis on one grade or performance.* There are situations in the educational system in which one performance may change the course of a student's educational life. An example is the series of scholarship examinations. Although such practices are common in Europe, no single test or performance should carry sufficient weight to cause extreme tension and frustration among the student body.

OCCUPATIONAL OPPORTUNITIES

The entire field of health sciences is rich in career opportunities which combine the excitement of exploding knowledge and a feeling of service to others. At present and also for the foreseeable future, there is a shortage of trained and qualified personnel in most areas of the health sciences, of which health education is a part. Furthermore, with the population increasing and with growing concern for the health needs of everyone, there will certainly be demands for more and more persons to become involved in health education as a career.

One thinks of health educators as being confined to formal educational systems, from the elementary schools to the universities. Far from it! Job opportunities exist in such voluntary health agencies as the American Cancer Society, the National Tuberculosis Association, and others. These organizations, which are supported by voluntary financial contributions and services, employ staff members at the national, state, and local levels. Since each agency is generally concerned with a specific health problem, trained personnel are hired to educate the public concerning that particular problem in an effort to combat or eradicate it.

There are also many opportunities in "official health agencies," the tax-supported arms of local, state, and federal government. Examples are city and county health departments, state health departments with their district offices, and the various divisions of the United States Department of Health, Education and Welfare (HEW). All employ health educators in various capacities in order to reach the public with their health messages.

Most of the state and national professional organizations employ health educators to make the public aware of certain health problems and their solutions. Professional associations are groups of individuals with a common background of service, a systematic curriculum and training, and some form of certification which legally allows them to practice their profession. Among the professional organizations employing health educators are the American Medical Association, the American Dental Association, and the American Alliance of Health, Physical Education, and Recreation.

CASE STUDY

At King High School the health classes were taught by physical education teachers and coaches who were certified in both fields. The regional accreditation visit revealed the lack of interest in this assignment by all but one of the teachers involved. The report of the accreditation team further revealed that this attitude toward health classes had permeated to the students.

After receiving the above report the superintendent had a conference with Mr. Jamison, the Department Head, concerning the negative report. He told Mr. Jamison that he was to resolve the problem before the next semester began and that at this time there seemed to be very little possibility of adding additional staff.

1. What are the essential issues in this case?
2. How can this problem be resolved?
3. What principles or policies are found in the above case study?

SELECTED REFERENCES

Anderson, C. L. *Community Health* (2d ed.). St. Louis, Mo.: C. V. Mosby, 1973.

Anderson, C. L., and William H. Creswell, Jr. *School Health Practices* (6th ed.). St. Louis, Mo.: C. V. Mosby, 1976.

Bucher, Charles A., Einar A. Olsen, and Carl E. Willgoose. *The Foundations of Health* (2d ed.). Englewood Cliffs, N.J.: Prentice-Hall, 1976.

Cornacchia, Harold J., Wesley M. Staton, and Leslie W. Irwin. *Health in Elementary Schools* (3rd ed.). St. Louis, Mo.: C. V. Mosby, 1970.

Haag, Jessie Helen. *School Health Program* (rev. ed.). New York: Holt, Rinehart and Winston, 1967.

Jenne, Frank H., and Walter H. Greene. *Turner's School Health and Health Education* (7th ed.). St. Louis, Mo.: C. V. Mosby, 1976.

Marcum, Everett C. "Operative Guidelines for College and University Departments," *School Health Review,* **1** (February 1970); 21–25.

Mayshark, Cyrus, and Leslie W. Irwin. *Health Education in Secondary Schools* (3rd ed.). St. Louis, Mo.: C. V. Mosby, 1972.

Mayshark, Cyrus, and Donald Shaw. *Administration of School Health Programs* (2d ed.). St. Louis, Mo.: C. V. Mosby, 1977.

Means, Richard K. *A History of Health Education in the United States.* Philadelphia: Lea and Febiger, 1963.

Miller, Dean F., and Susan Shunk. "A Survey of Elementary School Health Services with Emphasis on Preparation for Emergency Care Procedures of Sick and Injured Students," *The Journal of School Health,* **42** (February 1972): 114–117.

Nemir, Alma. *The School Health Program.* Philadelphia: W. B. Saunders, 1970.

Oberteuffer, Delbert, and Mary K. Beyrer. *School Health Education* (4th ed.). New York: Harper and Row, 1966.

Stiles, William W. *Individual and Community Health.* New York: McGraw-Hill, 1953.

Turner, C. E., Harriet B. Randall, and Sara Louise Smith. *School Health and Health Education* (6th ed.). St. Louis, Mo.: C. V. Mosby, 1970.

7

PUBLIC AND HUMAN RELATIONS

STUDY STIMULATORS

1. What has been the attitude of educators in general concerning the relationship with the public in the past?
2. What is the basic difference between publicity and public relations?
3. What are some basic principles upon which a program of public relations should be built in order to be successful?
4. What media are available for use in a good public relations program of a department of physical education and athletics?
5. Are there guidelines which may be of special value when meeting members of the working press?
6. In order to conduct a successful program of public relations in the areas of physical education and interscholastic activities, what groups or "publics" must be reached?
7. How has PEPI made an impact upon physical education in your state?

The most crying need in the humbler ranks of life is that they should be allowed some part in the direction of public affairs.

HENRIK IBSEN

Since physical education and athletics are an integral part of the whole school program, the first portions of this chapter will be devoted to public relations and the school. The materials are of a general nature and they apply equally to all phases of the school system. Physical education and athletics have enjoyed a favorable place in the relationships between schools and their publics. This in itself has uncovered additional problems for school administrators. In the latter portion of the chapter specific examples of interaction between the public and physical education and athletic programs are given. In this manner the authors hope to increase understanding of a rapidly developing responsibility of all school personnel. Schools can no longer ignore this facet of responsibility, its direction cannot be left to chance. Public relations training should be part of every administrator's professional training, since most schools will not be in the position to obtain the services of a professional public relations expert.

The business world, by necessity, has learned to communicate with the public. The educational world has not kept pace even though education is in every sense of the word "big business" in terms of money spent and products involved. This seems to be a paradox, since the basis of our society is the educational levels of its participants and the interaction of these participants in a free society. Humans have the capacity to transmit knowledge, desires, and feelings to others. This dynamic process of communications is fundamental for human society. Historically, those involved in education have tried to operate in a world of their own, isolated from the public to whom they owe their existence.

School personnel, as a group, have been suspicious of the communications media. They have been entirely too slow to provide the public with the information to which it is entitled. By law, schools are public business. Since the public owns the school, the problem is not to sell the school to the public but to inform it and to have the public participate in decision making in the school system, as do the stockholders in any business. The school personnel spend the citizens' money and mold their most precious possessions into products which must meet their approval. They have a right to know what is done with their money and their children, and they don't support that which they don't approve of or understand.

PUBLIC RELATIONS: AN INTERPRETATION

The public relations field evolved from publicity, and in the minds of many it still remains synonymous with it. Since public relations is a relatively new field of endeavor, there are more definitions of what it is *not* than concise definitions of what it is. A definition of school public relations must include the management function which sees the problems of the school in terms of public interest and initiates communication between the school and the public in order to inform the public about the school's program and thus gain its approval.

A school system cannot avoid public relations. Relations with the public may be either good, bad, or somewhere in between. The public has opinions about the school, its personnel, and its programs, including physical education and athletics. These opinions are formed from impressions gained by contact with students, school programs, and school personnel. Sometimes these impressions are formed by reading newspaper releases and by other less objective means. Unfortunately, the picture may not be in focus with that which actually exists.

Public relations must begin with the bold premise that the public has a right to know everything about the school and not just what the administration and the board of education wishes it to know.

The credibility gap exists in schools as it does in other arms of government service. To inform the public is dangerous business if the program or product is not good. But it is more dangerous to deceive the public, because sooner or later someone will discover the facts and bring them to light. Even a good program of public relations will not substitute for a good school program, nor will it replace poor policies which exist.

As has been stated above, school administrators have been and still are suspicious of the mass communications media. Even where the law demands open school board meetings, decisions are often made prior to these open meetings, which then become showcases. Educators often expect newspapers to use double standards, serving the schools as publicity medium and yet serving the public in its normal role. These two roles are not always compatible. Duty occasionally forces a reporter to bring out unpleasant facts about the schools. This does not enhance his or her position in later visits to the school, for educators often take criticism as a personal attack. Since many administrators have only a superficial knowledge of public relations at best, they behave as though they are in a special position until they need public support. In times of crisis, attitudes tend to change. Hastily conceived programs often fail when the public becomes difficult to convince. Administrators then become almost entirely defensive and lose their objectivity. The public is entitled to know the unvarnished truths of the school's position with respect to policies, finances, and programs. Hidden weaknesses fester and sooner or later erupt. If granted full command of the facts, the public could help in the solution of problems. According to Stiles, "Until individuals feel free to challenge established traditions and to freely propose alternate solutions without fear of incrimination, sound public and human relations do not exist in schools." [1]

The vital function of public relations is to establish an open channel so that the public will be sufficiently informed to make proper decisions.

The Role of Publicity

As expressed earlier in this chapter, public relations evolved from publicity and the two terms are still used synonymously. Public relations has long outgrown this role. Publicity is but one facet, one arm, of the process of relating one individual to another or to a

---

[1] Lindley J. Stiles, "Positive and Human Public Relations for School Personnel," *Virginia Journal of Education*, **69** (November 1965): 14.

group. In spite of one writer's remark that "publicity has its rightful place in the public relations program and its place is in the servant's quarters," publicity does play an important role. Its relationship to public relations is parallel to that between advertising and customer relations. Publicity trys to engender an interest, while public relations is the sustaining of a good relationship. Publicity is the dissemination of information about individuals or groups in order to attract the public's attention to an event, an outstanding performance, or the development of a new idea.

Publicity reflects present positions and practices. It may extol or justify, depending on whether the practices and positions are good or bad. Both praise and condemnation can be valuable in showing what is presently occurring or what is desired. A football coach may explain a series of losses by publicizing a series of key injuries. Similarly, the coach may explain some unusual success by the sudden and unexpected development of one of the young players.

The chief problem in school publicity, especially in the areas of physical education and athletics, is to secure, organize, and present information to the mass communications media. A cursory examination of any daily newspaper shows the enormous amount of space that is devoted to school sports news. The schools could not begin to buy this space in a competitive market.

Publicity can be as unfavorable as it is favorable. It can be subject to misinterpretation and misunderstanding. If it is overdone, it can bring out an unfavorable reaction from the group it is trying to influence.

Publicity cannot stand alone. It must be part of a total program of public relations.

PRINCIPLES OF PUBLIC RELATIONS FOR PHYSICAL EDUCATION AND ATHLETICS

It is an impossible task to try to isolate the many problems of public relations which confront the administrators of programs of physical education and athletics, since each setting makes for provincial problems.

The following is an attempt to develop a list of working principles which can be used to solve local problems.

Good public relations start with a good program. A teacher, coach, or administrator with an outstanding personality might sell an inferior or "paper" program for a short time. Sooner or later that person will be asked to produce. There is no substitute for a good program of physical education or athletics. No amount of "Madison Avenue" advertising will get the public to support an inferior program over a long period of time. The profession must start with a marketable product. Good programs can begin under severe restrictions and lack of support. Students, even young ones, are discriminating enough to know when they are given a quality program. It is surprising at times how rapidly the news of a good program spreads to other schools throughout the state and to professional associations throughout the nation.

A program of good public relations interprets the profession to the public. The single greatest problem in the field of physical education is the misconception of what "physical education" is really all about. A physical educator who asked ten lay people for a definition of physical education would receive ten different answers. If ten professionals were asked, almost as many different replies would be received. Even when professionals agree, they tend not to communicate such agreement to the public. It is little wonder that the lay public has a hazy picture of the discipline of physical education. Each person interprets physical education from his or her experience or from that of his or her children. Little is written in lay periodicals which might enlighten anyone who might be interested. Even academic colleagues are in the dark about the position of physical education in the academic spectrum.

The fastest means of beginning a public relations program is through the students. Use of students is the fastest and most intimate way for the school to contact parents. The center of the parents' interest in school is their *child;* therefore parents also feel a close relationship with the teacher. Even though the teacher may have 60 students, he or she is still *Johnny's* teacher or *Sue's* coach. The parents do not feel as close to the principal, and seldom is the term "Johnny's principal" heard. In an unpublished study, Van Winkle[2] found that when parents were asked "from what source do you get most information about your schools?" over 50 percent replied "from my child." No other source was greater than 10 percent.

The type of program, and how it is interpreted to the students, is the keystone of a good public relations program in physical education and athletics. All students should be told what they are expected to do and why they are doing it. This is the time when ob-

---

[2] Harold Van Winkle, "A Study of School-Community Information Programs in Northwest Ohio," (doctoral thesis, Indiana University, 1956).

jectives can be interpreted for the students in terms they can understand. They will then have an interest in becoming more skilled, and healthier, and in learning social values; or their interest may be entirely recreational. It is here that they form permanent opinions about the activity program, opinions they will relay to their parents.

The image of the profession is an important factor in the public relations program. What happens when the teacher moves onto the gymnasium floor and begins the lesson is more important than any other phase of public relations. The image of the school and the physical education program is determined by the people who make up the program and, once established, cannot easily be changed. What type of image do physical educators offer others in the school system? What have they done to remove the picture of the stereotyped man or woman physical education teacher? Van Winkle suggests that one way to improve the public image is for each individual in the profession to begin by making a self-inventory of the following:

> 1. Are you well groomed and attractively dressed, or are you in the sloppy sweatshirt group?
>
> 2. Check your personal habits. Do you smoke in front of your students, or anywhere in school? Are you seen in local bars? Do you use profanity? Have you let yourself become flabby and overweight through lack of exercise and self-control?
>
> 3. What about the quality of your teaching? Do you have your courses planned in advance for the semester with carefully determined objectives you want your students to reach, or do you improvise from day to day and on the spur of the moment?
>
> 4. Do you treat your students with kindness and understanding, but at the same time maintain discipline?
>
> 5. Are you well-read, or do you find the scholarly life a bore? Are you seen at concerts and dramatic productions, or do you limit your recreation to attending athletic contests?
>
> 6. How much attention have you or your departmental faculty given to curriculum? Has this attention consisted primarily of scheduling classes, rather than a thorough study of physical education in the total school program and in the lives of students? [3]

Physical educators and coaches have long taken a defensive stance against society and especially other educators who are critical of the field. A public relations expert once visited the author's

---

[3] Harold Van Winkle, "Improving the Image," *Journal of Health, Physical Education, Recreation, and Athletics*, **39** (February 1968): 43–44. Reprinted by permission.

class. He asked the class to give him ten things they wanted to bring before the public. The students wrote them on the chalkboard, and the public relations expert found that eight of them were negative or defensive. Is it not the time to show a positive image?

Good public relations involves cooperative planning. When a new program of activities or course of study is to be introduced, it is often wise to share it with a committee of parents before putting it into practice. Even though they are not experts, parents can give the layperson's reaction to the proposal. If a new athletic facility is needed, the resources of the community should be utilized. Before a good program of athletics or intramurals is eliminated because of lack of staff, space, or money, it is well to discuss the problem with the citizens of the community. They might be able to give some alternative solution, and if it becomes necessary to eliminate these activities, the school will have a sympathetic rather than a hostile citizenry.

A public relations program must be continuous to be effective. Often public relations is held in a state of suspended animation until there is a need for approval of either financing or change in administrative programs. This type of "fire alarm" public relations is not effective. Effective public relations is not an emergency but it helps to meet emergencies. It is not a transitory activity, it is a continuous one. It depends on the public, whose good will and understanding usually cannot be acquired quickly. Public relations is not a commodity to be purchased or brought out of storage in time to salvage a building program from defeat at the polls. Public relations involves the daily program of instruction and the mundane affairs of schools, as well as the crucial issues facing schools.

To keep a continuous program, local reporters may be in need of continued in-service programs which stress the purpose and practices of today's schools. There is a great turnover in those who cover the educational scene.

A public relations program must be based on honesty. The people who support the schools have a right to know the facts about them. Sound programs of public relations must tell the truth no matter how undesirable this seems to the administrators. Programs must deal realistically with citizens' questions about the conduct of the school. The abrogation of this responsibility causes a loss of confidence. Misconceptions and half-truths that are given to obtain short-term goals become expensive when they are exposed to the light of truth. Even such trivia as down-grading talents of players to harvest the glory in their future success cannot be condoned. Phony efforts to create such a frame of reference are transparent to most of the public. Brochures and publicity releases from some educational institutions have the creditability of a fairy tale.

A good program of public relations makes use of a variety of media. Public relations techniques make use of all existing communications media and sometimes invent new ones for a particular problem. This involves a skill which not all physical educators possess. One of the real problems is to select the proper media for specific phases of the program. Fortunately, both physical education and athletics lend themselves to most of the well-known media to a greater extent than do other academic disciplines. The administrator, the athletic director, and the physical educator must understand how public opinions are formed. They must understand how consensus is arrived at by the members of a group. In the latter, in addition to using mass media they may have to utilize face-to-face conversation with the power leaders of the group.

There are many well-established media which can be used. The person or persons involved or responsible for public relations in the department or school should learn the specific requirements of all media and the types of results which can be expected from each. It must be remembered that there is open competition from other educational institutions and from businesses, for the time and space available. The odds are always against one institution; therefore, in the words of one car rental company, physical education must "try harder."

So many kinds of media are available that it is impossible to explain them extensively. Some of the more commonly used ones for athletics and physical education are listed below, with a few words of explanation and caution.

Face-to-face discourse. This has frequently been shown to be the most effective instrument of persuasion. This begins on the playing fields and in the gymnasium with the students and can be extended to parents and other community groups. There are many opportunities to speak to parents during visitations to schools, at P.T.A. meetings, and at service club or church meetings. The face-to-face discourse includes also the associations physical educators have with their own colleagues and administrators. Much of this can be carried on through social or academic meetings, where an honest interchange of ideas takes place.

Reports or bulletins. One of the most inexpensive and effective means of reaching both students and parents is through handouts given to students. These may run the gamut from the grade reports to a notice of a future exhibition. Younger children are more apt to take materials home than are the high school students. Mailings to homes are expensive, and reports sent this way should merit this extra expense.

Open houses and exhibitions. The entire realm of physical activity lends itself to exhibitions or activity nights. New programs can be demonstrated to parents who can then see their children's place in the program. These exhibitions can be scheduled as special nights or they can become a program within another scheduled event, such as a P.T.A. meeting or at the half-time of a basketball game. Gymnastic and dance exhibitions have been especially effective in this type of arrangement. Exhibitions of this nature should portray the school program rather than something "dreamed up" for the special event.

Radio and television. Both these media are excellent for telling the story of physical education and athletics. Since activity is a visual art, television is a natural means for communicating with the public. Unfortunately, television time is at a premium and not available for many programs of lesser general public interest. Short film clips and interviews concerning up-coming events can be used effectively. Spot announcements on radio are much more available. Some local stations carry special programs which are for the sole purpose of publicizing coming events. In the use of both radio and television excellent planning is necessary.

Newspapers. The school competes with all facets of society for newspaper space. Since newspapers must cover all the news of the day, the physical educator and coach, together with the administrator, must determine what types of materials are acceptable. The more they know about the news and how to report it, the more successful they become in getting their news printed. The newspapers always have more news than they can print. To establish a good working relationship with the newspapers, school personnel should heed the following suggestions.

1. The school personnel should become acquainted with the newspeople with whom they have to work. Newspeople should be invited to see the program about which they are expected to write.

2. School personnel should become aware of the various departments of a newspaper. A good story sent to the wrong department may be lost, since there is a distinct difference between sports news, political news, and social stories.
3. Coaches should have score books and statistics available for ready reference in case of telephone calls regarding their sports.
4. Demands for retractions should be carefully considered, since the ensuing controversy may cause more damage than the original story.
5. Since reporters are seldom involved with policy making, school officials should not complain to the reporters concerning the newspaper's policy.
6. The newsperson has an obligation to the public to give the news as he or she sees it. Teachers, coaches, and administrators should expect to get an unfavorable story occasionally without considering it a personal attack.
7. Newspeople should be treated fairly. Stories should not be given freely to other newspeople when a particular one has worked hard to obtain it. If there are both evening and morning papers in the same locale, the big stories should be broken at alternate times so as to ensure fair coverage. Dated releases may be used to achieve this end.
8. The attempt to buy favorable stories with gifts and promises beyond what is common practice should be avoided.
9. "Off the record" statements should not be used too often. It is difficult to suppress some news items. Reporters will hold a story if the reason given is a reasonable one.
10. The best news media to use are local ones, since they are the base for local support of the programs. Large city and distant newspapers may add glamour to the public relations program, but will not help gain the support of the local citizenry.

Professional writing. Professional physical educators have not written enough about their profession, nor have they written for the proper media. The articles which are prepared are sent to professional periodicals. This is necessary to a point, but only professional physical educators read these periodicals. For good public relations the professional writings of physical educators must find their way into the broader or general education publications and then into the lay or popular magazines which filter into the homes. To date this has been done to a very limited extent. Lay magazines have the coverage which reach the people who should be informed about the programs of physical education in this country.

Miscellaneous media. Within the school there are a number of ways in which attention can be drawn to any facet of the physical education program. Among these are photographs, paintings or charts which, when placed in the proper setting, can draw the attention of students, faculty, and administration. The bulletin board centrally located should be utilized to show current intramural standings. Occasionally pictures of outstanding portions of the program can be placed in store windows or other places of business where they can be seen by the townspeople.

THE MANY PUBLICS MUST BE REACHED

The public relations experts, those who make their livelihood in the field, have known for many years that the "public" has many faces. Each field of endeavor has many different "publics" to which it must address itself. So it is with physical education and athletics. It is necessary to reach these "publics" and to communicate with them about the programs which are to be carried on in the schools. The following is a list of these "publics" which must be reached if any program of public relations is to succeed.

1. The *present students* must be reached because they carry home the message every day from the gymnasium and the field. Students who are given a good physical education program can become excellent press agents. They must be given quality programs, because when they become future parents and taxpayers they interpret the needs of the school in terms of their own past experiences. The next generation must share the cost of a poor program given to the present generation.

2. Other *teachers* in the system must be reached. They should be informed about the scope and nature of the present program and how it is related to their subject and the whole of the educational process. The information may be given to them through informal and social contacts or during committee or interdepartmental meetings. Many of these colleagues may be in positions to either endorse or reject curricular proposals in physical education.

3. The *administrative staff* must be reached since these are the people who endorse, interpret, and recommend programs and changes in programs to the board of education and the public.

It cannot be assumed that all principals or superintendents are knowledgeable in physical education.

4. The *general public* must be reached. These people include more than the parents who were mentioned earlier. The general public must pass the building and operating levies. It must also give support and approve the programs carried on in the school.

SPECIAL PROBLEMS OF PUBLICITY FOR ATHLETICS

Public relations and publicity take on additional significance in those states in which junior high school and high school athletic programs must be supported from funds other than tax revenue. Both public relations and publicity must be carefully planned and geared to the size of the program in order to guarantee that the budget will be met. There are a number of media available for these purposes. Since the media were discussed previously in this chapter, only specific examples will be repeated here to show how the athletic director or coach can reach the "publics" necessary.

1. *Preseason brochures* which list the squad members, their size, and grade level are almost mandatory. These can be as simple as mimeographed sheets or as complex as the large souvenir booklets sold at professional contests.
2. *Daily or weekly releases* giving vital statistics, physical condition, and personnel changes serve the purpose of attracting the public through newspaper copy.
3. A *downtown coaches' group* meeting weekly stimulates interest in the sport. The coach has a chance to meet people face-to-face, to answer questions, and in some instances to correct erroneous impressions about the game or sports program.
4. Formation of *knothole gangs* stimulates interest of a group who will support the program in the future or perhaps even join the program at a later date.
5. *Speeches at sports banquets* give the coach or athletic director a chance to be heard on a variety of subjects. The contributions of sports to the student and society is an example of one suitable topic.

RESPONSIBILITY FOR PUBLIC RELATIONS

There are very few administration line charts which show the responsibilities for public relations. Although the superintendent is responsible for public relations in an educational system, the duties normally fall into the hands of the building principal. Unfortunately, most building principals have only a layperson's knowledge of the techniques used in a good program. At times the burden of informing the public falls onto the teacher and coach if there are no provisions for a head of department or athletic director. In reality, all school and departmental personnel have a responsibility for establishing good public relations. From the secretary who answers the phone or greets the visitor to the janitor or groundskeeper who gives someone directions to the superintendent's office, all play a part. Internal public relations between these people and the personal contact they have is as important as external public relations. It is not always necessary for these relations to be pleasant or friendly to have good human relations. There are at times disagreements, but the lines of communication are still open. Criticism should not be taken as attack.

Since school systems cannot afford to hire public relations personnel, it is imperative that administrators and teachers study the techniques necessary to communicate their needs and programs to the public. Also, since problems of physical education and athletics are so widely misunderstood, it becomes doubly necessary for physical educators to become skilled in the arts of communication and human relations.

PEPI: Physical Education Public Information Project

One of the biggest public relations projects ever to be launched by a professional association was initiated by the American Alliance for Health, Physical Education, and Recreation at its convention in Detroit in 1971 when it voted to fund a pilot project for one year. Later that year the Alliance named Fay Biles, Kent State University, as the PEPI Director.

The entire project is based on a system of overlapping local and state coordinators who develop contacts with the local media to utilize materials developed by the national headquarters staff. Such material is formulated into an individualized public relations program based on local needs.

The focus of all this material is on five principal concepts which are indicative of what is termed the "new physical education." These concepts are:

1. A physically educated person is one who has knowledge and skill concerning his or her body and how it works.
2. Physical education is health insurance.

3. Physical education can contribute to academic achievement.
4. A sound physical education program contributes to development of a positive self-concept.
5. A sound physical education program helps an individual attain social skills.

Although the fruits of public relations must be viewed over a long period, the immediate results seem to be all positive. The program could easily develop into a model for other similar associations. Much of the spin-off from this project can be seen in an excellent summary article entitled "Speak Out" in the *Journal of Health, Physical Education, and Recreation* (October 1972). This article could well serve as a basis for a localized program of public relations.

CASE STUDY

Central City High School was embarking upon an extensive building program which would include physical education and athletic facilities. Mr. Collier, head of the physical education and athletic programs, together with his staff, evaluated the present program and determined that the bulk of the problems stemmed from the fact that the girls and boys both had to use the same floor space. Because of the varsity athletic programs, the girls' extracurricular program was practically nonexistent. Then, too, the coeducational clubs such as gymnastics and dance were without practice space.

From conversations with school administrators and townspeople, Mr. Collier had gathered that the majority of the people would endorse a facility which provided a large seating area for athletics and meetings. Without jeopardizing the position of the school in this time of emergency building, Mr. Collier and his teachers wished to obtain more teaching stations at the price of some permanent seating.

1. What are the essential issues in this case?
2. How can Mr. Collier and his staff achieve their purpose?
3. What principles of good public relations are found in this case study?

SELECTED REFERENCES

American Association for Health, Physical Education, and Recreation. "Speak Out: A Public Relations Guide for Professionals in Recreation, Health, Physical Education and Sports," *Journal of Health Physical Education Recreation,* **43** (October 72): 41–56.

Baley, James A. "Public Relations," *Journal of Health Physical Education Recreation,* **32** (November 1961): 27–28.

Canfield, Bertrand R. *Public Relations* (5th ed.). Homewood, Ill.: Richard D. Irwin, 1968.

Duke, Wayne. "Public Relations and Athletics," *Journal of Health Physical Education Recreation,* **30** (October 1959): 17–52.

Gallemore, Sandra L. "The Teacher: Key to an Effective Public Relations Program," *The Physical Educator,* **30** (May 1973): 66–68.

Hughes, William Leonard, Esther French, and Nelson Lehsten. *Administration of Physical Education for Schools and Colleges.* New York: The Ronald Press, 1962, Chap. 5.

Luffman, Helen E. "Use the Experts," *Journal of Health Physical Education Recreation,* **32** (November 1961): 29.

Marston, John E. *The Nature of Public Relations*, New York: McGraw-Hill, 1963.

Miller, Ben W. "Public Relations—A Professional Need," *Journal of Health Physical Education Recreation,* **32** (January 1961): 32.

Rice, Arthur H., Jr., "A 'Hypodermic Needle' Approach," *Michigan Education Journal,* **43** (January 1966): 6–9.

Shroyer, George. "Inform, Don't Let Them Guess," *Journal of Health Physical Education Recreation,* **39** (February 1968): 42.

Singer, Robert N. "Communicate or Perish," *Journal of Health Physical Education Recreation,* **39** (February 1968): 40–41.

Stiles, Lindley J. "Positive and Human Public Relations for School Personnel," *Virginia Journal of Education,* **69** (November 1965): 11–14.

Van Winkle, Harold. "Improving the Image," *Journal of Health Physical Education Recreation,* **39** (February 1968): 43–44.

Voltmer, Edward F., and Arthur Esslinger. *The Organization and Administration of Physical Education* (4th ed.). New York: Appleton-Century-Crofts, 1967.

Wiley, Roger C. "Physical Education Festival: A Public Relations Device," *The Physical Educator,* **17** (October 1960): 98–100.

8

EVALUATION OF STUDENTS, PROGRAMS, TEACHERS, AND ADMINISTRATION

STUDY STIMULATORS

1. What are some principles which underlie the grading of students in a physical education class?
2. Can a rationale be developed for the use of subjective grading?
3. Should the factor of improvement be considered in a student's grade evaluation?
4. How can teaching effectiveness be evaluated by the administration?
5. What are the strengths and weaknesses of having students evaluate instruction?
6. How can the administrator utilize the process of self-evaluation to improve his or her position?
7. What are the advantages and disadvantages of pass-fail grading?

Man is the measure of all things.

PROTAGORAS

The saying which prefaces this chapter could well be expanded to say that a human is also the "measurer" of all things. Evaluation is an inescapable fact of life. If this were not true, it is doubtful that much, if any, of the world's progress would have occurred. Since thoughtful evaluation is essential for intelligent change, whether it is in the field of nuclear physics or in education, some aspects of the problem need to be considered briefly.

Many examples could be cited of the fact that a human is by nature a measurer, an evaluator. Explicit in physical education are such examples as batting and fielding averages in baseball, shooting percentages in basketball, the number of tackles the football player successfully executes, and the number of laps the beginning swimmer can traverse before tiring. One might say that such measures are imposed by the coach or the teacher. True, but this does not negate the fact that, adult imposition aside, boys and girls compare themselves with other boys and girls. Witness the two youngsters who count the number of times each can hop on one foot while skipping rope, or the young children who vie for chinning honors on a low-hanging tree limb. Motivation to score higher or better is ostensibly an innate urge with most people.

If a human truly is an inveterate measurer, and if he or she in this case is the physical educator, what purpose should the innate evaluative inclination serve? Surely the supreme purpose of educational evaluation is to enhance learning. However, the improvement-of-learning concept is a complicated one revolving around several questions which must be addressed:[1]

1. Is learning enhanced if students are classified according to some criterion? If so, what is the criterion (criteria) and how can it (they) best be evaluated?
2. Must student needs be taken into consideration when trying to construct the best possible learning environment? If so, how should such needs be assessed?
3. Is the methodology of the instructor important in an optimal learning situation? If so, which pedagogical method is best? Under what conditions? Can the part that methodology plays in learning be reliably measured?
4. Can motivation for both student and teacher be stimulated through evaluative processes? How?
5. Can grades in physical education be justified? If so, what role does evaluation play in such justification?

The last point is the most emotional, if not the most provocative, one. Many educators quarrel with the use of evaluative measures to grade (mark) pupils. The use of report cards is a debatable topic and some educators, as well as parents and pupils, urge their complete abolition. Others argue only with the methods by which marks are determined and reported. The usual arguments against grades cite such factors as the following:

1. Grades provide artificial motivation.
2. Competition for grades has several undesirable aspects.
3. Grades reward fragmented learning.
4. Grades are too often accepted at face value.
5. Grades sometimes overlook exceptional effort by some pupils and a lack of effort by others.
6. Teachers do not grade objectively.
7. Teachers grade inconsistently.
8. Grades are sometimes based on personality factors.
9. Evaluation consumes too much of the teachers' time that might better be spent in preparing to instruct.

---

[1] Mary Jane Haskins, *Evaluation in Physical Education* (Dubuque, Iowa: W. C. Brown, 1971), pp. 2–3.

10. Emphasis is on evaluation by the teacher; pupils are not encouraged to evaluate their own work.
11. Pupils do not understand the basis on which they are graded.
12. Pupils study teachers as much as they study coursework to try to ensure a good grade.

Rationalizing the abolition of grades and report cards on the face value of such points is just as unintelligent as not recognizing the faults in present grading systems. For example, what is "natural" motivation? From whence does it come? How? Is it not better to motivate pupils artificially to do more acceptable work than to let them slide by with no effort at all? The example, although a polarity, is hopefully thought-provoking. What is the motivation of the salesperson who tries to sell more wares than the other salespeople employed by the company? Artificial? Natural? The behavioral sciences apparently do not have a satisfactory answer, since "... motivational theory is in its infancy, and techniques of evaluation are far from sophisticated."[2] Allport, for instance, believes that a motive is any internal condition in a person that induces action or thought;[3] however, he states that motives are, by nature, changing and spontaneous and that any acceptable concept of motivation must be pluralistic—allowing for motives of many types.[4] He describes as "functionally autonomous" those motives which, originally developed by any "tension," now seek new goals. As an example of this he cites a student's becoming absorbed in the study of a subject in which she or he originally enrolled only because it was required.[5] The motivational theory of Maslow, much accepted by educators, focuses upon a hierarchical structure of goals rather than on temporary needs, but it recognizes the place of unconscious motivation and acknowledges the fact that "any motivated behavior may satisfy many needs, while any one act may have many sources of motivation."[6] Thus, it would seem that so-called artificial motivation cannot be completely undesirable.

Regardless of which of the many theories of motivation is most acceptable, the fact cannot be overlooked that since education plays such a vital role in our society, the assessment of student

---

2 John F. Travers, *Learning: Analysis and Application* (New York: David McKay Co., 1965): p. 69.

3 Gordon W. Allport, *Pattern and Growth in Personality* (New York: Holt, Rinehart and Winston, 1961): p. 196.

4 *Ibid.*, pp. 220–226.

5 *Ibid.*, pp. 235–236.

6 Travers, *op. cit.*, p. 58.

achievement "ought to be regarded as of central importance to the whole educational enterprise."[7] Obviously, if evaluation is to be as meaningful as possible, factors in the educational enterprise other than the pupils need also to be evaluated. These include the teacher, the program, the facilities and equipment, and the administration. Clark and Beatty divide this concept into four levels:

> To be comprehensively useful, the school's program of evaluation must be organized at four levels. There are judgments to be made independently by (a) the individual student, concerning his becoming; (b) the teacher, concerning an individual relationship with each student; (c) the teacher and students, concerning how to organize all the relations which must be maintained in a class; and (d) all the resource people—administrators, supervisors, coordinators, counselors, researchers, lay boards, and citizens' committees—concerning the facilities the teacher uses to help the student toward his becoming effective.[8]

In summary, then, "the ultimate purpose of the whole process of evaluation is to provide feedback to guide every person who needs to learn and every person who needs to assist learning."[9]

Before proceeding to a treatment of pupil evaluation, it seems appropriate to define several terms.

Evaluation is the *art* of judgment. It can be applied to some predetermined value either qualitatively or quantitatively. According to Wilhelms and Diederich:

> . . . to do its fundamental task, evaluation must perform five tasks. It must:
>
> 1. Facilitate self-evaluation.
> 2. Encompass all the objectives.
> 3. Facilitate teaching and learning.
> 4. Generate records appropriate to various uses.
> 5. Facilitate decision-making on curriculum and educational policy.[10]

Measurement is but a technique of evaluation, and it usually

---

[7] John T. Flynn and Herbert G. Barber (eds.). *Assessing Behavior: Readings in Educational and Psychological Measurement* (Reading, Mass.: Addison-Wesley Publishing Co. 1967), p. 20.

[8] R. A. Clark and W. H. Beatty, "Learning and Evaluation," in *Evaluation as Feedback and Guide,* 1967 Yearbook. Fred T. Wilhelms, editor. (Washington, D.C.: Association for Supervision and Curriculum Development, 1967): p. 69. Reprinted by permission.

[9] F. T. Wilhelms and P. B. Diederich, "The Fruits of Freedom," *Evaluation as Feedback and Guide,* 1967 Yearbook. Fred T. Wilhelms, editor. (Washington, D.C.: Association for Supervision and Curriculum Development, 1967): p. 248.

[10] *Ibid.,* p. 234. Reprinted by permission.

results in quantitative data. It is the description of existing status without placing a value on it.[11]

Tests are instruments used to measure.

Grading or *marking* is a method by which evaluation is reported. Grading can be further divided into (1) *absolute* grading which considers only *achievement*, and (2) *relative* grading which takes into account achievement as related to *capacity*. There is much debate, too, about which of these is the better plan. This concept will be explored briefly when examples of evaluative plans are presented.

PUPIL EVALUATION

In spite of the many flaws in the existing methods used to report evaluation, the determination and reporting of pupil growth probably has greater potential for interpreting the school program, for securing cooperation between parents and educators, and for promoting the development of the pupil than does any other activity.[12] And, as Norsted [13] suggests, more can be said in favor of the wholesome effects of school marks than can be said of their deleterious effects. The trend toward a pass-fail marking system, largely a phenomenon of the 60s, is now seemingly decreasing in popularity as both parents and pupils seek more specific evaluative information than is included in a "pass." Similarly, mere anecdotal reports, although they can be quite specific, do not satisfy a natural inclination to compare oneself with some kind of standard. In other words, no alternative to grading has thus far been advanced which shows any real promise. Grading is a well-established and time-honored practice in most schools. (Eight of ten systems with enrollments of 300 or more issue report forms which use some type of scale, either A to F or numerical.) [14] Therefore, since most teachers are required to grade, it needs to be done as carefully and thoroughly as possible.

Much has been written decrying present marking practices in physical education which range from a total absence of grading to basing grades solely on such factors as attendance, participation, and showering. Pupils, parents, and administrators are dissatisfied with such practices and certainly the field of physical education

---

[11] Latchaw, Marjorie, and Camille Brown, *Evaluation Process in Health Education, Physical Education and Recreation.* (Englewood Cliffs, N.J.: Prentice-Hall, 1962): pp. 11–12.

[12] J. S. Ahmann and M. D. Glock, *Evaluating Pupil Growth* (Boston: Allyn and Bacon, 1959), p. 565.

[13] R. A. Norsted, "To Mark or Not to Mark?" *Journal of Education,* **121** (March 1938): 84.

[14] George B. Brain, "Student Evaluation," *Education Digest,* **33** (December 1967): 54.

will not and cannot gain respect until such practices are superseded by more justifiable ones. Basic to a concerted effort on the part of the profession to improve grading practices is an embracing of certain principles which are generally acceptable among leaders in the field. McCraw's list is perhaps representative:

1. Grades should be based on all the objectives. The major portion of the grade should be based on skill and/or fitness.
2. Grades should be based on achievement with ample consideration given to capacity and improvement.
3. The grading scheme should be consistent with that used in the rest of the school.
4. Grades should be based on performance in relation to objectives—not in comparison with others.
5. All teachers in the system should develop the plan for grading.
6. A variety of objective and subjective instruments should be used.
7. Evaluative instruments should not be used exclusively for grading. They can be used also for such purposes as class assignment, determination of needs, and motivation.
8. Students should be informed of the grading procedure.[15]

Although such a list is self-explanatory, some of the principles will be discussed at greater length.

Physical education is a multiobjective field. If *all* objectives are to be tested before assigning a final grade, can such a large number of them continue to be advocated? Can the statements of objectives be narrowed to only a few important and perhaps unique ones? If so, how few? how unique? Which objective, if any, is most important and therefore should receive the greatest weight in the grading process? It is not the purpose of this chapter to discuss objectives at any great length; therefore, no great attention is given to the three classifications of objectives (psychomotor, cognitive, and affective) nor to the current trend toward stating such objectives in terms of behavioral outcomes. However, as a basis for suggested grading plans, each of three broad objectives for the discipline of physical education are treated briefly.

The *physical* (psychomotor) objective is unique to the field of physical education. Several facets of the objective could be considered, but probably the ones which merit most consideration are

[15] Lynn W. McCraw, "Principles and Practices for Assigning Grades in Physical Education," *Journal of Health Physical Education Recreation,* **35** (February 1964): 24–25.

physical fitness and *skill development*. Presently many people in the field (and many outside the field) deem the fitness objective the most important one. Others vote for skill development. The chicken-and-egg controversy comes to mind when listening to the rationales for both these viewpoints. Is it better to make youngsters physically fit and hope that because they are they will use various game skills to maintain their fitness? Or, conversely, if youngsters are taught a sufficient amount of skill to make an activity enjoyable, will they participate in the activity often enough to ensure a high level of fitness? Obviously, each viewpoint has its justifications.

The *mental* (cognitive) objective also encompasses two main ideas: the ability to use *mental processes* quickly and well and the *emotional* health factor. Physical education, properly taught, is just as "academic" as other subject areas. The knowledge of how the body functions, the principles underlying movement, and the various game strategies are but examples of the academic aspects of physical education. The need to make decisions quickly and to react accordingly in a game situation can also be classified under the broad category of mental development. In addition, the releasing of tensions and pressures in a game situation adds to emotional stability.

The *social* (affective) objective has many ramifications and has been given a great deal of lip service by physical educators in general. However, if by social one means such things as desirable attitudes, courage, justice, fair play, and the like, then physical education can contribute as much, if not more, to this objective than any other field. Other fields tend only to verbalize about such values, whereas physical education puts them into actual practice. It is interesting to note in this connection, however, that there is little supportive research evidence that social learnings are inherent in the activities themselves.[16]

There is not universal agreement among leaders in physical education regarding the relative importance of each objective. Many argue that since the *physical* objective is unique to physical education, it must be the most important. Many others contend that the *social* objective is most important since it can be taught best in physical education. Others, particularly among the rising number of leaders in the field who urge programs worthy of academic respect, argue for the importance of the mental objective. Still others submit that all are equally important. Actual examples of various weightings will be shown later in this chapter.

---

[16] Thomas J. Sheehan, "The Construction and Testing of a Teaching Model for Attitude Formation and Change Through Physical Education" (Ph.D. dissertation, The Ohio State University, 1965), p. 1.

The principle that the grading scheme should be consistent with that used in the rest of the school perhaps needs elaboration. Some physical educators cite the larger number of classes taught by one individual in physical education, along with a larger enrollment in each class, as justification for grading less often if at all, or for awarding S's and U's instead of the usual letter grades. The authors feel strongly that if physical educators make a conscientious attempt to grade according to their objectives and to follow the school's grading plan, and if they keep the administration informed of these procedures, the administration, in turn, can be persuaded eventually to schedule physical education classes in terms of number and size—the same as other classes.

Finally, the principle that both objective and subjective testing instruments should be used may cause consternation among some teachers. As discussed below, subjective instruments are more prone to human error; however, this does not preclude their use. A well-qualified physical educator should know, for example, what constitutes good form and good playing. Provided he conscientiously grades subjectively, there is no reason to apologize for the procedure.

Techniques of Evaluation

It is assumed that the undergraduate student has taken a course in tests and measurements in physical education. Therefore, the treatment here is a brief one with many gaps. If the assumption is incorrect, the student should consult a text which treats the subject comprehensively.

The various types of evaluative instruments can be classified basically under two headings. *Objective* instruments are less dependent on the human element, and therefore the likelihood of error in measurement is greatly reduced. *Subjective* instruments are dependent on some formulation of an ideal concept against which pupils are measured. Since this concept may vary from day to day, the human element is a significant one.

Included among the types of objective tests are the following:

1. Skill tests in which the subject performs specific skills as well as possible. They may or may not be timed tests. If they are, the human element is a factor because of, among other things, the necessity to use a timing device.
2. Written tests in which only one answer is purported to be the best one.

3. Physical fitness tests in which the individual's achievement in the various components of fitness is measured.

Such tests may be *standardized*; i.e., the test itself has been refined through scientific procedures[17] and norms have been established. Norms may be established nationally, statewide, or locally.

Some subjective tests are:

1. Written tests of the essay type.
2. Written assignments such as term papers.
3. Playing ability tests in which the student is measured against the instructor's considered judgment of what constitutes good play. This type of test can be made more objective if specific criteria are predetermined. (See Figs. 1 and 2.)
4. Attitude inventories such as those of Wear[18] and McAfee.[19]
5. Sociometric devices such as sociograms which measure relationships among groups and identify cliques, pairs, gangs and "isolates."[20,21,22] If the use of such evaluative devices is completely unknown, a thoughtful treatment of the subject by Zajonc[23] is recommended.

Examples of Grading Plans

All authorities agree that pupil evaluation should be based on course objectives. General agreement on what these objectives are and the relative importance of each is nonexistent. In view of the fact that, theoretically, evaluation should be simple, feasible, etc., it seems that a list of objectives should be short, valid, and capable of being measured. The importance assigned to each will probably always remain an individual matter. Table I shows different schemes for grading based on the three categories of objectives discussed above. The weight assigned to each objective is dependent, at least

---

[17] Carl E. Willgoose, *Evaluation in Health Education and Physical Education* (New York: McGraw-Hill Book Co., 1961): p. 31.

[18] Carlos L. Wear, "Construction of Equivalent Forms of an Attitude Scale," *Research Quarterly,* **26** (March 1955): 113–119.

[19] Robert H. McAfee, "Sportsmanship Attitudes of Sixth, Seventh, and Eighth Grade Boys," *Research Quarterly,* **26** (March 1955): 120.

[20] Patricia Whitaker Hale, "Proposed Method for Analyzing Sociometric Data," *Research Quarterly,* **27** (May 1956): 152–161.

[21] Frances Todd, "Sociometry in Physical Education," *Research Quarterly,* **24** (May 1953): 23–25.

[22] Bryant J. Cratty, *Social Dimensions of Physical Activity* (Englewood Cliffs, N.J.: Prentice-Hall, 1967), pp. 59–74.

[23] Robert B. Zajonc, *Social Psychology: An Experimental Approach* (Belmont, Calif.: Wadsworth Publishing Co., 1966), pp. 92–98.

Ratings in Tennis (Beginners)

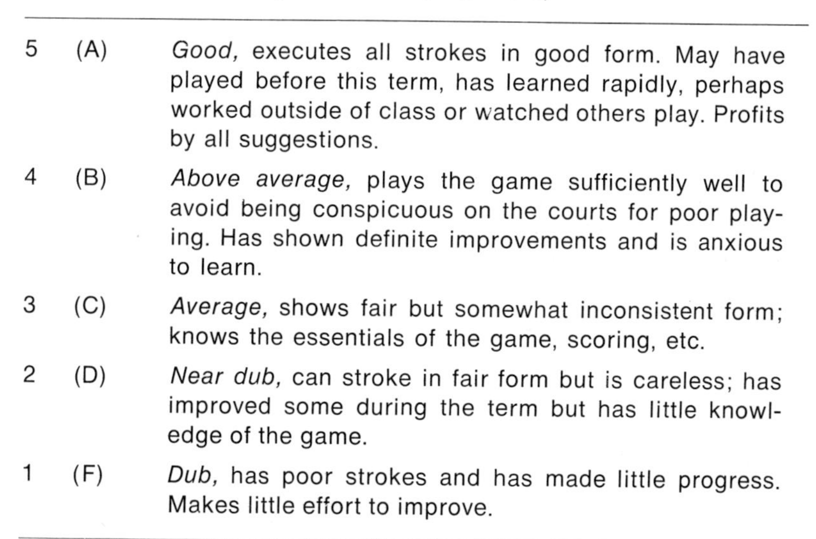

5	(A)	*Good,* executes all strokes in good form. May have played before this term, has learned rapidly, perhaps worked outside of class or watched others play. Profits by all suggestions.
4	(B)	*Above average,* plays the game sufficiently well to avoid being conspicuous on the courts for poor playing. Has shown definite improvements and is anxious to learn.
3	(C)	*Average,* shows fair but somewhat inconsistent form; knows the essentials of the game, scoring, etc.
2	(D)	*Near dub,* can stroke in fair form but is careless; has improved some during the term but has little knowledge of the game.
1	(F)	*Dub,* has poor strokes and has made little progress. Makes little effort to improve.

Fig. 1 Sample skill test (tennis). (Adapted from: M. Gladys Scott and Esther French, *Measurement and Evaluation in Physical Education* (Dubuque, Iowa: W. C. Brown Co., 1959), pp. 423–424.)

to some extent, on the educational level. For example, the social objective with its stress on attitude formation and the achieving of various social skills is much more important at the elementary than at the college level. For purposes of clarity and consistency, then, the plans presented here are considered only at the secondary level. Cited plans do not by any means exhaust the possibilities; they are merely examples.

Table 1

	Percentages			
Objective	Plan I	Plan II	Plan III	Plan IV
Physical (psychomotor)	40	33⅓	32	50
Mental (cognitive)	25	33⅓	12	25
Social (affective)	35	33⅓	56	25

In order to compute an actual grade, the following hypothetical situation is used for all plans.

Tom and Dick are two of the students in a tenth grade physical

Diagnostic Checklist—Basketball Skill

Date________________ Rater________________

Skill	G = Good F = Fair P = Poor	Player:			Player:			Player:			Player:		
		G	F	P	G	F	P	G	F	P	G	F	P
A. BALL HANDLING													
1. Handles ball lightly and easily													
2. Fingers spread on ball													
3. "Gives" when catching ball													
4. Avoids turn-overs													
B. BOUNCING													
1. Keeps head up													
2. Controls ball with finger tips													
3. Bounces only when necessary													
C. PASSING													
1. Uses short, quick passes													
2. Uses a variety of passes													
3. Fakes effectively													
4. Passes to space ahead of receiver													
5. Follows through after pass													
D. SHOOTING													
1. Focuses on target													
2. Follows through with arms and fingers													
3. Arc is high enough													
4. Avoids bad shots													
5. Shoots when opportunity is present													
E. GUARDING													
1. Uses sliding steps in all directions													
2. Shifts with each pass													
3. Low, stride position-hands up													
4. Not easily faked out of position													
5. Maintains correct position in defensive pattern													
6. Covers for teammates													
F. EVADING OPPONENT													
1. Uses feints to advantage													
2. Pivots effectively													
3. Moves into space to receive pass													
4. Breaks off cuts at right time													
5. Pulls opponent out, then breaks													
G. THINKS BASKETBALL!													
COMMENTS:													

Fig. 2 Sample skill test (basketball).

education class which has just completed a six-week unit of instruction in basketball. Tom is a gifted athlete and one of the few boys in his school who has ever made the varsity basketball team as a tenth grader. He is self-assured to the point of cockiness and sees little need in his "wasting my time playing basketball with the rinky-dinks in this class." Dick, on the other hand, although not a "motor moron," is essentially unskilled. Due to a combination of circumstances, he has had no organized physical education prior to the tenth grade. He is anxious to learn because he enjoys watching basketball and he feels that he will more easily become "one of the boys" if he learns to play the game acceptably. Mr. Smith, the instructor of the class, has amassed the following information about the two boys in each category of objectives.

Physical. Mr. Smith feels that both skill and fitness are equally important and he therefore assigns the same weight to each as a part of the overall physical objective. In specific basketball skill tests, as well as on playing ability, Tom scored the highest grade in the class. In addition, the basketball coach believes that many close games are won or lost on physical condition and he spends much time on this phase of the game. Consequently, Tom scored highly in this category also. Dick, realizing that his basic skills are not developed, spends time outside of class practicing shooting, dribbling, and other fundamentals. Although his individual skills are much improved, he is still largely inept in the game situation. He realizes the importance of fitness and works hard to build his own fitness level. Therefore, in Mr. Smith's grade book we find the following entries:

	Tom		Dick	
Skill	A	} A	C	} C−
Playing ability	A		D	
Fitness	A		B	
	A		C+	

At this point, the question of improvement enters the picture. Some physical educators theorize that the skill grade should be relative, based on capacity, or based only on improvement. There are at least three considerations which make this theory a bit untenable. The first is the practical one of measuring capacity, initial ability, and final achievement. In the typical two-day-per-week secondary school program, it becomes a matter of how much time can justifiably be spent on testing. The second consideration revolves around the "sand-bagging" technique. Some pupils, knowing they will be graded only on improvement, will purposely score poorly on the pretest. The third consideration has to do with the value placed on improvement. A skilled performer cannot be expected to achieve the same degree of improvement as the unskilled performer. For example, Tom improves from eight to ten successful shots out of ten free throw trials and Dick improves from zero to four. Who has improved to a greater extent?

A student who makes a sincere effort to improve usually will improve to some extent. Effort is a corollary of attitude. Therefore, perhaps improvement should be counted only on the attitude grade, and then perhaps only negatively, as explained below.

Mental. Mr. Smith considers only knowledge in this category and his grade is based on a comprehensive written test at the end of the six-week unit plus a short paper on the origin of basketball. In view of his varsity status, Tom figures he knows more than anyone else in the class about basketball and he sees no need to study for the test. In addition, his paper is a half-page of poorly written material gleaned from only one source. Dick hands in a well-written four-page paper in which he cites several sources and some conflicting ideas. He studies hard for the written test and consequently scores well on it.

	Tom	Dick
Test (75%)	C	A
Paper (25%)	D	A
	C−	A

Social. Mr. Smith makes it clear to the boys at the outset of the school year that he expects each student to attend regularly, to be in clean regulation costume, to shower after each session, and to exert a real effort to learn. These expressions of positive attitude are *expected* and therefore are not rewarded in his grading scheme. If the student does not exhibit such examples of good citizenship, his grade is cut, or he is rewarded negatively. Actually, then, we could say that each student starts with an "A" in this category. Mr. Smith also talked with Tom early in the basketball unit and tried to point out to him that he could show true leadership traits by assisting the boys in the class less physically gifted than himself and by teaching some strategy in his particular squad. However, Tom became cockier as the unit progressed, showed little patience with his peers, and tried to play the entire game himself when his squad was on the floor. It was obvious that his classmates, and particularly his squadmates, were fed up with him. Dick, because of his lack of skill, truly empathized with his peers who also were having difficulty in learning. He constantly shared hints with them, encouraged them to keep trying, and had a pat on the back for the boy who performed well. Result?

	Tom	Dick
Social	D	A

Now, using Table 2, the final grade in physical education for the six-week period, according to each grading plan, can be computed as in Table 3.

Depending on the weight or importance assigned to each category of objectives, Tom's final grade ranged from B− to C+, whereas Dick's ranged from B to B+. In this example it happens that Dick's final grade is better than Tom's in every instance. It seems reasonable to assume that Tom may voice an objection, but the proof is in Mr. Smith's grade book for all to see.

Before closing this part of the chapter, several additional points seem pertinent.

First, if the grading scheme is to remain simple and feasible, grades can be more easily computed if multiples of five are used in assigning weight to objectives. As can be seen from the various plans, percentages other than multiples of five do not alter the marks significantly.

Second, an "A" can be based on several different factors. In the hypothetical example, Mr. Smith assigned "A"s to the highest scores in his class. He could have chosen instead to use some predetermined standard (for example, 88% and above correct answers on a written test worth 100 points, or certain scores on a physical fitness test item, such as sit-ups, based on national norms). Finally, he could have based the assignment of "A"s on the highest percentage of improvement or on skill in relation to capacity. In a typical class in physical education, the first example is justifiable in most instances and is the most conducive to a simple plan of grading.

Third, too often in physical education the typical distribution of grades in the entire class runs from A to C, with a large preponderance of A's and B's and very few C's. If physical education is to continue to plead for respectability and status, the grades must be

Table 2 Weighted points for grade computation. (Chart computed by Burton Willeford, Firestone High School, Akron, Ohio.)

Letter grade*		Point value	Percentages																		
			5	10	15	20	25	30	35	40	45	50	55	60	65	70	75	80	85	90	95
			Weighted points†																		
	A	11	.55	1.1	1.65	2.2	2.75	3.3	3.85	4.4	4.95	5.5	6.05	6.6	7.15	7.7	8.25	8.8	9.35	9.9	10.45
	A−	10	.5	1.0	1.5	2.0	2.5	3.0	3.5	4.0	4.5	5.0	5.5	6.0	6.5	7.0	7.5	8.0	8.5	9.0	9.5
	B+	9	.45	.9	1.35	1.8	2.25	2.7	3.15	3.6	4.05	4.5	4.95	5.4	5.85	6.3	6.75	7.2	7.65	8.1	8.55
	B	8	.40	.8	1.20	1.6	2.0	2.4	2.8	3.2	3.6	4.0	4.4	4.8	5.2	5.6	6.0	6.4	6.8	7.2	7.6
	B−	7	.35	.7	1.05	1.4	1.75	2.1	2.45	2.8	3.15	3.5	3.85	4.2	4.55	4.9	5.25	5.6	5.95	6.3	6.65
	C+	6	.30	.6	.90	1.2	1.5	1.8	2.1	2.4	2.7	3.0	3.3	3.6	3.9	4.2	4.5	4.8	5.1	5.4	5.7
	C	5	.25	.5	.75	1.0	1.25	1.5	1.75	2.0	2.25	2.5	2.75	3.0	3.25	3.5	3.75	4.0	4.25	4.5	4.75
A	C−	4	.20	.4	.60	.8	1.0	1.2	1.4	1.6	1.8	2.0	2.2	2.4	2.6	2.8	3.0	3.2	3.4	3.6	3.8
B	D+	3	.15	.3	.45	.6	.75	.9	1.05	1.2	1.35	1.5	1.65	1.8	1.95	2.1	2.25	2.4	2.55	2.7	2.85
C	D	2	.10	.2	.30	.4	.50	.6	.70	.8	.90	1.0	1.1	1.2	1.3	1.4	1.5	1.6	1.7	1.8	1.9
D	D−	1	.05	.1	.15	.2	.25	.3	.35	.4	.45	.5	.55	.6	.65	.7	.75	.8	.85	.9	.95
F	F	0	0	0	0	0	0	0	0	0	0	0	0	0	0	0	0	0	0	0	0

* This chart enables the grader to use a plus and minus system or a straight A,B,C,D,F system.

† This chart enables the grader to use any *multiple of five* weighting. Example: Suppose the objectives are weighed as follows:

Skill—20%	B+	1.8
Fitness—30%	B−	2.1
Knowledge—25%	C	1.25
Social—25%	A	2.75
		7.90 or B

Table 3

			Plan I		Plan II		Plan III		Plan IV	
	Objective	Grade	Weight	Points	Weight	Points	Weight	Points	Weight	Points
Tom	Physical	A	40	4.4	33⅓*	3.5	32	3.4	50	5.5
	Mental	C−	25	1.0	33⅓	1.3	12	0.50	25	1.0
	Social	D	35	0.70	33⅓	0.65	56	1.15	25	0.50
	Total points			6.10		5.45		5.05		7.00
	Final grade			C+		C		C		B−
Dick	Physical	C+	40	2.4	33⅓	2.0	32	1.9	50	3.0
	Mental	A	25	2.75	33⅓	3.5	12	1.3	25	2.75
	Social	A	35	3.85	33⅓	3.5	56	6.1	25	2.75
	Total points			9.00		9.00		9.30		8.50
	Final grade			B+		B+		B+		B

* For all weightings which are not multiples of five, the points are estimated values only. If an instructor actually uses such weightings, the point values should be mathematically computed.

based on some kind of normal distribution and on achievement. The practice of giving A's to the student who shows up for class in a clean costume, participates, and then showers—regardless of achievement—cannot be abandoned too quickly. Algebra teachers do not give A's to the students who show up with textbooks and notebook, labor all period over a set of problems, and finally turn in neat papers on which the answers are incorrect. Nor should physical education teachers! The distribution of grades need not follow the normal curve exactly. Most teachers will skew such a curve somewhat.

Finally, marks are not always reported in letter grades as shown. Regardless of the system employed by the school, it can be transposed into the given examples. There seems to be a trend for marks to be reported with both a letter and a number, such as B^2, in which the letter represents achievement and the number represents other characteristics.[24] Some advocate the use of a separate report card since the multiobjectives of physical education are severely limited by a single symbol. Others suggest that the report card be expanded to include, in addition to a grade, an anecdotal report which assesses a student's achievement in comparison to his or her capacity and in comparison to others and to national norms.

Summary of Pupil Evaluation

The assignment of some symbol to denote the summation of evaluative procedures in education is a debatable topic. In spite of all the arguments against grading, the practice is a time-honored one, not likely to be replaced soon. Therefore, if physical education is to achieve status in the educational scheme, physical educators must evaluate the pupil consistently and well. The assignment of a normal distribution of grades, based on the achievement of the objectives of the field, is a necessary step in the right direction.

EVALUATION OF THE PHYSICAL EDUCATION PROGRAM

When one thinks of evaluating the entire physical education program, an immediate association may bring to mind the hurried preparation for a regional accreditation visit. Evaluation of the program including facilities, curriculum, staff, and administration should be a periodic, if not an annual, event. Self-evaluation brings insight into the strengths and weaknesses of a program which is necessary for the operation of any program.

---

[24] Miller K. Adams, "Principles for Determining High School Grading Procedures in Physical Education for Boys" (Ed.D. dissertation, New York University, 1960).

Administrators and teachers feel threatened whenever the words "accountability" and "evaluation" are even mentioned. If evaluation is treated as an ongoing educative process, the threat of evaluation is greatly diminished. Administrators and teachers should select a different set of performance objectives each year. These objectives then serve as the basis of the evaluation, although the evaluation should not be limited to these objectives.

Since physical education programs have more ramifications than most classroom subjects, these programs are in need of periodic evaluation. Baker[25] devised evaluating standards which she sent to state departments of education of the 50 states, Puerto Rico, and the District of Columbia. Replies were received from 45 states and excerpts from that part of the study dealing with secondary school physical education follow:

1. *Time allotment.* Recommended standard: Daily period of instruction equivalent to that in other subjects plus a regular intramural program.

Only 14 of the states responding reported that definitely 50 or more percent of the public secondary schools in their states met the standard of a daily period equivalent to that of other subjects; similarly, only 10 states met the standard of a regular intramural program.

2. *Space allotment.* Recommended standard: For senior high school, two teaching stations (each 48′ × 70′).

At the senior high school level only 20 of the states reported that definitely 50 or more percent of the schools met this space standard.

3. *Equipment.* Recommended standard: Equipment enough for a group of 30 to be active at one time. One piece of equipment per person (rackets, tennis balls), one piece of equipment per two persons (baseballs, softballs), one piece per four persons (basketballs, deck tennis rings).

Of the states responding, 11 reported that definitely 50 or more percent of the schools in their states provided as much equipment as the above mentioned standard.

4. *Program.* Recommended standard: Balanced and progressive program throughout.

Only 18 of the states responding reported that definitely 50 or more percent of the schools met this standard. Only in games, in-

---

[25] Gertrude M. Baker, "Survey of the Administration of Physical Education in Public Schools in the United States," *Research Quarterly,* **33** (December 1962): 632–36.

dividual sports, and self-testing activities did 50 percent of the states meet the standards.

5. *Personnel.* Recommended standard: Minor in physical education if teaching up to 49 percent of time; major in physical education if teaching up to 50 percent of time.

Of the states responding, 21 reported that the standard of a minor was definitely met in 50 or more percent while 30 states reported that the standard concerning a major was definitely met.

The Ohio Association for Health, Physical Education, and Recreation, in cooperation with the State Department of Education, has published an *Evaluation Criteria for Physical Education.* This is a self-appraisal checklist for secondary schools. The areas to be evaluated include philosophy and principles, organization and administration, class management, staff, curriculum, facilities and equipment, elective program, and special problems. That portion of the evaluation dealing with the staff is found in Fig. 3.

A self-evaluation scale such as the one shown in Fig. 3 tends to ensure an awareness of the limitations and weaknesses of a program. Without such an evaluation even a good program may begin to show signs of weakness without realizing it.

EVALUATION OF INSTRUCTION

Accountability is one of the major themes in education today. The work of administrators, staff personnel, and teachers in the public schools is being evaluated more intensely than ever before. The taxpayers who support the public school programs are demanding that those persons employed by the local school district perform at an acceptable level in the conduct of the educational program. In order to ascertain the level of performance of school-district employees, a program of evaluation is necessary.

In the school year 1977–78, the eleventh-grade students in all of the Florida high schools were given a series of performance tests. The results of these tests were widely discussed, not only in Florida, but throughout the nation. Now the Florida state legislature is considering a test of teacher competency, and this proposal is being attacked by most educational groups. However, it does point out the public interest in the evaluation of school programs and processes.

No modern public school system can progress without a valid means of evaluating employees. The development of an effective

Evaluation Scale

0 1 2 3 4

The Staff

Possible score = 40 points
Actual score = ___ points

1. Coaches of interscholastic athletics should possess a philosophy in harmony with the stated philosophy of the school's department of physical education and should meet minimum state requirements. ______

2. All physical education teachers meet state certification standards for teaching physical education in secondary schools. ______

3. Staff members are effective with respect to:
   a. planning and organizing class work ______
   b. establishing and maintaining fine student-teacher relationships ______
   c. a knowledge of the curriculum areas of physical education ______
   d. methods of teaching ______
   e. relationship with other teachers ______
   f. participating in community life. ______

4. Staff members are following a plan for personal and professional growth through participation in graduate work, workshops and conferences, meetings and conventions, and independent study. ______

5. The school has a definite well-organized in-service education program for improving the quality of instruction in the physical education classes. ______

Total______

Fig. 3 Evaluative criteria for physical education staff. (Courtesy of the Ohio Association for Health, Physical Education, and Recreation, *Evaluative Criteria for Physical Education*, 1987.)

evaluation program is a complex process. Central administration should appoint a committee of the best available administrators, teachers, and staff to develop an evaluation program to best meet the needs of the local school district.

Criteria must be established for evaluating the performance of an individual. These criteria will be different for teachers, administrators, and staff personnel. In the case of teachers the most common criteria are quality of teaching, personal characteristics, contributions to the school other than teaching, and contributions to the community.

Probably the most controversial of all the areas of evaluation is that of instruction, since it involves personal performance of both teacher and student. There is no clear-cut definition of teaching effectiveness. Beery pointed this out in the following words:

> One of the major barriers to experimental research in the field of teacher education has been the lack of satisfactory criteria of teaching success. Human traits are so elusive, teaching and learning are such complex processes, and the desired outcomes of teaching are so varied that no simple and objective measure of teaching effectiveness has yet been devised, if indeed it ever can be.[26]

There are a number of methods by which teaching effectiveness may be judged by an administrator. Most of these may apply to physical education as well as they do to classroom instruction. Some of these methods are:

1. correlation of student abilities and grades,
2. observations of teaching by a supervisor or superior,
3. quality of work in a subsequent course,
4. pre- and post-testing of students,
5. student's performance on standard tests,
6. student ratings of instruction.

All of the above have known inherent weaknesses. The authors believe in the process of self-evaluation including student ratings. Although student ratings are affected by the level of the students, expected grades, the personality of the teacher, and the nature of the course (required or elective), they cannot be ignored as a self-evaluative tool. Students are consumers and as such evaluate their teachers every time they leave the classroom or gymnasium.

---

[26] John R. Beery, "Does Professional Preparation Make a Difference?" *The Journal of Teacher Education,* **13** (December 1962): 386.

This evaluation reaches parents and eventually the administrator, if only by rumor.

There are a number of standard rating scales available to teachers and any teacher may easily devise an open-end questionnaire to suit his or her particular needs.

Teachers are constantly being evaluated as they appear before students. Self-evaluation is preventive professional evaluation similar to preventive medicine or preventive maintenance in industry.

EVALUATION OF ADMINISTRATION

The age of the infallibility of administrators is now a thing of the past. By the time poor administration is discovered, the program (or school) is in such condition that it takes a long time to recover. It is true that in a line-and-staff relationship the immediate superior is responsible for persons directly below him or her on an organizational chart. It is assumed that periodic evaluations are made under these circumstances. Whether or not formal evaluations are made, the people with whom she or he comes into contact do evaluate the school administrator even if only in a casual manner. The administrator is evaluated on how he or she relates to people both within and outside the school setting, on contributions in attaining the academic goals set by the school, especially on his or her ability to recruit and retain excellent faculty, and on his or her ability to manage fiscal affairs.

The authors again urge administrators to employ a self-evaluation form to determine their own effectiveness. One such tool devised by Slate shows promise in this area. His semantic-differential test lists 20 sets of adjectives or phrases. A partial listing of these is found in Fig. 4.

As suggested by the originator of this scale, the adjectives may be changed by the administrator to suit his or her own needs. This is a novel idea in an area in which evaluation is much needed.

CASE STUDY

The Physical Education Department of Wilson High School was having a meeting prior to the beginning of school. The subject under discussion was grading. Peter Albers, a teacher with several years experience, remarked that he was tired of trying to grade his students on a complicated grading scale which included, among others, the factor of improvement. He further defended his position by citing the fact that most other areas, such as mathematics, English, and history, consider only achievement as the basis for a grade. Mr. Albers continued that he was disturbed by the attempts

	Very	Quite	Slight	Slight	Quite	Very	
Competent	___	___	___	___	___	___	Incompetent
Satisfied	___	___	___	___	___	___	Frustrated
Speaks up	___	___	___	___	___	___	Clams up
Sincere	___	___	___	___	___	___	Insincere
Stubborn	___	___	___	___	___	___	Flexible
Close-minded	___	___	___	___	___	___	Open-minded
Unfair	___	___	___	___	___	___	Fair

Fig. 4 Semantic differential test. (From Leslie M. Slate, "How to See Yourself as Your Employees See You," *School Management* (June 1966): pp. 88–89. Copyright © 1966, Managing Publishing Group, Inc., Greenwich, Connecticut. Reprinted by permission.)

to grade on any social objective, since citizenship evaluations were a separate part of the student's report. He proposed that the group grade entirely on achievement.

In order to make the grading process simpler for the entire staff, Mr. Albers suggested that they immediately adopt his proposal.

1. What are the essential issues in this problem?
2. What should be the course of action of the staff?
3. What grading principles might be derived from this case study?

SELECTED REFERENCES

Adams, Miller K. "Principles for Determining High School Grading Procedures in Physical Education for Boys." Ed.D. dissertation, New York University, 1960.

Ahmann, J. S., and M. D. Glock. *Evaluating Pupil Growth.* Boston: Allyn and Bacon, 1959.

Allport, Gordon W. *Pattern and Growth in Personality.* New York: Holt, Rinehart and Winston, 1961.

Baker, Gertrude M. "Survey of the Administration of Physical Education in Public Schools in the United States," *Research Quarterly,* **33** (December 1962): 632–636.

Beery, John R. "Does Professional Preparation Make a Difference?" *The Journal of Teacher Education,* **13** (December 1962): 386–395.

Brain, George B. "Student Evaluation," *Education Digest,* **33** (December 1967): 52–54.

Clark, R. A., and W. H. Beatty. "Learning and Evaluation," in *Evaluation as Feedback and Guide,* 1967 Yearbook. Edited by Fred T. Wilhelms. Washington, D.C.: Association for Supervision and Curriculum Development, 1967.

Cratty, Bryant J. *Social Dimensions of Physical Activity.* Englewood Cliffs, N.J.: Prentice-Hall, 1967.

Flynn, John T., Herbert Garber (eds.). *Assessing Behavior: Readings in Educational and Psychological Measurement.* Reading, Mass.: Addison-Wesley, 1967.

Hale, Patricia Whitaker. "Proposed Method for Analyzing Sociometric Data," *Research Quarterly,* **27** (May 1956): 152–161.

Hall, J. Tillman, et al. *Administration: Principles, Theory and Practice with Applications to Physical Education.* Pacific Palisades, California: Goodyear Publishing, 1973.

Haskins, Mary Jane. *Evaluation in Physical Education.* Dubuque, Iowa: W. C. Brown, 1971.

Kirby, R. F. "Improvement: A Factor in Grading," *Physical Educator,* **27** (December 1970): 150–151.

Latchaw, Marjorie, and Camille Brown. *Evaluation Process in Health Education, Physical Education and Recreation.* Englewood Cliffs, N.J.: Prentice-Hall, 1962.

McAfee, Robert H. "Sportsmanship Attitudes of Sixth, Seventh and Eighth Grade Boys," *Research Quarterly,* **26** (March 1955): 120.

McCraw, Lynn W. "Principles and Practices for Assigning Grades in Physical Education," *Journal of Health Physical Education Recreation,* **35** (February 1964): 24–25.

Melograno, Vincent J. "Evaluating Affective Objectives in Physical Education," *The Physical Educator,* **31** (April 1974), 8–12.

Norsted, R. A. "To Mark or Not to Mark?" *Journal of Education,* **121** (March 1938): 81–84.

Scott, Gladys M., and Esther French. *Measurement and Evaluation in Physical Education.* Dubuque, Iowa: W. C. Brown, 1959.

Sheehan, Thomas J. *An Introduction to the Evaluation of Measurement Data in Physical Education.* Reading, Mass.: Addison-Wesley, 1971.

Sheehan, Thomas J. "The Construction and Testing of a Teaching Model for Attitude Formation and Change Through Physical Education." Ph.D. dissertation, The Ohio State University, 1965.

Slate, Leslie M. "How to See Yourself as Your Employees See You," *School Management* (June 1966): pp. 88–91.

Smith, B. C., and H. A. Lerch. "Contract Grading," *Physical Educator,* **29** (May 1972): 80–82.

Todd, Frances. "Sociometry in Physical Education," *Research Quarterly,* **24** (May 1953): 23–24; 36.

Travers, John F. *Learning: Analysis and Application.* New York: David McKay, 1965.

Wear, Carlos L. "Construction of Equivalent Forms of an Attitude Scale," *Research Quarterly,* **26** (March 1955): 113–119.

Wilhelms, F. T., and P. B. Diederich. "The Fruits of Freedom," in *Evaluation as Feedback and Guide,* 1967 Yearbook. Edited by Fred T. Wilhelms. Washington, D.C.: Association for Supervision and Curriculum Development, 1967.

Willgoose, Carl E. *Evaluation in Health Education and Physical Education.* New York: McGraw-Hill, 1961.

Zajonc, Robert B. *Social Psychology: An Experimental Approach,* Belmont, Calif.: Wadsworth, 1966.

PART II

PHYSICAL EDUCATION

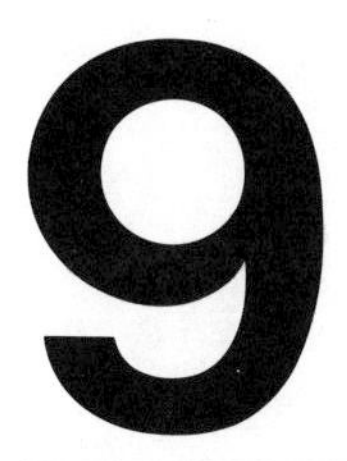

THE BASIC INSTRUCTION PROGRAM

STUDY STIMULATORS

1. What excuses for absence from physical education classes should be honored?
2. What are the advantages and disadvantages of the different methods of roll taking in different sized physical education classes?
3. How can the teacher make effective use of leaders' clubs in the conduct of classes?
4. What kinds of records should be kept in the conduct of a typical physical education program?
5. What is the case for requiring a set uniform for the physical education student?
6. How should students be grouped for the most effective instruction in physical education?

What makes men good is held by some to be... instruction.

ARISTOTLE

The physical educator must build a program based on a sound philosophy, a meaningful aim, and significant objectives. Then as the program develops, she or he must be concerned with the myriad of administrative details necessary to keep the program operating in the most effective manner possible and must constantly strive for program improvement. This chapter is concerned with the administrative details in the development and conduct of the instructional class program in physical education.

THE SCOPE OF THE PROGRAM

The basic instructional program of physical education should be offered daily in all grades, one through twelve. Also, there should be at least two additional years of appropriate instruction in physical education at the college level if the youth of our nation are to be physically educated. The following are suggested types of activities for each level of education:

Primary level (Grades 1 through 3). Rhythms, games of low organization, relays, stunts and self-testing activities, story plays, games, mimetics, basic movement, apparatus, aquatics, winter sports.

Elementary level (Grades 4 through 6). Rhythmic activities, games of low organization, relays, tumbling, stunts, individual self-testing activities, athletic games of low organization, team sports, aquatics, outdoor education, camping, winter sports, basic movement.

Junior high school (Grades 7 through 9). Games and relays, individual and dual sports, team sports, dance—folk, square, social and modern—aquatics, tumbling and stunts, gymnastics, outdoor education, camping, winter sports, combatives.

Senior high school (Grades 10 through 12). Lifetime sports, team sports, tumbling, gymnastics, apparatus, dance—folk, square, social, and modern—aquatics, games and relays, combatives, outdoor education, camping, winter sports.

College and university. Emphasis on individual carry-over types of activities such as wrestling, gymnastics, tennis, swimming, handball, squash, square dance, social dance, modern dance, golf, fencing, badminton, archery, bowling, horseback riding, ice skating, body conditioning, and self-defense.

Curriculum Development

A major responsibility of physical education administrators and staff members is curriculum development and curriculum change. Determining what to include in the curriculum is a major challenge. The job of all educators is to help all students reach their maximum potential. One means of achieving this goal is to provide a relevant curriculum.

A physical education curriculum which will meet the major needs of students should include an appreciation and understanding of the value of physical activity, physical fitness, physical skills development, successful group participation and the opportunity to learn a desirable value system.

Curriculum construction is a complex task which requires the knowledge of both recommended curriculum as revealed by research and the various states' standards. The development of the curriculum for the basic instructional program of physical education is central to the effective administration of this program. Regardless of the educational level, the modern physical education program must be thoroughly planned as a course of study. The total physical education staff should take part in selecting the activities to be offered in the curriculum. There are many factors involved in making curricular decisions. The philosophy, aim, and objectives of the program, as well as the facilities and equipment available, staff competencies, budget, class size, time allotment, and community interests affect curricular planning. Other factors of importance in the selection of course content are student interest, student needs, and the activities known to be valid from past experience of physical educators.

Course of Study Development

The development of the course of study is a cooperative endeavor involving all the physical education instructors, supervisors, and the curriculum specialist (if the school district employs a person in this capacity). The school principal should be consulted concerning areas of the course of study which affect other departments in the school, and should be kept informed of progress made.

The written course of study should contain the philosophy of the physical education department, the immediate and long-range objectives, activities to be offered, time schedule, order in which activities will be presented, motivating and teaching techniques, adapted program, evaluation techniques, audiovisual aids, and a bibliography.

Regardless of the academic level, the total program should be planned first. This should be followed by the more specific details of yearly, monthly, weekly, and daily plans. A wide variety of progressive activities should be offered and duplication avoided.

There are excellent reference materials available for curriculum and course-of-study development (see the selected references at the end of this chapter). Samples of courses of study are available in the Instructional Resources Centers of most universities.

Scheduling

The manner in which physical education classes are scheduled is one of the major factors in determining the success of the program. The scheduling of physical education classes is conditioned by the attitude of school administrators toward the importance of physical education in the total school program. The physical education instructor should present his or her ideas about the best scheduling plan to the school administrators with due regard for the master schedule of classes.

All students should be scheduled in physical education classes. Provisions should be made for the physically handicapped student and the slow learner, as well as for the normal student. Consideration must be given to the number of students to be scheduled and to the number of teachers and teaching stations available. The schedule should be planned for the total school year.

There are many schedule plans in use in physical education programs in public schools today. These plans include a daily period of physical education, a two-day-per-week program, and a three-day-per-week program. Still other plans are physical education twice a week on a double period basis; coeducational physical education twice a week on a double period basis; physical education combined with health education on a two- or three-day basis; and the newer concept of modular or flexible scheduling which is discussed later in this chapter. In some cases, physical education is scheduled for double periods. Flexibility in scheduling is now being given much consideration. The merits of the above plans are not discussed, since practical considerations of the local situation often outweigh theoretical considerations.

Teaching Loads

Equalizing teaching loads is an important administrative practice. Teaching loads vary greatly among school districts. Recommended national standards, established by the National Education Association, suggest that every teacher should have two free periods per day. Often the teachers in special subject areas, including physical education, are overlooked when free periods are assigned. Free time in the school day is just as important for planning and preparation of physical education programs as for other subjects.

Most physical education instructors are scheduled for extra duties after school hours. These duties include coaching athletic teams, conducting intramural programs, conducting recreation programs, coaching cheerleading groups, and serving as advisors to various clubs. There are two prevalent methods used by school districts to compensate teachers for performing extra duties. One is to give the teacher additional salary for the extra work; however, usually this salary is not commensurate with the responsibility and time involved. The second method is to reduce the teacher's instructional load or provide released time from the normal school day. Many physical education authorities subscribe to reduced instructional load or released time on the basis that no person, no matter how well paid, can work productively and efficiently for an excessive number of hours.

Classification of Students

Physical education is taught most effectively when students are classified into groups that are similar in maturation level and skill ability. The random scheduling of students into physical education classes regardless of growth, development, skill attainment, or year in school is a deterrent to good teaching and learning. The most practical solution to the scheduling of classes is by grade level, but for this to be effective there must be rigid compliance.

If students are scheduled by grade levels, further classification within each physical education class by motor ability facilitates instruction, since it makes better provision for individual needs.

Some secondary schools have adopted the nongraded plan of scheduling students. This means that students are placed in phases according to their ability in each specific subject in the school curriculum, regardless of the usual freshman, sophomore, junior, senior classification. One plan is to have five phases, with the best students in Phase 5 and the least proficient students assigned to Phase 1. Thus, a student might be in Phase 4 in English, Phase 3 in mathematics, and Phase 2 in physical education. In physical education, students are originally placed in phases according to the results of a general motor-ability test. This plan has flexibility in that students may be moved from one phase to another as soon as they improve sufficiently. (A discussion of physical education in the nongraded school is presented later in this chapter.)

A classification system used in some graded schools is known as tracking. Tracking is a method of placing students of similar academic ability at specific grade levels in the same classes. For example, the best students in the tenth grade are on one track, those of average ability on another track, and those with the least ability on still another.

Classification is not as important in physical education at the elementary level as it is at the secondary level. However, it should be a concern of the elementary school physical education instructor, and appropriate steps should be taken to classify pupils in whatever manner seems most advantageous.

Class Size

Class size has a profound effect on the manner in which physical education classes are taught. Obviously, the method of instruction is decidedly different in small and large classes. Traditionally, physical educators have believed that physical education classes should be similar in size to those in the other disciplines in the curriculum.

Some physical educators have stated that no physical education class should have more than 35 students per instructor, with remedial and adapted classes being limited to 20 students. A more feasible plan is to determine class size by the number of teaching stations, the various levels of ability of the students, the number of instructors, and the activity being taught.

Dressing and Showering

One of the details in the administration of the basic instructional program is the development and implementation of proper procedures for dressing and showering. Dressing for class in the appropriate physical education costume and showering after class are an integral part of the upper elementary and the secondary school physical education experience.

If dressing and showering are to be a satisfying experience for students, locker and shower room facilities must be adequate in terms of the number of lockers, space for dressing, adequate shower heads for peak loads, toweling area, drainage of water, and sanitation. In addition, adequate time must be allowed for showering and dressing. Girls have the additional problem of drying their hair; therefore, a sufficient number of hair dryers for peak loads should be provided.

Supervision of the locker room is important, since there is always the possibility of "horseplay" and possible injury to students. Therefore, a member of the physical education staff should supervise the locker room—directly or by means of student leaders. The development of proper attitudes by students towards locker room conduct is important.

A major problem in the administration of the locker room program is the provision and handling of towels. The simplest, but least desirable, method is to have each student bring a towel from home each day he or she has a physical education class. Other methods range from having each student bring a towel from home at the beginning of the year from which a "towel pool" is established, to having towels provided by the school and washed by a commercial laundry at a minimum cost to each student. In the case of a towel pool, the towels can be laundered at school if the school has the necessary equipment and personnel. Ideally, the school provides and launders towels.

Physical Education Uniforms

Appropriate dress for physical education classes is essential for proper conduct of the program. Uniforms range from no prescribed outfit, so long as students change from their regular clothing, to a specific prescribed outfit manufactured by a gymwear company.

In elementary school physical education programs, if it is not feasible to require a prescribed uniform, the pupils may slip on jeans or slacks which provide the freedom necessary for physical activity. For pupils in the upper elementary grades through senior high school, a prescribed uniform is suggested. The prescribed uniform may be

1. a uniform prescribed only in terms of shorts and a blouse for girls and a T-shirt for boys,
2. a uniform prescribed in terms of a specific color shorts and blouse for girls and T-shirt for boys,
3. a specific prescribed uniform, manufactured by a gymwear company.

Justification for requiring a prescribed uniform for all pupils is based on expense (it is much less expensive over a period of time), nondiscrimination by socioeconomic status, better class morale, better appearance of the class, and safety and comfort.

There are several methods of selling uniforms to students. One method is for the physical education department to purchase the uniforms in large lots and then sell them to the students. This is the most economical method, since profit is not a concern. If this system is used, it should be arranged so that excessive staff time is not consumed and the handling of money is not a problem.

Procedures for maintenance of clean uniforms are a constant administrative problem. In the public schools the most frequently used method is to place the responsibility on the student. The uniform is laundered at home and frequent uniform inspections are made by the physical education instructor. Some schools have laundry facilities for washing and drying uniforms; however, this requires equipment and personnel beyond the scope of most public schools.

The type of physical education uniform prescribed and the method of purchase depends on the attitude of the school administrators towards physical education, the economic status of the parents, and whether or not parents have been educated to the fact that a good quality uniform can be purchased more economically if uniforms are purchased from one of the companies specializing in physical education uniforms.

A problem that arises in some communities is what to do about students who cannot afford to purchase physical education uniforms. This problem might be solved by appealing to community service clubs for help or by maintaining a pool of unclaimed uniforms.

Taking the Class Roll

Since time for activity in physical education classes is limited, methods of roll taking should be used which take as little time as possible. However, to be effective, the method must ensure accuracy. Policies on who takes the class roll and when and where it is taken must be established. The class roll may be taken by the instructor, assistant instructor, student leader, or squad leader. The roll may be taken at the beginning of the class period, after the class is underway, or at the end of the class period. Attendance can be checked in the locker room, on the gymnasium floor, or at the site of outdoor activities.

Included among the numerous ways in which the class roll may be taken are the instructor's calling the class roll alphabetically (this is at least desirable for it is too time-consuming), roll call in the locker room, numbers painted on the gymnasium floor (each student is assigned a number to stand on when the roll is checked), recitation of assigned numbers, the squad leaders' checking of roll and reporting it to the instructor, roll check as towels are issued, the signing of a register, and tag boards. Each of these methods has both advantages and disadvantages.

Excuses

There should rarely be excuses from the required physical education program. If the physical education program is properly conceived, there are appropriate activities for all students. Permanent excuses, if granted, should come from only the school or family physician.

Temporary excuses are a much greater problem to the physical educator. The most common reasons for temporary excuses are illness, injury, field trips, and participation in interscholastic athletics.

If students are excused from physical education classes for illness or injury, the length of time should be noted in writing by the physician (see Fig. 1). The central administrative office of the school should have "readmit to class" slips which permit the student to return to class. Reasons for the absence should be noted and in the case of illness or injury the time when the student may return to active class participation should be indicated. The physical education instructor must not permit class participation prior to

Temporary Physical Education Excuse Form
Gahanna–Lincoln High School

Date________________

Please excuse____________________from active physical education

for________________________due to____________________
(number of days) (reason)

I recommend:

Dress:____________________
Rest:____________________
Shower:____________________
Modified activity:____________________

____
(Medical Authority)

Fig. 1 Temporary physical education excuse form. (Courtesy of Gahanna-Lincoln High School, Gahanna, Ohio.)

the time noted, since to do so might aggravate the injury or illness and result in teacher liability.

The excusing of participants in interscholastic sports from the physical education class should not be condoned. Even on game days the athlete should be in class, although he or she may be excused from participation if the activity is of a strenuous nature which might cause injury or undue fatigue.

Records and Reports

An essential part of the administration of the basic instructional program of physical education is the development and maintenance of records. Records should never be kept for records' sake; therefore, basic questions must always be asked regarding the necessity for particular records. Are the records functional? Do they have a practical application for the basic instructional program?

Some kinds of records used in the administration of the basic program and their uses are:

1. health records: health evaluation of the student;
2. accident reports: legal value (see Fig. 2);
3. grade records: report card grades, for students and parents, and for guidance purposes;

Jefferson Local Schools
Gahanna, Ohio

Major Accident Report Form—to be Filed in Main Office

1. Name:__________Home address:__________
2. Grade:____Sex: M : F : Age:____Date:________
3. Place of accident: Time: A.M.____P.M.____
4. Nature of injury, part of body injured:__________
5. Description of accident: How did it happen? What was student doing? Where was the student? List specifically unsafe acts and unsafe conditions existing. Specify any tool, machine or equipment involved.____
6. Teachers on duty when accident occurred:________
7. Did teacher see accident happen: No______Yes______
8. Immediate action taken:____By (name)________
   First aid treatment____By (name)________
   Sent to school nurse____By (name)________
   Sent home____By (name)________
   Sent to physician:____By (name)________
   Physician's name________
   Sent to hospital:____By (name)________
   Name of hospital:________
9. Was parent notified? Yes____When____How____
   No ____Why Not?________
10. Name of person notified________
    By whom?________
11. Attest: 1. Name________2. Address________
    2. Name________2. Address________
12. What recommendations do you have for preventing other accidents of this type?________

Principal________Teachers________

Fig. 2 Major accident report form. (Courtesy of Jefferson Local Schools, Gahanna, Ohio.)

4. attendance records: for attendance reports to principal's office;
5. locker, locks, and basket assignments: for orderly check out and check in of lockers, locks, and baskets;
6. equipment issue records: to help prevent the loss of equipment (see Fig. 3);
7. uniform issue records: to help prevent the loss of uniform items (see Fig. 3);
8. equipment inventory record: to aid in planning for the purchase of needed equipment and supplies.

The number and kinds of records vary from school to school. Records are necessary for the preparation of departmental reports which are frequently requested by school administrators. An annual report, a comprehensive account of all departmental activities for the year, is a necessity.

Safety

Provision for the welfare and safety of students who participate in physical education classes is a prime duty of the physical education instructor. The instructors should receive the necessary knowledge and understanding of a good safety program for physical education in their professional preparation. Obviously, instructors should always be present during class time and should take all precautions necessary to prevent the occurrence of accidents. Each activity in the physical education program contains elements of danger which must be recognized in advance and for which plans must be made. For example, spotters should be provided for gymnastic classes, lifeguards should be available during swimming instruction, and mats should be provided for wrestling classes.

The personal safety of the student begins with the physical examination. Only by having complete knowledge of the physical condition of the boys and girls, together with specific recommendations of a medical doctor, can the instructor know what experiences are suitable and what limitations must be placed on the physical activities of individual class members.

Today's physical educator has a background in such areas as anatomy, physiology, growth and development of youth, as well as an understanding of appropriate activities for the various levels of maturity. Therefore, she or he can plan a program of physical education that will be the safest possible. In addition, the instructor can help ensure safety by teaching proper methods of performing

Blank High School Department of Physical Education
and Athletics

Name (print): ____
(Last) (First) (Middle)

Locker No.__________ Homeroom__________

I hereby accept full responsibility for the following uniforms and/or items of equipment checked out to me:

Equipment	Size	Equipment	No.
Blouse			
Navy Shorts			
White Shorts			
Leotard			
Swim Suit			
Towel			
Signature			

Address______________________________Phone__________

Fig. 3 Equipment and uniform issue form.

physical activities. The instructor is handicapped in teaching skills if classes are so large that individual instruction is limited.

Frequent inspection of facilities and equipment is essential to the safety program. Apparatus, ropes, mats, and other protective equipment must be checked to ensure that they are in good order. Repairs should be made immediately.

In spite of all the safety precautions that physical educators take, accidents do happen. Policies and procedures must be established in advance to handle any accident that might occur. First aid should be administered judiciously. Accident forms should be available in the director's office so that all details of the accident can be recorded. The recorded facts of the accidents may be indispensable if there is a liability case. Many cities have police or fire department emergency squads that are available in case of serious injury. Injured students should be moved in private vehicles only as a last resort. The legal ramifications of safety provisions are discussed in Chapter 4.

Student Leadership

Student leadership should be an integral part of the modern physical education program. Advantages accrue to both the physical educator and the student in the well-planned student leadership program. Properly trained and supervised student leaders can aid the instructor in many of the routine tasks involved in class instruction. For students who are interested in physical education and who possess leadership potential, there are excellent opportunities to use these abilities. It is important to emphasize that the students should be assigned leadership roles only in physical education classes other than the ones in which they are enrolled.

Selection of student leaders should be based on well-established guidelines: the potential leader should petition for membership in the leaders' group; selection should be based on the student's scholastic record, demonstrated interest and ability in physical education (such ability to be evaluated on the basis of results of skill and written tests), and recommendations of teachers outside of physical education.

The potential student leader in physical education should serve as an apprentice, performing such duties as monitoring the locker room, shower room, and instructor's office. Student leaders should wear a distinctive costume. Each student leader should be evaluated every grading period by the instructor to whom he or she is assigned and by the leaders' club adviser.

If a physical education leaders' group is established, a well-planned training program should be provided to enable the student leaders to be as effective as possible in their assignments. Generally the students selected should be juniors or seniors in high school, ninth graders in junior high schools, and sixth graders in elementary schools.

Student leaders may assist the instructor in a variety of ways in the conduct of the physical education program: planning the program, getting equipment ready for the program, assisting in class instruction, demonstrating skills, officiating, keeping records, aiding in skill-testing activities, and returning equipment after classes.

Teaching of Classes

The well-conceived physical education program of today begins with a written course of study which establishes an overall plan for the conduct of the program. This includes a written syllabus for each years' total activity offerings, unit plans, weekly plans, and daily lesson plans.

The modern physical educator should adopt neither the strictly formal nor the strictly informal approach to teaching. In the formal approach to teaching physical education, the instructor controls all class activities and all movements of individual members of the class are executed by a response to the command of the instructor. At the other end of the continuum, the totally informal approach, the instructor relinquishes complete control of the learning situation. Both approaches are out of tune with currently accepted teaching practices. The learning of physical education skills is best achieved in classes in which some freedom of action is permitted. Students should be provided adequate time to practice the skills presented by the instructor, both under the guidance of the instructor and on their own. Class routine should be organized in order that students will know what their responsibilities are.

Since a discussion of methodology does not fall within the province of this book, the reader who wants further information should refer to books dealing specifically with the topic, including Mosston's excellent contribution.[1]

Motivation

Motivating students to learn is a basic problem and a challenge for all teachers. While most young people are inherently interested in physical activity and learning physical skills, the physical education instructor must use every means available to motivate his or her students to want to learn. There are numerous motivating techniques available to the physical education instructor. Examples of some of these are the following:

---

[1] Mosston, Muska, *Teaching Physical Education: From Command to Discovery* (Columbus, Ohio: Charles E. Merrill Books, 1966).

A well-organized and administered program. Student motivation will be enhanced by a physical education program that has been well planned and one which provides competent instruction, adequate facilities and equipment, and sufficient time for the learning and practicing of specific skills. Each class will be a challenge to the student if new materials are presented in the proper progression and at the appropriate time.

Classification of students into homogeneous groups. Another means of student motivation is to place students of similar ability in groups. This technique provides an opportunity for students to learn skills and to compete with students who are at the same level of skill achievement. Reasonable possibilities for success are thus provided.

Extensive use of visual aids. Use of visual aids in the teaching of physical education is another motivating technique. Probably the most readily available sources of material of this type are the various pictures, graphs, charts, and drawings which the teacher can use to make attractive bulletin boards. In addition, many more sophisticated aids are available such as loop films, slides, overhead transparencies, projectors, movies, and even instant playback equipment.

Opportunity for team membership. Team membership usually provides a strong incentive for students to do their very best. Most students wish to contribute to the success of their team and to receive peer and adult acceptance as worthy team members.

Well-administered tournaments. Well-planned tournaments in physical education classes with appropriate schedules and good officiating also motivate students to put forth their best efforts.

Physical education demonstrations for the community. Physical education demonstrations have much value in motivating students. When individuals realize that the skills learned in physical education classes are to be demonstrated to the community, they strive for the best performance possible.

Trips to observe skilled performers. Trips to colleges or to professional events to witness highly skilled performers in physical education and sports activities provide incentive for students to emulate the skilled individual. Firsthand viewing of good athletes often leaves lasting impressions that probably cannot be obtained in any other way, including via television.

Credit and grades for physical education. Credit and grades for participation in physical education classes are a strong motivating factor, as they are in all disciplines in the curriculum. Unfortunately, credit and grades for some students are the only motivation for complying with physical education course requirements. However, when the grading system is properly conceived and a fair and honest appraisal of each student's class performance is provided, credit and grades become a positive means of motivation.

Discipline

Most educators agree that the first prerequisite to the teaching-learning process is an orderly class under the guidance of a teacher. There is no one best way for a teacher to conduct the class. There are a variety of methods and techniques available, and while one method or technique of conducting a class may work very well for one instructor, it may be a total failure for another. Teachers should handle classes and discipline in terms of their own personality and the personality of the class.

While there is no one best way to conduct classes and handle discipline, there are guidelines that have been established over a long period of time and that are helpful to all teachers, especially beginning teachers. First of all, teachers must believe in themselves and have confidence that they can handle their classes and any discipline problem that might arise. Self-control is a must, for if teachers do not have self-control, they cannot expect to control others. If teachers know their subject well and establish routines for class conduct which the students understand, many potential discipline problems will be eliminated. Successful teachers establish good rapport with their students early and convey to them the feeling that they are working for the same goals and that they are, in effect, partners in the search for knowledge.

In establishing relationships with his or her classes, the beginning teacher may be at a disadvantage in comparison with the experienced teacher. The experienced teacher's reputation has been determined, while the new teacher's has not. Most educators agree that the first day of a new term is crucial; it is then that the teacher must establish the fact that he or she is serious about the teaching-learning process. It is much better for the new teacher to be firm at the beginning and relax a bit at a later time than to permit disorder among students during the early days of classes and then attempt to get order by "getting tough." The teacher usually finds that this latter procedure does not work and that discipline problems only multiply.

Some excellent suggestions for the handling of discipline are made by Schain:

Establishing Preventive Discipline

1. Teacher-pupil relationship. Good rapport must be established between teacher and students.
2. Lesson planning. Teach your lessons interestingly and effectively.
3. Starting the lesson. Stand in front of the class and wait for absolute attention.
4. The teacher's voice. Variations and shadings of the voice can be an aid to discipline.
5. Class participation can be a factor in discipline. Enlist as many students as possible in the lesson.
6. Use of praise. When students do something worthwhile and noteworthy, praise them publicly.

Basic Guides to Corrective Discipline

1. The teacher is primarily responsible for classroom discipline.
2. Violations of discipline must not be ignored.
3. Punishment should follow any infraction.
   a) The punishment should fit the crime.
   b) Punishment should be immediate and definite.
   c) Punishment should be impersonal.

Do's for Corrective Discipline

1. Use the power of silence.
2. Be consistent in your manner and treatment of infractions.
3. Change the seat of chronic troublemakers as soon as you notice the problem.
4. Be prepared to change class activity if necessary.
5. Make use of parents.
6. Keep a record of disciplinary interactions.
7. Use the resources and help of the school personnel.

Don't's for Corrective Discipline

1. Don't threaten.
2. Don't lose your temper.

3. Don't use sarcasm.
4. Don't make issue with students in public.
5. Don't send students out of the room for misbehavior.
6. Don't reward bad behavior.
7. Don't use assignments as a punishment for poor discipline.
8. Don't punish the whole class for individual infractions.[2]

These suggestions are not a panacea for preventive and corrective discipline; however, they may be helpful to the beginning teacher. In addition, it cannot be stressed too strongly that the wisdom of using physical education activities such as running laps or doing push-ups as punishment is very questionable.

Evaluation

In the basic instructional program of physical education, there are four types of evaluation: evaluation of students, evaluation of teachers, evaluation of the administration, and evaluation of the program. All are necessary and all must be carefully planned and implemented if the basic instructional program is to be effective. These four types of evaluation are discussed in detail in Chapter 8.

Team Teaching

The team-teaching concept for physical education is gaining acceptance in many of the larger junior and senior high schools, as well as in some elementary schools. Team teaching is a means by which two or more staff members plan together and teach together in an effort to improve instruction. The advantages are many. Reams and Bleier discuss the advantages of team teaching:

> Team teaching, combined with flexible scheduling, offers the greatest advantage over traditional programs. However, team teaching within the boundaries of the traditional time schedule still provides an instructional environment with opportunities for improvement of the physical education program. The primary advantages are:
>
> 1. Instructor-pupil ratio may be varied with the type of activity, ability level, or facilities available.
> 2. The department is able to utilize the talents and interests of individual staff members to the best advantage.
> 3. The pupil has the benefit of the talent of several instructors rather than being limited to one person during an entire year.

---

[2] Adapted from Robert L. Schain, *Discipline, How to Establish and Maintain It* (Englewood Cliffs, N.J.: Prentice-Hall, 1961): pp. 22–42. Reprinted by permission of the Publishers, Lieber-Atherton, Inc.

4. Adaptation to abilities can become a reality rather than a desire. Each level should have specific lesson plans based on the general abilities of that group. This enables the pupils to better establish goals for their progression through the physical education program.

All of the advantages of team teaching are not directly related to the pupils, but they do improve the total program and this eventually affects the individual pupil. These include:

1. Flexibility, although limited by the regular class period, can be gained by varying the level of instruction and adjusting the time spent on developing skills according to the ability of the group.
2. A cohesion of staff members can be obtained that is nearly impossible to achieve under the traditional program. The instructors play an integral part in the function of each class. This means that all policies should be group policy.
3. Supervision and control become easier. It has often been the policy to assign instructors specific areas of between class supervision, such as locker room, office and outside areas. However, there is a feeling by the pupil that only his instructor must be obeyed. In the team approach, there is no one instructor.
4. Variety in instruction is accomplished through the rotation of groups. No instructor will be working with the same ability level all year. Each new group necessitates a new approach.[3]

Evergreen Park Community High School in suburban Chicago, Illinois, has adopted the team-teaching concept. A brief description of their program follows (see Fig. 4).

All students of the same grade level are scheduled into a single class. This arrangement produces a schedule of four classes meeting during the day. A team of four instructors is assigned to each of the classes. All physical education instructors are scheduled to meet in a common planning period which takes the place of a fifth class. This arrangement is justified because teachers are handling the same number of classes as before.

The team-teaching concept has advantages for class organization. The large group technique is utilized for such things as warm-ups, instruction, special programs, and tournaments. Each class period begins with the large group before it is broken down into the smaller segments determined by the nature of the activity.

On Monday of each week the large group meets in the school auditorium for a health instruction lecture. All questions are reserved for the four small group health discussions which meet on assigned days of the week (see Fig. 5).

---

[3] David Reams and T. J. Bleier, "Developing Team Teaching for Ability Grouping," *Journal of Health Physical Education Recreation,* **39** (September 1968): 50–51. Reprinted by permission.

Period	1	2	3	4	5	6	7
Class	Freshman P.E.	Sophomore P.E.	Planning Period	Lunch	Senior P.E.	Junior P.E.	Conference
Team	Inst.*I Inst. II Inst. III Inst. IV	Inst. I Inst. II Inst. III Inst. IV	All	All	Inst. I Inst. II Inst. V Inst. III	Inst. I Inst. II Inst. V Inst. III	All

* Instructor.

Fig. 4 The program schedule. (From Marvin I. Clein, "A New Approach to the Physical Education Schedule," *Journal of Health Physical Education Recreation*, **33** (November 1962): 34. Reprinted by permission.)

For physical education activities, the large group is also broken down into four smaller groups; however, this may be modified since

<table>
<tr><th>Group</th><th>Monday</th><th>Tuesday</th><th>Wednesday</th><th>Thursday</th><th>Friday</th></tr>
<tr><td>"A"
Ability group</td><td rowspan="4">Health Lecture Auditorium
Inst. IV</td><td>Health,
Inst. IV</td><td>Fund. of Soccer,
Inst. III</td><td>Fund. of Soccer,
Inst. III</td><td>Fund. of Soccer,
Inst. III</td></tr>
<tr><td>"B"
Low on physical fitness test</td><td>Weight training,
Inst. II</td><td>Health,
Inst. IV</td><td>Weight training,
Inst. II</td><td>Conditioning games,
Inst. II</td></tr>
<tr><td>"C"
Ability group</td><td>Fund. of Soccer,
Inst. III</td><td>Fund. of Soccer,
Inst. III
Asst. II</td><td>Health,
Inst. IV</td><td>Fund. of Soccer,
Inst. III
Asst. I</td></tr>
<tr><td>"D"
Fall sports participants</td><td>Advan. Soccer Skills,
Inst. I</td><td>Advan. Soccer Skills,
Inst. I</td><td>Advan. Soccer Skills,
Inst. I</td><td>Health,
Inst. IV</td></tr>
</table>

Fig. 5 Sample class organization, grade 10. This figure illustrates ability grouping and teacher specialization. (From Marvin I. Clein, "A New Approach to the Physical Education Schedule," *Journal of Health Physical Education Recreation*, **33** (November 1962): 34. Reprinted by permission.)

the size of the group is generally determined by the type of activity or by the abilities of the students. Regrouping may take place at any time because of changing emphasis in the program of instruction.[4]

The Nongraded School Physical Education Program

One of the newest curriculum and scheduling plans in the secondary schools is the nongraded school plan. The nongraded school concept includes new ideas for physical education programs which are progressive and should be understood by all physical educators.

An example of a school system that has adopted the nongraded plan and flexible scheduling for its high school is the Athens, Ohio, Public School System. A description of the physical education program follows.

All students in all subjects including physical education are placed in phases based on nationally recognized standardized tests. General guidelines for placing students in the specific phases are:

Phase 1. Courses offered at this level are designed to help students who are *quite deficient* in basic skills and feel the need for considerable help and attention. Class enrollments will be smaller so that more teacher time can be spent with individual students.

Phase 2. Courses at this level are designed for those students who are *somewhat deficient* in basic skills and who will profit from additional help with those skills.

Phase 3. Courses at this level are designed for those students who are achieving at an *average level.*

Phase 4. Courses at this level are designed for students who desire to study a subject in depth.

The physical education staff of Athens, Ohio, High School has followed the general guidelines for phasing in establishing the physical education curriculum. The criterion for phasing is the percentile score achieved by the student on the American Association for Health, Physical Education, and Recreation Youth Fitness Test. Phase 1 is for students who placed in the 0th percentile to the 25th percentile; phase 2 is for those in the 26th to the 40th percentile; phase 3 is for students in the 41st to the 60th percentile: and phase 4 is for those in the 61st to the 100th percentile.

---

[4] Marvin I. Clein, "A New Approach to the Physical Education Schedule," *Journal of Health Physical Education Recreation,* **33** (November, 1962): 36. Reprinted by permission.

All students are required to take two years of general physical education, and they may elect advanced physical education courses for the other years in school.

General physical education: phase 1 (one year, one half credit). This course provides students with the basics for good movement skills necessary for participation in individual, dual, and team activities. Emphasis is on a personalized approach to meet the needs and desires of each student.

General physical education: phase 2 (one year, one half credit). This course offers an opportunity for students to improve their physical fitness through concentrated effort and individual attention. Secondly, students can increase their ability and knowledge in track and field, gymnastics, dance, individual, dual, and team sports. A third segment of this course is concerned with learning and enjoying a variety of leisure-time skills.

General physical education: phase 3 (one year, one half credit). This course presents students with the opportunity to continue building toward efficient skills in individual, dual, and team sports, gymnastics, dance, as well as in track and field activities, with increased stress on actual competition. Emphasis is still placed on strengthening each individual through a program of exercises, weight lifting, etc. A wide variety of leisure-time activities is an important part of the course content.

General physical education: phase 4 (one year, one half credit). The fourth phase of general physical education focuses on striving for excellence in physical conditioning. Students are given the opportunity to develop skilled performance in the individual, dual, and team sports, and become outstanding in gymnastics, dance, track and field. By exposure to a variety of recreational carry-over activities, this course gives each student a sound basis for continuing interest and participation.

Electives

Electives are offered to both boys and girls in the junior and senior years in beginning swimming, social dancing, advanced gymnastics, and advanced physical education (for those students who have achieved success in physical education and desire to pursue their interest further.)

Modular or Flexible Scheduling

A vital part of the nongraded school program is the concept of modular or flexible scheduling. Athens, Ohio, High School has adopted modular scheduling to provide maximum flexibility in scheduling and greater opportunities for individualized instruction.

In the modular system the school day is divided into periods of time called "modules." In the case of Athens, Ohio, High School, the school day commences with a ten-minute homeroom period followed by 27 fifteen-minute modules and ending with another ten-minute homeroom period. A class period may be two or more modules in length. Time requirements among the various subjects taught vary considerably to meet individual student needs and in respect to total time in class per work needed, optimum length of class meetings, and frequency of meeting times. The modular schedule allows sufficient flexibility to accommodate these differences. Typically, most students and teachers have a different schedule each day during the week. This is known as a "weekly cycle." Once established, the weekly cycle remains stabilized throughout the year. This type of schedule allows for the scheduling of students and teachers for large group instruction (50 to 350 students) and small group instruction (10 to 15 students).

In summary, modular scheduling is strongly student-centered without being detrimental to content of courses. Its purpose is to offer the student increased learning opportunities and substantially more responsibility and freedom, and to provide each student with a schedule tailored to his or her individual needs. Figure 6 shows how the physical education staff of Athens, Ohio, High School has adopted modular scheduling for their physical education program.[5]

SPECIAL EDUCATION AND MAINSTREAMING

Educators today are concerned about providing the best possible educational opportunities for all youth, including those classified as exceptional. Dunn categorizes 12 types of exceptional children:

1. Educable mentally retarded
2. Trainable mentally retarded
3. Gifted
4. Emotionally disturbed

---

[5] The material used to describe the nongraded high school program and the physical education program of Athens, Ohio, High School is used with the permission of the administration of Athens, Ohio, Public School System.

	Days per week	Modules per class meeting	Total time per class meeting
I. Required courses			
A. Phases 1–4	3	4	60 minutes
	1	2	30 minutes
II. Elective courses			
A. Advanced dance	3	3	45 minutes
B. Advanced gymnastics	3	4	60 minutes
C. Advanced physical education	3	4	60 minutes
D. Beginning swimming	3	4	60 minutes
E. Physical education leadership	3	4	60 minutes
	1	2	30 minutes
F. Social dancing	2	3	45 minutes

Fig. 6 Number of modules for physical education classes (Athens, Ohio, High School).

5. Socially maladjusted
6. Speech-impaired
7. Hard of hearing
8. Deaf
9. Partially seeing
10. Blind
11. Crippled
12. Chronically ill.[6]

Recent federal legislation has helped mobilize school administrators at all educational levels to develop educational programs and facilities that will best meet the needs of these 12 categories of exceptional children. Professional physical educators are as involved as any other group of educators in planning meaningful educational experiences for exceptional children.

[6] Lloyd M. Dunn, ed., *Exceptional Children in the Schools* (New York: Holt, Rinehart and Winston, 1963), p. 44.

The term "special education" is commonly used to refer to the kinds of educational experiences essential to meet the needs of exceptional children. Kirk defines special education as that additional service, over and above the regular school program, that is provided for an exceptional child to assist in the development of his or her potentialities and/or in the amelioration of his or her disabilities.[7] Thus special education is not a total program entirely different from that prepared for the education of the ordinary child. Rather, "special education" refers only to those aspects of education that are unique and/or in addition to the regular program for all children.[8]

The major thrust today in special education is "mainstreaming," or the process of maintaining or returning an exceptional child to the regular classroom for part or all of the school day, to give the child opportunities to be involved with nonhandicapped children, and to participate in normal school day activities. This definition also applies to physical education activities for the exceptional child.

It is important to note that mainstreaming is not designed to abolish existing special education classes or services, but it must be considered as an alternative to better meet the needs of certain groups of exceptional children who are capable of performing reasonably well in the regular classroom.

Each decision regarding mainstreaming a student should be made on an individual basis by a knowledgeable group of concerned persons, including psychologists, parents, special education teachers, regular teachers, and the student if he or she is mature enough to express an opinion. The principal consideration in placing exceptional children in regular classroom situations is the total welfare of the student.

Special education authorities recommend that placement of the exceptional child in the regular classroom or physical education class occur during the first quarter of the school year, in order to be the least disruptive possible to the child. It is further recommended that mainstreaming of exceptional children into regular classrooms occur before grade 10; after this, the adjustment is difficult, since the student would have spent all of his or her previous school time in special education classes.

The progress of children who are mainstreamed should be evaluated frequently by the placement group. Determinations can then

---

[7] Samuel A. Kirk, *Educating Exceptional Children* (Boston: Houghton Mifflin, 1972), p. 37.

[8] *Ibid.*, pp. 34–35.

be made as to the feasibility of the child's remaining in the normal classroom or returning to special education classes.

In discussing the physical education program for exceptional children, Daniels and Davies state that

> the exceptional child needs and should have normal developmental experiences whenever he can benefit from them. Frequently the limitations of the child are such that special provisions or arrangements must be made in order that he may be protected while his special needs are being met. Thus, every possible effort should be made to have him participate in the standard play activities with normal groups. At other times, special planning and arrangements will have to be worked out in accordance with his best interests.[9]

The federal Department of Health, Education and Welfare has sponsored legislation passed by the United States Congress to ensure that handicapped children obtain an education in the most normal setting possible. The two key laws pertaining to the education of the handicapped are: (1) Public Law 93–112, Section 504 of the Rehabilitation Act of 1973, and (2) Public Law 94–142, Education for all Handicapped Children Act of 1975. Section 504 of the Rehabilitation Act of 1973 provides that "no otherwise qualified handicapped individual . . . shall, solely by reason of his handicap, be excluded from the participation in, be denied benefits of, or be subjected to discrimination under any program or activity receiving federal financial assistance." The regulation, which applies to all recipients of federal assistance from HEW, is intended to ensure that federally assisted programs and activities are operated without discrimination on the basis of handicap. As providers of services, recipients are required to make programs operated in existing facilities accessible to handicapped persons, to ensure that new facilities are constructed so as to be readily accessible to handicapped persons, and to operate their programs in a nondiscriminatory manner.[10] Section 504 thus represents the first federal civil rights law protecting the rights of handicapped persons and reflects a national commitment to end discrimination on the basis of handicap.[11]

Public Law 94–142 states that "the purpose of this Act is to assure that all handicapped children have available to them . . . a free appropriate public education which emphasizes special education

---

[9] Arthur S. Daniels and Evelyn A. Davies, *Adapted Physical Education,* 3rd ed. (New York: Harper & Row, 1975), p. 323.

[10] *Federal Register,* Vol. 42, No. 86, May 4, 1977, p. 15.

[11] *Ibid.*

and related services designated to meet their unique needs, to assure that the rights of handicapped children and their parents or guardians are protected, to assist states and localities to provide for the education of all handicapped children, and to assess and assure the effectiveness of efforts to educate handicapped children.[12]

In order to qualify for financial assistance, a state must demonstrate that it has established procedures to ensure that to the maximum extent appropriate, handicapped children, including those in public or private institutions or other care facilities, are educated with children who are not handicapped and that special classes, separate schooling, or other removal of handicapped children from the regular educational environment occurs only when the nature or severity of the handicapped is such that education in regular classes with the use of supplementary aids and services cannot be achieved satisfactorily.[13] More specifically, as stated in Part 121a.307:

(a) *General.* Physical education services, specially designed if necessary, must be made available to every handicapped child receiving a free appropriate public education.

(b) *Regular physical education.* Each handicapped child must be afforded the opportunity to participate in the regular physical education program available to non-handicapped children unless:
   (1) The child is enrolled full time in a separate facility; or
   (2) The child needs specially designed physical education, as prescribed in the child's individualized education program.

(c) *Special physical education.* If specially designed physical education is prescribed in a child's individualized education program, the public agency responsible for the education of that child shall provide the services directly, or make arrangements for it to be provided through other public or private programs.

(d) *Education in separate facilities.* The public agency responsible for the education of a handicapped child who is enrolled in a separate facility shall insure that the child receives appropriate physical education services in compliance with paragraphs (a) and (c) of this section.

The Report of the House of Representatives on Public Law 94–142[14] includes the following statement regarding physical education:

> Special education as set forth in the Committee bill includes instruction in physical eduaction, which is provided as a matter of course to all non-handicapped children enrolled in public elementary and

---

[12] Public Law 94–142, 94th Congress, 5.6, November 29, 1975, p. 773

[13] *Ibid.*, p. 781.

[14] House Report No. 94–332, p. 9 (1975).

secondary schools. The Committee is concerned that although these services are available to and required of all children in our school systems, they are often viewed as a luxury for handicapped children.

The Committee expects the Commissioner of Education to take whatever action is necessary to assure that physical education services are available to all handicapped children, and has specifically included physical education within the definition of special education to make clear that the Committee expects such services, specially designed where necessary, to be provided as an integral part of the educational program of every handicapped child.[15]

CASE STUDY

Bill Hardy and Jane Elkins sat in the physical education office at the end of another school year. Both were concerned about the lack of progression in the activities within their program. They agreed that in most cases the materials available for activities were extensive enough to permit proper progression. At this point Elkins spoke up: "How can we consider a progression within activities when the administration allows any student from ninth to twelfth grade to sign up for any class? Under these conditions any student might take the advanced section of an activity before he had taken the elementary section." Hardy replied, "Perhaps if we could come up with a satisfactory plan of classes for next year, the principal might consider altering the method of scheduling pupils in physical education."

1. What issues are involved in this case?
2. What solutions are possible?
3. Are there any principles or policies which evolve from this case?

SELECTED REFERENCES

Adams, R. "P.E.'s a Child Feeling O.K. About Himself," *Instructor,* **83** (March 1974): 64–65.

Albertson, L. M. "Physical Education or Physical Indoctrination?" *Physical Educator,* **31** (May 1974): 90–92.

American Alliance for Health, Physical Education and Recreation. *Assessment Guide for Secondary School Physical Education Programs.* Washington, D.C.: The Association, 1977.

American Association for Health, Physical Education, and Recreation. *Organizational Patterns for Instruction in Physical Education.* Washington, D.C.: AAHPER Press, 1971.

Anderson, D. R. "Are We Making Procrustean Beds of Our Secondary School Physical Education Programs?" *Journal of Health Physical Education Recreation,* **43** (November 1972): 36.

---

[15] *Federal Register,* Vol. 42, No. 163, August 23, 1977.

Anderson, E. W. "Individual Differences: A Basic Principle for Physical Education," *Physical Educator,* **30** (October 1973): 128–129.

Annarino, A. A. "IIP: Individualized Instruction in Physical Education," *Journal of Health Physical Education Recreation,* **44** (October 1973): 20–23.

Annarino, A. A., and S. Otto. "Curriculum Development," *Physical Educator,* **34** (March 1977): 51–54.

Avedisian, C. T. "Planned Programming Budgeting Systems," *Journal of Health Physical Education Recreation,* **43** (October 1972): 37–39.

Bain, L. L. "Description of the Hidden Curriculum in Secondary Physical Education," *Research Quarterly,* **47** (May 1976): 154–160.

———. "Instrument for Identifying Implicit Values in Physical Education Programs," *Research Quarterly,* **47** (October 1976): 307–315.

Balazs, E. K. "Candid Look at Physical Education," *Journal of Physical Education,* **72** (January 1975): 93–94.

Bennett, J. "Modules and Movement," *Journal of Health Phsyical Education Recreation,* **41** (April 1970): 48–49.

Bertel, H. "Try What? Introduction of a New Activity in the Physical Education Class," *Journal of Health Physical Education Recreation,* **45** (May 1974): 24.

Bourdreaux, C. "Physical Education as Preparation for Adulthood," *Journal of Health Physical Education Recreation,* **43** (January 1972): 29.

Bucher, Charles A. *Administration of Health and Physical Education Programs, Including Athletics* (5th rev. ed.). St. Louis, Mo.: C. V. Mosby, 1971.

———. *Methods and Materials for Secondary School Physical Education* (3rd ed.). St. Louis, Mo.: C. V. Mosby, 1970.

———. "What's Happening in Education Today?" *Journal of Health Physical Education Recreation,* **45** (September 1974): 30–32.

Caldwell, S. F. "Toward a Humanistic Physical Education," *Journal of Health Physical Education Recreation,* **43** (May 1972): 31–32.

Chavez, R. "Confidence in Working With Exceptional Children Can Be Gained in a Laboratory Setting," *Journal of Health Physical Education Recreation,* **44** (October 1973): 65–67.

Check, J. F. "Is Creative Teaching for the Physical Educator in Vogue?" *Physical Educator,* **28** (December 1971): 192–195.

Cutler, S. Jr. "Nongraded Concept and Physical Education," *Journal of Health Physical Education Recreation,* **45** (April 1974): 30–31.

Daughtrey, Greyson, and John B. Woods. *Physical Education and Intramural Programs: Organization and Administration.* Philadelphia: W. B. Saunders, 1976.

———. *Physical Education Programs: Organization and Administration.* Philadelphia: W. B. Saunders, 1971.

Davis, H. "Physical Education and its Contribution to Equality in Education," *Journal of Physical Education,* **70** (May 1973): 110–111.

———. "What Does the Future Hold for the Black Physical Educator?" *Journal of Health Physical Education Recreation,* **43** (January 1972): 65–66.

Dewitt, R. T., and Ken Dugan. *Teaching Individual and Team Sports* (2nd ed.). Englewood Cliffs, N.J.: Prentice-Hall, 1972.

Dintiman, George B., et al. *Comprehensive Manual of Physical Education Activities for Men.* New York: Appleton-Century-Crofts, 1970.

Ernst, L. "Sprint to Lifetime Sports," *Education Digest,* **39** (November 1973): 50–53.

Everts, C. "Firsthand Experiences for Future Physical Educators," *Journal of Health Physical Education Recreation,* **43** (October 1972): 40.

Fait, Hollis F. *Physical Education for the Elementary School Child: Experiences in Movement* (2nd ed.). Philadelphia: W. B. Saunders, 1971.

Fins, Alice. "Sex and the Principal: A Long Look at Title IX," *NASSP Bulletin* (September 1974): 53–62.

Fordham, Sheldon L., and Carol Ann Leaf. *Physical Education and Sports.* New York: Wiley, 1978.

Freischlag, J., and R. McCarthy. "Community-University Cooperative Physical Education Programming for the Retarded: El Paso, Texas," *Physical Education,* **32** (March 1975): 11–13.

———. "Competency-Based Instruction," *Journal of Health Physical Education Recreation,* **45** (January 1974): 29–31.

Frost, Reuben B. *Physical Education: Foundations, Practices, Principles.* Reading, Mass.: Addison-Wesley, 1975.

Frost, Reuben B., and Stanley J. Marshall. *Administration of Physical Education and Athletics: Concepts and Practices.* Dubuque, Iowa: W. C. Brown, 1977.

Gallahue, D. L. "Aims of Physical Education," *Physical Educator,* **33** (December 1976): 170.

Gerstung, R. "Philosophy of Physical Education," *Physical Educator,* **31** (March 1974): 41.

Geyer, C. "Physical Education for the Electronic Age," *Journal of Health Physical Education Recreation,* **43** (April 1972): 32.

Graham, G. M. "Bridge Between What Is and What Could Be," *Physical Educator,* **32** (March 1976): 14–16.

Grebner, F. "Voluntary Participation in Physical Activities," *Physical Educator,* **32** (March 1975): 24–25.

Green, L. "What Is Competency-Based Education?" *Journal of Health Physical Education Recreation,* **44** (October 1973): 87.

Grieve, A. "Try It, You'll Like It: Format for Physical Education Curriculum Guide," *Journal of Health Physical Education Recreation,* **43** (May 1972): 34–35.

Hale, Patricia. *Individual Sports: A Textbook for Teachers.* Dubuque, Iowa: W. C. Brown, 1974.

Harper J., and J. M. McKenzie. "Improving Interracial Professional Relationships in Physical Education," *Journal of Health Physical Education Recreation,* **46** (September 1975): 22–23.

Hartman, B., and A. Clement. "Adventure in Key Concepts: Ohio Guide for Girls Secondary Physical Education," *Journal of Health Physical Education Recreation,* **44** (March 1973): 20.

Healey, J. H., and W. A. Healey. *Physical Education Teaching Problems for Analysis and Solution.* Springfield, Ill.: Charles C Thomas, 1975.

Hill, B. "Physical Education and the Classroom," *School and Community,* **61** (May 1975): 23+.

Hook, A. J. "Computer Monitored Physical Education," *Journal of Health Physical Education Recreation,* **44** (September 1973): 24–25.

Hunsicker, P., and G. Reiff. "Youth Fitness Report: 1958–1975," *Journal of Health Physical Education Recreation,* **48** (January 1977): 31–33.

Johnson, J. H. "Punishment and Pain in Physical Education Classes," *School and Community,* **57** (May 1971): 44.

Johnson, M. L. *Functional Administration in Physical and Health Education.* Boston: Houghton Mifflin, 1977.

Kaesgen, N. C., and C. Pincombe. "Junior High Course," *Journal of Health Physical Education Recreation,* **45** (September 1974): 94.

Kaufmann, D. A. "Taking the Guesswork out of Skill Instruction," *Journal of Physical Education,* **71** (September 1973): 9.

Kelly, B. J. "Getting it all Together: The Integrated Learning Semester; Sport and Human Values," *Journal of Health Physical Education Recreation,* **45** (October 1974): 32–35.

———. "Implementing Title IX," *Journal of Physical Education and Recreation,* **48** (February 1977): 27–28.

Kelly, N. "Think Before You Move: Primary Grades," *Instructor,* **83** (August 1973): 58.

Kizer, D. L. "Physical Education Teaching Methods Made Meaningful," *Journal of Health Physical Education Recreation,* **45** (June 1974): 50.

Klammer, O. "Teaching Aids for Large Classes," *Journal of Health Physical Education Recreation,* **42** (March 1971): 71.

Knight, R. F., and S. Scott. "Ohio–Michigan Conference on Curriculum Improvement in Secondary Physical Education," *Journal of Health Physical Education Recreation,* **41** (January 1970): 57–60.

Larson, Leonard A. *Curriculum Foundations and Standards for Physical Education.* Englewood Cliffs, N.J.: Prentice-Hall, 1970.

Lawson, H., and B. Lawson. "Alternative Program Model for Secondary School Physical Education," *Journal of Physical Education and Recreation,* **48** (February 1977): 38–39.

Lewis, C. G. "Contract Teaching: Symposium," *Journal of Health Physical Education Recreation,* **45** (October 1974): 36–47.

Lewis, G. T. "Student Behavior: A Rationale for Elective Physical Education," *Physical Educator,* **31** (October 1974): 127–128.

Locke, F., and D. Lambdin. "Personalized Learning in Physical Education," *Journal of Physical Education and Recreation,* **47** (June 1976): 32–35.

McGee, R., and F. Drews. *Proficiency Testing for Physical Education.* Washington, D.C.: American Association for Health, Physical Education and Recreation, 1974.

McKinney, W. C., and P. M. Ford. "What Is the Profession Doing About Education for Leisure?" *Journal of Health Physical Education Recreation,* **43** (May 1972): 49–53.

Mallios, H. C. "Physical Educator and the Law," *Physical Educator,* **32** (May 1975): 61–63.

Martin, J. E. "What Is a Senior Leader?" *Physical Educator,* **30** (December 1973): 191.

Matthews, Donald K. *Measurement in Physical Education* (4th ed.). Philadelphia: W. B. Saunders, 1973.

Moser, D. L. "Good Discipline Is a Product of Good Teaching," *Journal of Health Physical Education Recreation,* **42** (June 1971): 23.

Moss, J. K. "Recess Is Not a Physical Fitness Program," *Teacher,* **91** (December 1973): 28–30.

Munson, C., and E. Stafford. "Middle Schools: A Variety of Approaches to Physical Education," *Journal of Health Physical Education Recreation,* **45** (February 1974): 29–31.

Myers, C. R. "Physical Education Management, Mismanagement, or Where Do I Go From Here?" *Journal of Physical Education,* **72** (November 1974): 42–45.

Negley, H. H., and W. T. Paynter. *Motion and Direction: Physical Education Curriculum Guide, Grades K-12.* Indianapolis: Indiana State Department of Public Instruction, 1976.

Norred, R. G. "Relating to Administrators," *Journal of Health Physical Education Recreation,* **45** (June 1974): 24–25.

"Now Physical Education; Symposium," *Journal of Health Physical Education Recreation,* **44** (September 1973): 23–32.

O'Donnell, L. E. "Experience Based Contracting in Elementary Physical Education," *Physical Educator,* **33** (October 1976): 135–139.

Oversket, L. "Coeducational Lottery System," *Journal of Health Physical Education Recreation,* **44** (September 1973): 27–28.

Park, R. J., and B. A. Heisler. "School Programs Can Foster Creativity Through Physical Education," *Education,* **95** (Spring 1975): 225–228.

"Physical Education and the Law," *Journal of Health Physical Education Recreation,* **45** (October 1974): 24–29.

Polidoro, J. R. "Affective Domain: The Forgotten Behavioral Objective of Physical Education," *Physical Educator,* **30** (October 1973): 136–138.

Pucci, T. G. "Physical Education vs. Interscholastic Athletics in the School in the Middle," *Physical Educator,* **30** (December 1973): 185–187.

Reed, J. S. "High School Cycling Program," *Journal of Health Physical Education Recreation,* **44** (November 1973): 13.

Rhea, H. C. "Modern Curriculum?" *Physical Educator,* **34** (March 1977): 26–27.

Saeger, E. "Man Behind the Scenes," *Physical Educator,* **31** (May 1974): 81.

Schwarzkopf, R., and G. Morris. "Obesity and the Forgotten Child," *Physical Educator,* **34** (March 1977): 12–14.

Seefeldt, V. "Middle Schools: Issues and Future Directions in Physical Education," *Journal of Health Physical Education Recreation,* **45** (February 1974): 32–34.

Seidel, Beverley L., and Matthew C. Resick. *Physical Education: An Overview.* Reading, Mass.: Addison-Wesley, 1972.

Seidel, Beverley L., *et al. Sports Skills: A Conceptual Approach to Meaningful Movement.* Dubuque, Iowa: W. C. Brown, 1975.

Seidentop, Daryl. *Physical Education: Introductory Analysis.* Dubuque, Iowa: W. C. Brown, 1972.

Shore, J. "Rotate to Participate," *Journal of Health Physical Education Recreation,* **45** (April 1974): 32.

Singer, R. "Systems Approach to Teaching Physical Education," *Journal of Health Physical Education Recreation,* **45** (September 1974): 33–36.

"Statement of Basic Beliefs About the School Programs in Health, Physical Education, and Recreation," *Journal of Health Physical Education Recreation,* **44** (June 1973): 22–24.

Stringfellow, M. E. "Competency Based Instruction in Measurement and Evaluation," *Journal of Physical Education and Recreation,* **47** (September 1976): 50–51.

Thomas, J. "Scheduling in Elementary School Physical Education," *Physical Educator,* **27** (October 1970): 131–132.

Tillman, Kenneth G. "Student Participation in Departmental Responsibilities," *Journal of Health Physical Education Recreation,* **45** (June 1974): 59–60.

Trecker, Janice L. "Sex Stereotyping in the Secondary School Curriculum," *Phi Delta Kappan,* **55** (October 1973): 110–112.

Vannier, Maryhelen, and Hollis F. Fait. *Teaching Physical Education in Secondary Schools.* Philadelphia: W. B. Saunders, 1975.

Willgoose, Carl E. *Curriculum in Physical Education.* Englewood Cliffs, N.J.: Prentice-Hall, 1969.

Wrenn, J. P., and A. M. Love. "Whither Thou Goest, Physical Education?" *Physical Educator,* **30** (October 1973): 139–141.

Ziatz, D. H. "How Do You Motivate Students to Learn?" *Journal of Physical Education and Recreation,* **48** (March 1977): 26.

10

FINANCE AND BUDGET

STUDY STIMULATORS

1. How do the states give financial support to local schools? What is the basis of this support?
2. What is the result of prohibiting the expenditures of state funds for athletics, as most states do?
3. What is the purpose of the budget for a department of physical education?
4. What are some principles to be followed in the proper construction of a budget?
5. What are sources of income for a program of interscholastic athletics?
6. What suggestions could be made for the proper conduct of concessions at athletic contests?
7. What is the advantage of an outside audit?
8. Should income from the boys' varsity program help to defray the expenses for the girls' varsity program?

How pleasant it is to have money!

ARTHUR HUGH CLOUGH

FINANCING PUBLIC EDUCATION

The financing of public education in the United States becomes more difficult each year. Most local school districts find that funds derived from local taxation are insufficient to meet local school needs. Thus, state funds are necessary to supplement local school monies. In recent years, there has been a trend to turn to federal sources for additional aid to local school districts in order that the youth of this country might be provided with the quality of education they deserve. In many states, school consolidations are the means used to provide larger school districts; these mean more students and therefore more tax money available to provide an enriched curriculum, enlarged teaching staffs, and better facilities.

Each of the 50 states in the United States is responsible for providing a system of public education within its borders. There is also a responsibility to finance the public education program. Although the major responsibility for fiscal support for the schools rests with the various state governments, local governments and the federal government also share in the financing of public schools.

Until comparatively recent times, the financial support of public schools was provided by local school taxes. Gradually, over the years, however, increasing amounts of financial support have shifted from local school districts to the states and, to a lesser degree, the federal government, as it became apparent that in most cases local funds were inadequate to finance public education. Also, it became obvious that there was a great variance in the ability of individual school districts to pay for their education programs.

These factors, along with the concept that there should be equal educational opportunity for all children of school age in each state, led to increasing state financial support for education.

Another factor that led to increasing the state's percentage of financial support for public education was that many state departments of education established minimum educational standards for school districts to improve the quality of education in the districts. Many school districts could not meet the standards without additional state aid, so the states, quite often, provided the necessary funds. It should also be noted that the inability of local school districts to meet state standards often led to consolidation of two or more small districts into one to comply with the minimum standards.

Although the trend has been to increase state aid for local school districts, the funds provided by the states are not uniform, ranging from approximately 30 percent to approximately 70 percent. (One exception is the state of Hawaii, where the public education system is 100 percent state-supported.)

State funds for support of schools are derived from several sources, including state monies from the general funds and earmarked state taxes, as well as from state property taxes. In many states the principal source of tax revenue is from sales and gasoline taxes. Many years ago Texas developed a unique method of providing funds for the support of public school education. The state legislature enacted the Permanent School Fund, to be financed by revenues produced on land owned by the state. These funds may not be spent, but revenues from their investment are distributed annually. In Texas money from this source provided a substantial portion of the total cost of public education.

States use various methods for determining the basis for apportioning funds to the local school districts; they include average daily attendance, aggregate days of attendance, school enrollment, the school census, and the method that many considered to be the best—the number-of-weighted-pupils concept, which is commonly known as the foundation program. This program provides for state and local sharing of the cost of education in local school districts.

Attempts to equalize educational opportunities in states for all students by means of the foundation programs of financing education evolved over a period of years in this century through the work originally of Edward P. Cubberly and then Harlan Updegraff, George D. Strayer, Robert M. Haig, and Paul R. Mort. Their ideas resulted in the Strayer-Haig-Mort, or Foundation Program, Model. This formula involves the following steps:

1. Compute the ability of each school district to pay for its own program.
2. Deduct from the cost of that program the amount that will be available in the district from a required levy on the equalized valuation.
3. Make the difference available to the district from state funds.[1]

According to Johns and Morphet, adaptations of this formula currently are used to apportion more than 60 percent of all state funds that are apportioned to local boards for the financing of schools.[2]

The foundation program of financing public education requires that local school districts provide their share of the fund to finance public education programs. In most cases state funds provide a minimum program which can be enriched by local monies. Authorities on the foundation concept of financing public education maintain that the input of local funds into the financing of public education increases local interest. The principal problem with local funds for public schools is the great inequities in the tax base in local school districts. The primary source of local financial support for schools comes from property (advalorem) taxes. Local governments have equalization boards that assess property taxes. The authority to assess property taxes at the local level is derived from the state government. Some states establish limitations on local school property taxes.

According to Johns and Morphet, there has been no trend in recent years to increase the severity of property tax limitations. A few states even have relaxed them somewhat. Tax limitations range from less than five mills (a mill is a unit of monetary value equal to 1/1000 of a dollar) on the true value of property to no limit to the taxes that may be voted (e.g., in California, Connecticut, Maryland, Massachusetts, New Hampshire, New Jersey, Tennessee, and Vermont). (However, there are limits to the taxes that may be levied in these states without a vote of the people.) [3]

Capital improvements are usually financed by bond issues which must be approved by a vote of the citizens. Most states authorize

---

[1] Roe L. Johns and Edgar L. Morphet, *The Economics and Financing of Education*, 2d ed. (Englewood Cliffs, N.J.: Prentice-Hall, 1969), p. 249.

[2] *Ibid.*

[3] *Ibid.*, p. 214.

boards of education to issue bonds. Bond payments are usually spread out over a 20- to 25-year period. Most states place a limit on bonded indebtedness; however, the usual practice is to make that limit high enough to permit the school districts to meet their school building needs.

Following are excerpts from the state of Texas School Foundation Program, a typical state program for financing public school education in the United States:

> STATE POLICY. It is the policy of the State of Texas that the provision of public education is a state responsibility and that a thorough and efficient system be provided and substantially financed through state revenue sources so that each child shall have the opportunity to develop to his/her full potential. It is further the policy of this state that the value assigned to each school district for the purpose of determining the district's local share of its guaranteed entitlement under the Foundation School Program shall be equitably determined notwithstanding the various types of wealth within each district so that no class of property is unfairly treated.
>
> OPERATION OF SCHOOLS. (a) Each school district must provide for not less than 175 days of instruction for students and not less than 10 days of inservice training and preparation for teachers for the 1977–1978 school year and not less than 175 days of instruction for students and not less than 8 days of inservice training and preparation for teachers for each school year thereafter.
>
> COMPENSATION OF PROFESSIONAL AND PARAPROFESSIONAL PERSONNEL. (a) A school district must pay each employee who is qualified for an employed position classified under the Texas Public Education Compensation Plan set forth in Section 16.056 of this chapter not less than the minimum monthly base salary, plus increments for teaching experience, specified for the position.
>
> (b) Salaries shall be paid on the basis of a minimum of 10 months' service, which must include the number of days of instruction for students and days of inservice training and preparation for personnel required by Section 16.052 of this code. The days of inservice training and prepartion required herein shall be conducted by local boards of education under rules and regulations established by the State Board of Education that are consistent with the state accreditation standards for program planning, preparation, and improvement.
>
> EDUCATION PROGRAM PERSONNEL. (a) Education program personnel units shall be allotted to each school district on the basis of the district's current average daily attendance for the best five six-week reporting periods of the school term.
>
> (b) Each school district shall be allotted personnel units on the basis of the district's average daily attendance in education programs as follows:

(1) one personnel unit for each 18.5 students in average daily attendance in kindergarten and grades 1 through 3;

(2) one personnel unit for each 21 students in average daily attendance in grades 4 through 6;

(3) one personnel unit for each 20 students in average daily attendance in grades 7 through 9; and

(4) one personnel unit for each 18 students in average daily attendance in grades 10 through 12.

A school district may use its personnel units for any combination of personnel classified under the Texas Public Education Compensation Plan which the district feels will best meet the needs of the students in the district, provided that the total of the number of personnel units for each position chosen multiplied by the personnel unit value for that position specified on the salary schedule, does not exceed the total number of personnel units to which the district is entitled under the provisions of this section. The commissioner, with the approval of the State Board of Education, shall establish minimum standards for staffing patterns for all personnel.

A district need not employ personnel for the full number of personnel units to which it is entitled.

Section 16.104, Texas Educational Code, as amended, is amended to read as follows:

COMPREHENSIVE SPECIAL EDUCATION PROGRAM FOR HANDICAPPED CHILDREN. The commissioner of education, with the approval of the State Board of Education, shall develop, and modify as necessary, a statewide design for the delivery of services to handicapped children in Texas which includes rules for the administration and funding of the special education program so that an appropriate public education is available to all handicapped children between the ages of 3 and 21 by no later than September 1, 1980. The statewide design shall include, but may not be limited to, the provision of services primarily through local school districts and special education cooperatives, supplemented by a regional delivery structure and special allotments for districts impacted by residential or hospital placements.

Section 16.151. OPERATING COST ALLOTMENT. Each school district shall be allotted $110 for each student in average daily attendance during the 1977–1978 school year and $115 for each student in average daily attendance each school year thereafter.

Section 9. Subsections (c), (g), (h), and (i) of Section 16.206, Texas Education Code, as amended, are amended to read as follows:

(c) For the 1977–1978 school year, allowable total base costs of maintenance, operation, salaries, depreciation, etc., for each bus shall be:

72 capacity bus	$5,701 per year
60–71 capacity bus	5,492 per year
49–59 capacity bus	5,283 per year
42–48 capacity bus	5,074 per year
30–41 capacity bus	4,866 per year
20–29 capacity bus	4,657 per year
15–19 capacity bus	3,821 per year
1–14 capacity bus	161 per pupil per year.

Section 16.252. LOCAL SHARE OF PROGRAM COST. (a) For the 1977–1978 school year and each year thereafter, each school district's share of its guaranteed entitlement under the Foundation School Program shall be an amount equal to the product of an index rate of .0018 multiplied by the full market value of property in the district or the product of an index rate of .00205 multiplied by the index value of property determined pursuant to Section 11.86 of this code, whichever amount is smaller.

Section 16.303. REQUIRED LOCAL EFFORT. In order to receive equalization aid, the district must raise its local fund assignment.

Section 16. Chapter 11, Texas Education Code, as amended, is amended by adding Subchapter F to read as follows:

SUBCHAPTER F. SCHOOL DISTRICT TAX ASSESSMENT PRACTICES BOARD.

Section 11.71. PURPOSE. It is the policy of this state to ensure equity among taxpayers in the burden of school district taxes and among school districts in the payment of state financial aid to schools. The purpose of this subchapter is to promote that equity by providing for uniformity in the tax appraisal and assessment practices and procedures of school district tax offices, for improvement in the administration and operation of school district tax offices, and for greater competence among persons appraising and assessing school districts' taxes.

Section 11.72. SCHOOL TAX ASSESSMENT PRACTICES BOARD. (a) The school tax assessment practices board is established. The board consists of six members appointed by the governor with the advice and consent of the senate. A vacancy on the board is filled in the same manner for the unexpired portion of the term.

Section 11.82. REPORTS OF SCHOOL DISTRICT VALUES. (a) Each office assessing property for school district taxes shall file an annual report listing the total market value and the total assessed value of taxable property in the district and other information required by the board.

(b) The report shall be on a form prescribed by the board and shall be delivered to the board before a date prescribed by the board.

As integral parts of the total education programs of the schools, physical education and athletic programs are also plagued with financial difficulties. Physical education and intramural programs are generally financed by tax money in the same fashion as English, mathematics, science, or any other area of the curriculum. However, this is usually not true of interscholastic athletic programs. While some local school districts have a policy of supplementing gate receipts with tax money to finance the interscholastic athletic program, most school districts in the United States must still depend solely on income from interscholastic contests to meet expenses. It is hoped that in the future more states will follow the lead of the state of New York in legally recognizing that athletics are a part of physical education, thus permitting local school districts to use tax money for the support of interscholastic athletic programs. All teachers should have a knowledge of the financial and budgeting system in public schools, since they must function within its framework.

Since funds for physical education and interscholastic athletics are usually limited, it is incumbent upon physical education and athletic directors to make wise use of available funds in order that students may receive the maximum benefit possible from these educational programs. Professional preparation programs in physical education should provide future teachers and coaches with knowledge in sound business practices. Many graduates from these programs will eventually become directors of physical education and athletics, and they should know the techniques of bookkeeping, of accounting procedures, of preparing budgets, and of making financial transactions. At least one institution is offering graduate work in sports administration and an integral part of this curriculum is devoted to teaching students how to handle the financial aspects of athletic programs.

The remainder of this chapter deals with three major topics: (1) the budget process, (2) financial management of physical education, and (3) financial management of athletics.

THE BUDGET PROCESS

The budget is basic to financial management in any field of endeavor. A budget is a written estimate of anticipated income and expenditures. Budgets are prepared for a year in advance and for educational institutions the fiscal year is the unit of time from the first day of July to the following June 30th. Since most public schools in the United States operate on a September-to-June calendar, the fiscal year plan enables the administrative officers of the school to be aware of the funds available to operate their programs. For public schools, budgets are usually prepared in March and April, well ahead of the beginning of the fiscal year. The budget should be a carefully prepared document based on all financial information available and on the needs of the school program. Once the budget is prepared and approved, it serves as a guide for the spending of funds. The budget provides the administrator with the means of avoiding deficits and of making an equitable distribution of the funds available for the instructional program.

In beginning the preparation of a budget, the administrator must first collect information. The best guide is the budgets prepared in previous years. These budgets are a source of information pertaining to income and expenditures over a period of several years. They also indicate the accuracy of past financial planning and serve as a guide in the planning of the next year's budget. If the person responsible for preparing the budget is in a new school with no previous budgets available, he or she should consult personnel in schools of comparable size in comparable communities about their budget preparation. Also, he or she might contact other school administrators who have reputations for being knowledgeable in budget preparation. A budget planner who is in a large city school system might solicit aid from personnel in the central business office or from administrators in another school in the system.

In addition to using previous budgets as a guide, the administrator should be aware of the department's needs—for example, whether additional personnel are needed, whether new activities are to be offered in the curriculum, and whether new facilities, supplies, and equipment are necessary. The superintendent of schools can provide information regarding the total school district's financial picture while the school principal can inform the department head of the overall financial situation in the school. All of this information should be valuable to the director of physical education and athletics in budget preparation. With this background information, the budget maker can devote attention to the specific items of income and expense for the coming year.

After all staff members have been consulted regarding their special needs and all necessary information assembled, the information must be classified. There should be separate physical education and athletic budgets. Since the only source of physical education funds is the board of education's allocation, there is only one figure on the income side of the physical education budget. Physical education expenditures may be classified under the following headings: equipment, supplies, maintenance, repairs, and major permanent improvements. To ensure flexibility, the department head should have discretionary funds available to take care of items not covered. Another means of classification of expenditures for the physical education budget is by major program areas: boys' physical education, girls' physical education, intramurals, and recreation programs. Included under each of these major program areas are such subheadings as equipment, supplies, maintenance, repairs, and major permanent improvements.

Income for the athletic program comes from a variety of sources, and there are a myriad of expense items. There should be two major headings in the athletic budget: income and expenses. Under income, each specific sport in the program should be listed and the anticipated income for that sport posted. Under expenses, each specific sport should be listed together with the anticipated expenditures. (See the example given in Fig. 1.)

Varsity Athletics
Korb Senior High School

Sport	Expenses	Income
Football	$6000.00	$8500.00
Basketball	2797.00	3000.00
Baseball	400.00	—
Golf	200.00	—
Tennis	150.00	—
Track	100.00	—
Training room	500.00	—
Miscellaneous	200.00	—
Total	$10,347.00	$11,500.00

Fig. 1 Composite varsity athletic budget.

The second step in the budgeting procedure is to itemize the anticipated expenditures within the budget separately for each sport. An example drawn from the preceding illustration using the sport of basketball is shown in Fig. 2.

The third step in the budgetary procedure is to establish a control card for each sport on which each expenditure is recorded at the time the bill is paid. Either the purchase order number (P.O.

Korb Senior High School

Sport: Basketball		Year
Item	Anticipated expenditures	Actual expenditures
Officials	$ 362.00	
Transportation	390.00	
Uniforms	500.00	
Physical exam	50.00	
Awards	200.00	
Motion pictures	250.00	
Scorers	45.00	
Auxiliary police	150.00	
Balls	150.00	
Cleaning (uniforms)	150.00	
Scouting	100.00	
Printing (programs)	150.00	
Medical	50.00	
Meals	150.00	
Clinics	100.00	
Totals	$2797.00	

Fig. 2 Itemized expenditures in a single sport within the budget.

No.) or the voucher number (V. No.) should be recorded, as shown in Fig. 3. The balance for each sport is readily available. Ready reference may be made to the anticipated expenditures, which were discussed above. Further reference to vouchers and purchase orders is made in Chapter 11.

After the budget has been completed by the director on the forms provided by the local school district, it is presented to the school principal to be included with the budgets prepared by heads of the other departments in the school. The athletic budget may be routed to the business manager for athletics and/or the athletic council for approval prior to presentation to the principal. The principal then presents the school's budget to the superintendent of schools. The superintendent of schools then considers the budgets for all schools in the school district, makes any necessary revisions, and presents the school district budget to the board of education for final approval. Revisions may be made by the board of education. Once the budget is finally approved and funds allocated, the monies may be spent after the fiscal year begins.

Varsity Athletics

Sport Basketball

Account No. 126 Sheet No. 1

Amount Budgeted $3000.00

Date	P.O. No. or V. No.	Vendor	Credit or debit	Balance $3000.00
Dec. 1, 1974	1278	National Sporting	$450.00	$2550.00
Dec. 7, 1974	1279	Dr. R. A. Jones (exam)	50.00	2500.00
Dec. 11, 1974	1280	Upstate Sporting Goods	135.00	2365.00
Dec. 16, 1974	1282	Universal Printing	146.68	2218.32
Jan. 3, 1975	1281	County Officials Association	96.00	2122.32

Fig. 3 Example of control sheet for individual sports within the budget.

It is the obligation of the person or persons responsible for administering the physical education and athletic budgets to be prudent in the spending of the allocated funds. While the budget is only an estimate of income and expense, it is expected that the departments will not spend more than the sums allotted. It should be noted that emergency circumstances may make it necessary to obtain additional funds in some area. There should be some flexibility in the budget so that money can be transferred from one area of the budget to another. Also, there should be a contingency or sinking fund available for emergencies.

Complete records of all income and expenditures must be kept by the director of physical education and the director of athletics. The director of athletics must account for every penny of income. A journal record of all income and expenditures must be kept. Each expenditure is itemized under the appropriate subheading. This tells the budget administrator what the money has been spent for, the cost of the item, and the amount of money remaining in that account. In the larger school systems the central accounting office will provide the individual schools in the district with a monthly balance sheet for each department in the school. This is an additional aid to the director in administering his budget.

PPBS: Planning, Programming, Budgeting Systems

The process described in the previous paragraphs is the traditional line-item budget system in use for decades. However in 1961 the Rand Corporation developed a conceptual approach to budget decision-making and installed it in the Department of Defense. In the following years, business and government agencies adopted it readily because it seemed to be an efficient system. In the first decade after its inception education utilized it only to a minimum degree. Now, however, schools in the public sector of education, especially higher education, are being forced to adopt the system while those in the private sector are adopting it as an improvement in the budgeting process.

What is PPBS? It is a budgeting system which adds the elements of planning and programming into the budget picture in order to help the budget decision-maker. It provides types of information not available under other budgeting and planning systems now in use. It is different from the traditional approach which may be influenced by the salesmanship of the proposer of the budget. However the former method will continue to be used as part of the process in state-supported schools since legislatures allocate monies on the basis of expenditures rather than on objectives. Even here such agencies as boards of regents are basing some judgments on programs and attainment of objectives through such measurements as student credit-hours or degrees.

The steps in PPBS involve planning as its first stage. Both institutional and departmental objectives and goals are planned and developed. These are stated in attainable standards and differ from the theoretical or ideal aims the organization strives to attain. The second step is to identify the programs through which these objectives or goals will be reached. The programs may be divided into sub-programs (athletics to specific sports). At this point the input (revenue: gate receipts, concessions) and output (expense: meals, travel, etc.) become very specific. A further step may be to integrate the entire program. Each unit then submits a proposed budget that includes both direct and overhead cost together with its income derived from all sources such as state subsidy, fees, grants, etc.

Physical education and athletics share the same problem common to most of education—it is difficult to identify the outputs (products) of the system. The graduate is a product of a number of departments rather than one. The quality of the graduate is extremely difficult to ascertain. Then, too, research and public service are difficult to measure. Physical education and athletics do not have tangible products as their only output since many "products" cannot be precisely or immediately measured. Many of our so-called "values" are in this category. Be that as it may, the trend in the future will be toward this style of budgeting. PPBS encourages measurable data but when such data are not possible it encourages an identification and explanation of what is not measurable. It is designed to develop and present information in the best possible manner in order to aid management (higher administration) in making the best possible allocation of limited resources for which many units are competing. When projected revenue does not equal the expected expenditures, the higher support levels must be justified. For instance, major pieces of equipment may break down unexpectedly or some high priority class such as those adopted for handicapped subjects may be justified, even those that have small enrollments.

Finally, the traditional method of budgeting will continue to be used as a base for departmental operations. Yet within the next decade both athletics and physical education will be called upon to justify requests for the competing dollar through a system of planning, programming, and budgeting. Although PPBS is not computer based (it can be used with or without computers), the larger institutions will use computers to give decision-makers information more readily. The administrator should become familar with the literature on this subject. The articles by Avedisian, Farmer, and Crumrine and Frazier found in the selected bibliography are well worth perusing.

FINANCIAL MANAGEMENT OF PHYSICAL EDUCATION

The only physical education income in most public school systems is derived from tax monies that are allocated by the board of education. The principal of the school allocates a sum of money for the physical education program in the same manner that funds are allocated for any other instructional program in the school. Since there is no problem of estimating income, and since there can be no transfer of funds between them, physical education and athletic budgets should be prepared separately.

Physical education program expense items are varied, but can be categorized under equipment, supplies, maintenance, repairs, and major permanent improvements. *Equipment* includes items of a semipermanent nature: parallel bars, hurdles, volleyball standards. *Supplies* are expendable equipment: baseball bats, field-hockey sticks, table-tennis balls, and handballs. Under *maintenance* would be put expenses for the maintenance of the swimming pool, tennis court, the football and soccer fields, and of refinishing the gymnasium floors. *Repairs* include such items as repairing stadium bleachers, tennis nets, and basketball backboards. *Major permanent improvements* are the addition of such things as a quarter-mile track, a swimming pool, or a wrestling facility.

Expendable supply needs are determined by inventory. Some items will be worn out and beyond use; other items may be retained for further use. Supplies to be purchased are the difference between usable items and the needs of the program the next year.

The physical education director should maintain a current list of new equipment needed and equipment to be repaired. Repairs should be included in the budget and made as soon as possible.

Major permanent improvements that the physical education director and the staff think are necessary must be approved by the school principal. Such improvements usually involve large sums of money and the director will have to justify the need. This should be done in writing and in detail. It may take considerable time to obtain the permanent improvements desired.

It should be noted that teachers' salaries are a part of the total school budget and are not of concern in financial management of the physical education department.

FINANCIAL MANAGEMENT OF INTERSCHOLASTIC ATHLETICS

The financial management of interscholastic athletic programs is a complex process. Many school personnel are involved; however, the overall administration of interscholastic athletic finances should be centered in one individual. There are many methods of handling athletic finances, and no one method is best, but sound guidelines are available regardless of the size of the school and the program.

Source of income. Interscholastic athletic income is derived from several sources including funds from the board of education, gate receipts from athletic contests, income from state tournament competitions, sale of season tickets to students and general public, guarantees for away games, gifts, radio and television rights, and concessions. The booklet "Successful Financial Plans for School

Athletic Departments"[4] offers many ideas for raising money for interscholastic athletic programs. Some of the more popular ventures include ads in sports programs, school carnivals, queen contests, having civic groups sponsor contests, Christmas tree sales, basketball free-throw contests, after-game dances, selling student directories, a class fund-raising plan, gymnastic shows, noon-hour movies, auctions, a school candy sale, a variety of basketball games, and selling birthday calendars, and league schedule booklets. Raising funds for interscholastic athletic programs by means of fund-raising activities is questioned by many educators; however, if boards of education cannot or will not provide the funds for the interscholastic athletic program, if the program is felt to be an important school and community activity, and if sufficient funds cannot be obtained by the usual means, then the persons responsible for the interscholastic athletic program have little choice but to engage in fund-raising activities.

Guarantees are another form of interscholastic athletic income. A guarantee is a sum of money received for participation in an away game. It may be a percentage of the gate receipts or a specific sum. When schools are traditional rivals, or members of a conference playing at home on alternate years, guarantees may be omitted. Other conferences specify a flat guarantee to cover expenses of the visiting team. If the game is a nonconference one, without a return agreement, a guarantee is generally given to the visiting school. Guarantees should always be in writing.

Expenses. A variety of expense items are involved in administering an interscholastic athletic program. A typical example is shown in Fig. 3, the budget for basketball. This is not an exclusive list. Other sports will naturally include other items.

Admission prices. When admission prices are charged, the fee for students should be nominal. If gate receipts are the only means of financing the program, adult admission prices should be appreciably higher than student prices. It is not unreasonable to expect the income from adult ticket sales to finance the bulk of the program.

Season tickets. It is a wise plan to offer season athletic tickets to both students and adults. Season tickets ensure reasonable income despite weather conditions and make funds available for

---

4 "Successful Financial Plans for School Athletic Departments." (River Grove, Ill.: Wilson Sporting Goods Company, 1961.)

early season expenses. They also assure the school a guaranteed minimum level of support.

Of the several types of season tickets, the booklet form is probably the most advantageous because, among other things, it reduces the chances of complete loss or theft.

Student activity tickets. The student activity ticket is in reality an extensive application of the athletic season ticket. The activity ticket is designed to supply funds and to admit students to all school activities for which a fee is charged. Activities that a student activity ticket may cover are all home athletic contests, special assemblies, dances, plays, debates, concerts, subscriptions to school papers, school parties, and the school yearbook.

Students may buy an activity ticket in one of two ways: by paying the total purchase price at the start of the school year, or on the installment plan. Issue, payment, and bookkeeping for activity tickets may be handled in the various homerooms.

The student activity plan has the advantage of bringing the finances of all student activities together into a general fund, and guarantees operating expenses for each activity.

The administration of the general fund should be placed in the hands of a committee or board. A student representative from each activity involved should be represented on the board, with a faculty member in charge.

Concessions. Students and adults attending interscholastic athletic contests enjoy refreshments as a part of their entertainment. Providing refreshments through concession stands is one facet of the administration of interscholastic athletic contests. Decisions must be made regarding the school organization that will assume the responsibility for concessions and the disposition of profits.

Some interscholastic athletic departments operate the concessions at games and use the profits to help finance the athletic program. Other school-connected groups which operate concession stands include student clubs, football mothers, athletic boosters club, band mothers, and band boosters. Profits may be used to finance interscholastic athletics, the school band, general school activities, or all of these activities. The major problem with using school or school-related groups is that they may not be knowledgeable in the operations of concessions. Thus the service may not be satisfactory and profits not as great as they might be with a more efficient operation. The major advantage is that all profits remain with the school for school use.

Some large high schools have found it advantageous to place the operation of concessions at interscholastic athletic contests with commercial organizations. Bids can be requested and the organization which makes the best bid in terms of profit to the school awarded the contract. A percentage of net receipts rather than a specific sum arrangement is best for all concerned. When commercial organizations operate concessions, the athletic director is relieved of the problems involved. Also, service is usually better with professional management. Regardless of who operates the concessions, prices should be kept at a reasonable level. Well-operated concession stands can be of benefit to the school in terms of both crowd enjoyment and provision of additional funds for operating the interscholastic athletic program and/or other areas of the school program.

Control of interscholastic athletic funds and the accounting procedure. The success with which an interscholastic athletic budget functions depends to a large extent on careful control and a satisfactory accounting system. The accounting system provides a record of actual income and actual expense. Occasionally a board of education has its accounting division handle all high school activity financial transactions; but usually secondary schools handle their own accounting procedures. High schools establish their own bank accounts and monies are spent only on order of the school principal or other authorized school official.

The secondary school principal, except in the smaller schools, is seldom in charge of the accounting functions, but, however, often has ultimate responsibility for, and control of, interscholastic athletic funds. The administrator should understand that the accounting system serves to restrict the expenditures to income received, that unanticipated tendencies in cost and income will be revealed in time to revise the budget, that it protects the administrator, athletic director, and coach from charges of carelessness and misuse of funds, and that much information for drafting the athletic budget is secured from the accounting system.

The accounting system varies from school to school according to size and school organization. Some schools have a faculty member in charge of finances and accounting for all student activities while others have a separate faculty treasurer for athletic and nonathletic activities. The person in charge should be bonded. Whatever method is used, the accounting procedure is similar.

Game reports. Many high school athletic directors prepare an after-home-game report providing all pertinent information about the contest (score, attendance, weather, etc.). A special form should be prepared. A financial report should be included with information on all income (ticket sales by category) and all expenses (officials, ushers, police, ticket sellers). Game reports should be filed for future reference.

Expense reports. There are two kinds of expense reports: team and personal. Away-from-home athletic contests involve various kinds of expenses such as transportation, meals, lodging, and tips. A special form should be prepared on which all expenses can be recorded. This report is valuable to the persons responsible for keeping financial records.

In performing their duties, athletic directors and coaches must travel to clinics, meetings, and to other schools to scout opponents. They should be reimbursed for travel at a specified amount per mile if they use their own automobiles and for meals and lodging. Some schools use a per diem system for reimbursing staff for travel expenses.

The audit. Sound business practice requires an annual audit of interscholastic athletic funds. The audit should be made by an outside auditing firm. The audit protects those responsible for administering athletic funds from any possible suspicion in the misuse of funds.

The annual report. Many school systems prepare an annual athletic financial report. This report is published in local newspapers for community information and knowledge. The schools and the interscholastic athletic program belong to the citizens of the community. They should be kept informed, since this kind of communication builds public trust and confidence in the schools.

FINANCING GIRLS' INTERSCHOLASTIC ATHLETIC PROGRAMS

Although the girls' place in sport is gaining wider recognition, the development of girls' interscholastic athletic programs is sporadic in the United States. Some school systems have done nothing to further the girls' athletic program; other school districts have enlarged all aspects of the program.

Previously, the financing of girls' interscholastic athletics was haphazard at best. If girls' athletics received funds from local school districts at all, they were minimal. In many cases girls had to raise their own funds by bake sales, candle sales, candy sales, car washes, and other promotional activities.

In 1973, *Sports Illustrated* presented a series of articles on women's sports which discussed, among other things, the financial inequity between boys' and girls' interscholastic athletic programs. For example, one high school in Syracuse, N.Y. in 1969 budgeted $90,000 for boys' sports and a mere $200 for girls' sports; when, in 1970, the school board had to reduce the monies spent for athletic programs, all the girls' funds were cut while the boys' fund received $87,000. In Pennsylvania, the Fairfield area school district budgeted $19,980 for the total athletic program in 1972–73; of this amount, $460 was spent on the girls' program. Many inequities exist in the amount paid to women officials and women coaches, and it is not unusual for girls to have to sponsor various money-making projects in order to underwrite their programs.[5]

A 1974 survey of the financing of interscholastic competitive sports for girls in seven of the larger cities in Texas revealed a variety of patterns of support. Support ranged from none in the 1973–74 budget in three school districts to $3,000 per year per high school in one school district for equipment and supplies. Coaches of girls' secondary school track teams received additional salaries of between $400 and $588. The athletic director in one school district stated that he would be going to the Board of Education to request funds for the girls' interscholastic athletics in the 1974–75 budget. Another athletic director indicated that the 1974–75 budget would provide funds for equipment and supplies for the girls' athletic program.[6]

Many school districts in the United States have expanded their girls' interscholastic athletic programs and are providing reasonable financing. One example is the El Paso Independent School District, Texas. High school girls compete in tennis, swimming, track and field, volleyball, basketball, cross country and golf, sponsored by the Texas University Interscholastic League (U.I.L.). They also compete in gymnastics, a sport which is not U.I.L.-sponsored. In addition, the El Paso Independent School District sponsors junior high school, intermediate school, and elementary school interscholastic sports in basketball, track, and volleyball for girls.

---

[5] "Sport Is Unfair to Women," *Sports Illustrated* (May 28, 1973): pp. 90–91.

[6] Corpus Christi Independent School District, Texas, Survey, U.I.L. Competitive Sports for Girls, January, 1974.

There is one budget for interscholastic athletics for the El Paso Independent School District (boys' and girls' interscholastic athletics combined). The income is derived from the school district's general operating budget and gate receipts. This figure includes women coaches' salaries, awards, officials, equipment, insurance, and travel. Figure 4 shows the pay scale for the women physical educators who coach girls' varsity sports at the high school level. For the 1978–79 school year, the salary scale for men and women coaches is the same when the same sport is offered for both boys and girls.

Sport	Varsity coaching salary at the high school level
Volleyball	$ 850
Basketball	1700
Track	1000
Cross Country	600
Golf	700
Gymnastics	700
Swimming	800
Tennis	1500

Fig. 4 Salary scale for women coaching girls' interscholastic sports in the El Paso Independent School District, El Paso, Texas. (Reprinted by permission of the El Paso Independent School District, El Paso, Texas.)

CASE STUDY

The past several years were difficult for Willie Jordon, the department head and athletic director of Wharton High School. All teams had hit a down cycle during this period. Revenue was at an all-time low. Before, the football team had usually shown a profit and helped to finance the nonpaying spring sports. In the past two years the football team, because of poor seasons, had barely broken even at the gate.

Mr. Jordon was concerned about the fact that in several sports the equipment was in poor condition and in some instances was unsafe. A decision had to be reached soon. There seemed to be several alternatives, but none of them was very simple. As he reviewed the matter, he told his staff that either new sources of income had to be found or a curtailment of the program would be mandatory.

1. What issues are revealed in the above case?
2. What solution(s) should be recommended?
3. What principles are found in the above case study?

SELECTED REFERENCES

Avedisian, Charles T. "Planning Programming Budget Systems," *Journal of Health Physical Education Recreation,* **43** (October 1972): 37–39.

———. "PPBS—Its Implications for Physical Education," *Journal of Health Physical Education Recreation,* **43** (October 1972): 111–118.

Breeding, B. "Funding Intercollegiate Sports Programs in the Intermountain Area: Sports Competition for Women in Six States Bordering the Rocky Mountains," *Physical Educator,* **28** (October 1971): 133–134.

Cass, J. "First Things First: Financially Strapped Philadelphia School Board Accepts Donation to Finance Football," *Saturday Review,* **54** (October 16, 1971): 75.

Crumrine, J. P., and D. H. Frazier. "The Application of Program Budgeting in Collegiate Athletics and Recreation: Alternate Program Structures," *Administration Theory and Practice in Athletics and Physical Education.* Chicago: The Athletic Institute, 1973, pp. 17–41.

Daughtrey, Greyson, and John B. Woods. *Physical Education Programs: Organization and Administration.* Philadelphia: W. B. Saunders, 1971.

———. *Physical Education and Intramural Programs: Organization and Administration.* Philadelphia: W. B. Saunders, 1976.

Farmer, James. "Why Planning, Programming, Budgeting Systems?" *Monogram.* Boulder, Colorado: Western Interstate Commission for Higher Education, 1970.

Frost, Reuben B., and Stanley J. Marshall. *Administration of Physical Education and Athletics: Concepts and Practices.* Dubuque, Iowa: W. C. Brown, 1977.

Grebe, K. R., and K. Leslie. "Coaching Salaries: Approaching Equality?" *Physical Educator,* **33** (October 1976): 126–128.

Green, M. "Prestige and Finance," *Physical Educator,* **29** (October 1972): 127–130.

Herman, W. L. "But Where's the Money Coming From?" *Journal of Physical Education and Recreation,* **47** (October 1976): 17.

Johnson, M. L. *Functional Administration in Physical and Health Education.* Boston: Houghton Mifflin, 1977.

Keller, Irvin A., and Charles E. Forsythe. *Administration of High School* Athletics (5th ed.). Englewood Cliffs, N.J.: Prentice-Hall, 1972.

National Association of College Directors of Athletics and Division of Men's Athletics, American Association for Health, Physical Education and Recreation. *Administration of Athletics in Colleges and Universities.* Washington, D.C.: The Association, 1971.

Murphey, E., and M. Vincent. "Status of Funding of Women's Intercollegiate Athletics in AIAW Charter Member Colleges and Universities," *Journal of Health Physical Education Recreation,* **44** (October 1973): 11–12.

Smith, D. "Highlights Film Sells Stadium Seats for Football Season," *College Management,* **6** (November 1971): 22–23.

11

EQUIPMENT AND SUPPLIES

STUDY STIMULATORS

1. How are supplies distinguished from equipment? Why should they be budgeted separately?
2. What are the purposes of requiring bids when the costs are listed above a stated minimum?
3. What considerations should be given to a local dealer?
4. What are the essentials in an equipment room in a secondary school?
5. What principles should be followed when purchasing equipment?
6. What is the case for a school-issued uniform for the physical education program?

Give us the tools, and we will finish the job.

WINSTON CHURCHILL

The administration of physical education and athletic equipment and supplies has always been an important function of directors of physical education and/or athletics. This function has increased in importance with each passing year for the following reasons:

1. Public schools are accepting greater responsibility for providing equipment and supplies for students' participation in physical education and athletics.
2. The variety of physical education and athletic activities has increased.
3. Physical education and athletic equipment and supplies have become more sophisticated and greater selections of all types of equipment and supplies are available.
4. The cost of physical education and athletic equipment and supplies has greatly increased. Therefore, it is the obligation of the person or persons responsible for the purchase of such equipment and supplies to be knowledgeable regarding their purchase, use, accounting, and maintenance in order to obtain the greatest value possible for each dollar spent.

Certain basic factors should be considered in the administration of equipment and supplies. The school administration should appoint a specific person or persons to be responsible for such administration. The purchase of supplies and equipment for physical education and athletics is based on the needs of these programs and more specifically on the activities offered. Sufficient amounts of equipment should be purchased to provide optimum activity for all students. Only quality equipment and supplies should be purchased, since this more nearly ensures greater satisfaction during use as well as greater longevity. Specifications should be established and bids requested for the purchase of major items which involve large sums of money. The safety and protection of participants should always be considered when supplies and equipment are purchased. To facilitate repair and replacement of physical education and athletic uniforms, the color, style, and design should be standardized. In the remainder of this chapter, the administration of equipment and supplies is discussed under two major headings: (1) purchase, and (2) care and maintenance.

THE PURCHASE OF EQUIPMENT AND SUPPLIES

Included among the necessary subjects to be considered under the purchase of equipment and supplies are the purchaser, the inventory, the requisition, the purchase order, the voucher, specifications, bids, and the local dealer.

The purchaser. The position of the person responsible for the purchase of physical education and athletic equipment and supplies varies from school to school. In smaller institutions equipment and supplies are usually purchased by the director of physical education and/or athletics with the approval of the principal and/or superintendent. In larger institutions this function may be performed by a purchasing agent in the central business office or, in the case of athletics, by a faculty athletic manager, subject to the approval by the athletic council or principal. Buying in quantity results in great savings. The director of physical education and/or athletics should be consulted on the purchase of all equipment and supplies if the materials are purchased by another person. Coaches of specific sports know what equipment is necessary for their teams, and their practical experience with athletic goods enables them to make valuable suggestions and recommendations in regard to their purchase.

The inventory. An itemized inventory of the equipment and supplies on hand, together with the condition of each, is essential to intelligent purchasing. Such an inventory should be taken at least once a year, since it is used to determine what items must be purchased for the next year. It is best to inventory the equipment and supplies for each athletic team at the end of the season. By comparing the year's inventory with the previous end-of-the-season inventory plus the record of any equipment and supplies purchased since then, all equipment can be accounted for. This total list reveals what equipment and supplies are available for the next season, what items need to be repaired or replaced, and what new equipment and supplies need to be purchased. The coach of each sport should inventory the equipment for his or her activity, which will provide complete first-hand information. A copy of the physical education inventory should be placed in the hands of the principal. The athletic equipment and supplies inventory should be made available to the faculty manager of athletics as well as the principal. An example of a workable inventory for either physical education or athletic equipment and supplies is shown in Fig. 1. Not only does this reveal the amount and condition of specific equipment and/or supplies, but it also provides a record of what needs to be ordered by a certain target date. The explanation for the difference between the times that basketballs and pinnies are needed is that pinnies are used in most team sports and therefore they are needed when school starts in the fall for a unit in soccer. Items such as this should be assigned to only one activity for inventory purposes.

As indicated above, in large school systems where several schools need the same type of equipment, a great savings occurs through purchasing in large quantities. Usually this function rests with a purchasing agent who has readily available the latest quoted prices on specific items, names and addresses of vendors and the like. The El Paso, Texas, Public School System, which uses a central purchasing system for its eleven senior and eighteen junior high schools, is an example of this (see Fig. 2).

Basing their decision on inventories, the individual school physical education directors and athletic directors, with the principal's approval, request that the administrators in the central office order specific items of needed equipment. Request forms are provided for use by the directors in the individual schools (see Fig. 3).

The requisition. In school systems where all purchases are made through a central purchasing department, requisition forms are used. The director of physical education and/or athletics uses the requisition form to order the items needed and indicates the items needed, the amounts, description of the items, and the costs. The requisition form may need to be sent to the principal for ap-

Blank High School
Department of Physical Education
Inventorier Mary Smith (Instructor)

Activity: Basketball (Girls) Date: 6/12/74

Equipment Record

Date of Inventory	Item	No.	Condition (no. of each)				To be discarded	Lost or unaccounted for	Additional number needed	Date needed
			Unused	Good	Fair	Poor				
6/1/74	Basketballs	11	2	4	2	1	2		5	11/1/74
6/1/74	Glasses guards	6	0	3	1	1		1	3	11/1/74
6/1/74	Pinnies									
	Red	8	0	4	4				4	9/1/74
	Blue	10	2	4	3	2			2	9/1/74
	Green	5			2	2			12	9/1/74
	Officiating	4		4					—	—
6/1/74	Medicine balls									
	18 inch	1		1					—	
	24 inch	1		1					—	

Fig. 1 Sample inventory record.

EL PASO PUBLIC SCHOOLS

Storeroom Requisition—Physical Education Supplies & Equipment

School __________ Code No. __________ Principal __________ Date __________

Issued □ Total Cost Acct. No. 6391 $ __________

Returned For Credit □ Total Cost Acct. No. 6636 $ __________

Stock No.	Item		Quan.	Blank	Stock No.	Item		Quan.	Blank	Stock No.	Item		Quan.	Blank
40000	ARCHERY Arm Guard	ea.			40590	Softball	ea.			41191	Jump Rope, Plastic 7′	ea.		
40010	Arrow	doz.			40600	Soft Softball	ea.			41192	Jump Rope, Plastic 8′	ea.		
40020	Bow	ea.			40650	TENNIS Balls	doz.			41193	Jump Rope, Plastic 9′	ea.		
40030	Bow Strings	ea.			40660	Net Tapes	ea.			41194	Jump Rope, Plastic 16′	ea.		
40040	Quiver, Ground	ea.			40670	Raquet, wooden	ea.			41220	Pinnies, tie waist	ea.		
40050	Shooting Tab	ea.			40671	Raquet, steel	ea.			41230	Quoits	set		
40060	Target	ea.			40720	TABLE TENNIS Balls	doz.			41240	Shuffleboard	set		
40070	Target Face	ea.			40730	Net	ea.			41250	Soccer Ball, leather	ea.		
40080	Target Stand	ea.			40740	Net clamps	set			41255	Soccer Ball, rubber	ea.		
40110	BADMINTON Nets	ea.			40750	Paddles	set			41260	Tetherball & Cord	ea.		
40120	Racquet	ea.			40820	TINIKLING Blocks, 24″	ea.			41300	Utility Ball 5″	ea.		
40130	Shuttlecocks	ea.			40821	Blocks, 60″	ea.			41310	Utility Ball 8″	ea.		
40180	BASKETBALL Junior	ea.			40822	Bamboo Poles	ea.			41320	Weights, 110 lb.	set		
40190	Regular	ea.			40830	TRACK Blank Cartridges, 22	box			41830	Cage Ball, 36″	ea.		
40200	Nets, cord	set			40831	Blank Cartridges, 32	box			41350	Roller Skates, Clamp	pr.		
40210	Nets, steel	set			40840	Discus, Jr.	ea.			41360	Gym Bowl	set		
40220	Scorebook	ea.			40850	Discus, High School	ea.			41370	Paddle Tennis Paddle	ea.		
40270	FOOTBALL Ball, Elementary	ea.			40860	High Jump, Crossbar	ea.			41371	Paddle Tennis Balls	doz.		
40280	Ball, Regular	ea.			40890	Pistol, 22cr	ea.			41380	Miniature Fleece Balls			
40290	Ball, Reg. Int. Game	ea.			40900	Shot, 6 lb.	ea.			41390	Hose for ball inflator	ea.		
40300	Goal line flags	set			40910	Shot, 8 lb.	ea.			41400	Towels 40″ x 20″	doz.		
40305	Flag football belts	ea.			40915	Shot, 12 lb.	ea.			41410	Hula Hoop	ea.		
40310	Tackling Dummy, hand	ea.			40940	Steel Tape, 100′	ea.			41420	Nylon Rope (foot) $^{1}/_{4}$″	ft.		

Code	Item	Unit			Code	Item	Unit			Code	Item	Unit		
	GAMES					VOLLEYBALL								
40360	Checkers	set			41000	Leather Ball	ea.			41421	Nylon Rope (50′ length) 5/8″	ea.		
40370	Chinese Checkers	set			41010	Rubber Ball	ea.			41430	Gold Balls	doz.		
40380	Clue	ea.			41020	Nets	ea.			41440	Golf Balls, Practice	doz.		
40410	Monopoly	ea.			41030	Pole-volley-tetherball	ea.			41441	Whistle	ea.		
						MISCELLANEOUS					P.E. EQUIPMENT			
40420	Scrabble	ea.			41060	Award Certificate	ea.			40760	Table Tennis Table	ea.		
	SOFTBALL													
40470	Bases, canvas	set			41080	Ball Inflator	ea.			40870	Hurdles	ea.		
40480	Bases, rubber	set			41090	Ball Repair Kit	ea.			40880	Jump Standards	ea.		
40490	Bat, 125 B, Boys	ea.			41100	Bat, Plastic	ea.			40891	Pistol, 32 cr.	ea.		
40510	Bat, 54, Girls	ea.			41110	Bean Bag	ea.			40920	Split Timer	ea.		
40520	Bat, 57, Girls	ea.			41119	Beaters, Drum				40930	Starting Blocks	ea.		
40540	Bat, 75 Ft. Elem.	ea.			41130	Croquet	set			41040	Portable Standards	set		
40545	Bat, 125 Y, Boys	ea.			41139	Drum, Dance				41140	Dry Line Marker	ea.		
40550	Catcher's Mitt, Girls	ea.			41150	Field Hockey Kit				41210	Mat Hangers, wall	set		
40551	Catcher's Mitt, Boys	ea.			41160	Fun Ball, Plastic 4″	ea.			41270	Timer Kodak	ea.		
40560	Chest Protector, Girls	ea.			41170	Horseshoes, Rubber	set			41280	Tumbling Mat 5′ x 10′	ea.		
40561	Chest Protector, Boys	ea.			41171	Horseshoes, Steel	set			41450	Parallel Bar Replace	ea.		
40570	Home Plate	ea.			41180	Indian Clubs	pr.			33720	Stop Watch, Junghans	ea.		
40580	Mask	ea.			41190	Jump Rope No. 10 Sash	hk.							

To Be Filled In By
Originator Of Requisition

FUND	FUN.	ACCT/OBJ.	SUB. OBJ.	SCHOOL/ ORIGN.

P.E. SUPPLIES

FUND	FUN.	ACCT/OBJ.	SUB. OBJ.	SCHOOL/ ORIGN.

P.E. EQUIPMENT

DO NOT WRITE BELOW THIS LINE	FOR ACCOUNTING USE ONLY	Requisition approved:
Merchandise Received		
150 bks, in quad.-25. 6-72. Req. 11160		Asst. Supt. or other Authority Nº 2193

Fig. 2 Physical education supplies and equipment form. (Courtesy of El Paso Independent School District, El Paso, Texas.)

BROWARD COUNTY PUBLIC SCHOOLS
Division of Instruction
Department of Secondary Education

School Name__________ Date__________

Principal__________ Athletic Director__________

APPROVED LIST OF BASKETBALL EQUIPMENT

Item No.	Description	Quantity	Last Bid Price	Total
1	*Basketballs – Leather* Spalding 100 – No Other Bids CONFERENCE BALL		16.88	
2	*Basketballs – Rubber* Voit XB-20 Heavy or Equal		7.50	
3	*Training Ball – Leather* Wilson B1284 Training Ball, Heavy or Equal		15.35	
4	*Basketball Nets* Wilson B1950 (120 Thread-Cotton) Rawlings BN120 (120 Thread-Cotton) Spalding 66-101 (120 Thread-Nycott)		1.95	
5	*Rebound Ring* Wilson B9910 Spalding 66131 or Equal		3.45	
10	*Ankle Weights (soft pack)* 3 lb. Voit TA 30 or equal		3.05	
11	*Shoes – Basketball* Pro-Ked High____ U. S. Royal Low____ MK 220 High MK 224 Low Loose lined upper and gum rubber sole or equal		6.60	

Fig. 3 Basket ball equipment, individual school request form. (Courtesy of Broward County, Florida, Public Schools.)

proval, or it may be permissible to send it directly to the purchasing department for approval, rejection, or revision. If the requisition is approved, a purchase order is prepared and the item is purchased. Directors and coaches should anticipate needs well in advance and submit requisitions early in order to give the purchasing department adequate time to complete the transaction. Generally, at least three copies of the requisition are made, one for the originator of the requisition, one for the principal, and one for the purchasing agent. An example of a requisition form is shown in Fig. 4.

BROWARD COUNTY BOARD OF PUBLIC INSTRUCTION (Form No. A6) REQUISITION

SPECIAL APPROVAL (COUNTY LEVEL)

SUPERINTENDENT

ASST. SUPERINTENDENT

(1) SCHOOL/DEPT. ______ NO. ______

(2) DELIVER TO (FULL ADDRESS INC. ZIP CODE) REQ. NO. ______

(3) ATTN. OF ______

REQUESTING PERSON DATE ______

PRINCIPAL OR DEPT. HEAD DATE ______

DIVISION HEAD DATE ______

(4)	(5)
SOURCE OF FUNDS	ACCOUNT NUMBER

(6) IF EQUIPMENT REPLACEMENT –

TD # ______

SEC. RPT. DATE ______

(7) CLASSIFICATION HELPS (INFORMATION REQUIRED ON BOTH LINES)

TYPE OF ITEM (I. E. LIBRARY BOOKS, EQUIPMENT, TEXTBOOKS) ______

AREA OR DEPARTMENT (I. E. GENERAL SCHOOLS USE; SCIENCE; BAND) ______

(8) SPECIAL COMMENTS:

(9) QUANTITY	DESCRIPTION AND SPECIFICATIONS (TYPE DOUBLE SPACE)	UNIT PRICE	ESTIMATED AMOUNT

BASIS FOR UNIT PRICE

RECENT PURCHASE ☐ CATALOGUE ☐ COMMUNICATION ☐ ESTIMATE ☐ TOTAL $

(10) SUGGESTED SUPPLIER:

NAME ______

ADDRESS ______

CITY & STATE ______

FOR COUNTY LEVEL USE ONLY

PURCHASING:
SO. NO.

PO. NO.

BID NO.

ACCOUNTING:

FUND	ACCT. NO.

REQ. NO. ______

SERIAL NO. ______

AMOUNT ______

DATE ENC. ______

COUNTY, FLORIDA, PUBLIC SCHOOLS

Fig. 4 Requisition form. (Courtesy of Broward County, Florida, Public Schools.)

Purchase orders. Purchasing should be handled in a business-like manner. This requires the use of purchase order blanks. Order blanks should be uniform in size, usually $8\frac{1}{2}'' \times 11''$, to permit ease in filing. Such blanks give the physical education and/or athletic director, the purchasing agent, and the administrator a record of all purchases.

Purchasing procedures vary from school to school. If the superintendent or principal does the ordering, purchase orders made out in duplicate in different colors are sufficient. The original copy is sent to the firm with whom the order is placed and the second copy is kept in the administrator's office. In large school systems where a purchasing agent in the central business office is the buyer, the number of copies of the purchase order varies with the needs of the organization; in some cases as many as seven copies are made, each in a different color (the original copy going to the vendor with duplicate copies to the accounting office, purchasing department, receiving department, originator, property control, and a second copy to the purchasing department when the order is completed). This procedure provides a system whereby everyone concerned with the purchase order is informed and accurate records can be kept. One person should be responsible for all purchase orders and all such orders should be numbered consecutively. This makes it possible to account for all orders placed. Fig. 5 shows a sample purchase order form.

The voucher. A voucher is a school system's own form on which it can be billed. The voucher, in duplicate, is sent to the vendor with the purchase order. When the order is received and the voucher returned by the vendor and found to be in order, the bill is paid. One copy of the voucher is filed with the purchase order. This indicates that the bill has been paid. The second copy is returned to the vendor with payment. Uniform vouchers are valuable to purchase departments because of the ease in filing.

Specifications and bids. When purchasing in quantity, specifications for each item to be purchased should be prepared. Thus it is necessary for physical education and athletic directors to be familiar with quality, materials, style, price, reputable companies, and many other details, in order to prepare proper specifications for items to be placed on bids. For some items, specifications may be brief and concise, for others they must be made in detail. If specifications are to be established for a basketball, all that may be needed is the manufacturer's name and catalog number. If it is

BOARD OF PUBLIC INSTRUCTION, BROWARD COUNTY, FLORIDA
1320 S. W. 4th STREET
FORT LAUDERDALE, FLORIDA

PURCHASE ORDER NO. ______

DATE ______

DELIVER TO

BILLING INSTRUCTIONS

CHARGE TO AND SEND INVOICE IN DUPLICATE TO:
BOARD OF PUBLIC INSTRUCTION, BROWARD COUNTY
P. O. BOX 8369
FORT LAUDERDALE, FLORIDA 33310
Above purchase order number must appear on invoice.

THIS PURCHASE EXEMPT FROM FEDERAL EXCISE, STATE SALES, AND TRANSPORTATION TAXES.

NOTE: Please ship all materials prepaid.

	Quantity	DESCRIPTION	Unit Cost	TOTAL

COUNTIES ARE EXEMPT FROM FEDERAL EXCISE TAX, TRANSPORTATION TAX AND STATE SALES TAX. DO NOT INCLUDE THESE TAXES ON YOUR INVOICE. EXEMPTION CERTIFICATE WILL BE SIGNED UPON REQUEST. FLORIDA SALES TAX EXEMPTION CERTIFICATE NO. 03-00004-03-16.

TOTAL	
Discount	
TOTAL	

Bid No.	Fund	Account Number	Req. No.	Serial No.

VENDOR MUST FOLLOW BILLING INSTRUCTIONS, SEE ABOVE

E. A. MOSER, PURCHASING AGENT

VENDOR

BOARD OF PUBLIC INSTRUCTION,
MYRON L. ASHMORE, SUPERINTENDENT

Fig. 5 Purchase order form. (Courtesy of Broward County, Florida, Public Schools.)

a trampoline, more details are needed such as size, cost, material, and construction. Some larger school systems appoint committees of physical educators or athletic coaches to prepare specifications. Obviously, specifications are necessary if the dealer is to bid intelligently on specific equipment and supply items. When specifications are prepared, the term "or equal quality" is usually added in case dealers need to substitute a brand other than the one requested in order to provide supplies and equipment needed by the school system.

Most public school systems have established policies regarding bids. If the items to be purchased are above a certain amount of money, bids must be requested. The figure varies widely. Some school systems require bids on all purchases over $100, while other school systems set the figure at $300, $500 or even $1000. Usually at least three bids are required. Purchasers must advertise for bids and any dealer may bid on the items to be purchased. Time limits for bidding are established and a specific time to open the bids is announced. The dealers who are awarded the bids are notified and it is recommended that unsuccessful bidders also be informed of the results since this is a good public relations gesture. All dealers then know what prices the competition is offering for comparable products. Usually the lowest bid is accepted; however, unusual circumstances may alter this policy. For example, some school systems give preference to local dealers.

The local dealer. Local dealers often expect school authorities to purchase equipment and supplies from them. When the local stores are not able to provide the quality, price, and service that can be secured from outside sources, equipment should be purchased from these outside firms. The school official in charge of purchasing is obligated to get the greatest value possible with the funds available. Preference should be given to local dealers when they offer equal value or when their bid is close to the minimum bid. This practice can be defended on the basis of better service and encouragement of local support of schools.

Other purchasing considerations. Certain other factors should be considered when equipment is to be purchased. A definite time schedule should be established with deadline dates for the purchase of equipment for fall, winter, and spring *athletic* equipment. For example, spring sports equipment and supplies should be purchased by October 15, fall equipment and supplies by February 15, and winter sports equipment by May 15. Also a definite date, for example April 15, should be established for the purchase of *physical education* equipment and supplies for the following school year. Early buying provides the purchaser more time to meet the needs of the program and to study and research items to be purchased so that proper specifications can be determined. It also provides the dealer and the manufacturer more time to fill the order, and gives the purchaser more time to exchange unsatisfactory items.

While the aim of the physical education and/or athletic director is to provide the best equipment and supplies possible, in sufficient quantity to provide the optimum experience for the students, the director must always consider carefully the financial status of the school physical education and athletic program. Physical education programs are usually financed by general school funds and a specific budget is provided. Athletic programs are financed in numerous ways, but in most instances the principal source of revenue is gate receipts. Persons responsible for the financial operation of these programs, particularly the purchase of supplies and equipment, must not spend more than the school can afford to pay. Operating these programs at a financial loss creates serious problems for all concerned and should be avoided if at all possible.

Equipment and supplies should be purchased only from reputable dealers. Most such dealers provide legitimate discounts to public schools when bills are paid within a certain time limit.

One means by which athletic departments can save a considerable amount of money is to standardize athletic uniforms in terms of type, style, and color. This means that fewer replacement uniforms will have to be purchased each year. If type, style, and color are changed every few years, the overall amount spent on uniforms will rise rapidly and unnecessarily.

In schools in which funds for physical education and athletic equipment and supplies are limited, a priority list should be established in terms of value and importance to the program. If the priority list is followed, those areas of the program that have the greatest needs will have those needs met first.

Examples of recommended types and quantities of equipment are found in Tables 1 and 2.

THE CARE AND MAINTENANCE OF EQUIPMENT AND SUPPLIES

All the advantages of careful and intelligent purchasing are of no avail unless equipment and supplies are properly cared for and maintained. Therefore, directors of physical education and/or athletics must give careful consideration to the development of policies

Table 1 Basic Supplies and Equipment Recommended for Elementary Schools* (The quantities listed should be considered the minimum necessary for an adequate instructional program for a class of thirty pupils.)

Supplies	Quantity	Supplemental supplies and equipment	Quantity
Basketballs	5	Bowling pins	1 set
Soccerballs	5	Wands	30
Volleyballs	5	High jump standard	1
Footballs	5	High jump crossbar	1
Playground balls		Softball bases	1 set
Rubber 8 inch	15	Relay batons	4
Rubber 5 inch	15	Drum	1
Softballs	20	Plastic tape (different colors)	1 set
Softball bats	12	Trampoline	1
Tennis balls	40	Bean bags	30
Jump ropes	40	Balance beam	1
Plastic balls and bats	5	Portable standards & nets	4
Tumbling mats	2		
Air pump	1		
Tape line	1		
Stop watch	1		
Record player	1		
Records	—		
Pinnies (four colors)	4 sets		

*Adapted from the *Physical Education Course of Study*, The Protestant School Board of Greater Montreal, Canada, 1966, pp. V1–V2.

and procedures that will ensure maximum use of all equipment and supplies.

The equipment room. The care of equipment depends essentially on some well-organized system of handling it. The first requirement is a room in which equipment is stored and from which it is issued. This should be adjacent to the locker and drying rooms. The room should be large enough to store all physical education and athletic equipment and to allow for possible future expansion. In larger schools there may be two separate rooms for the storing and issuing of equipment, one for physical education and one for athletics, particularly when the two programs are administered separately.

The equipment room must be a secure place, with provisions for locking doors and windows. Proper lighting, heating, and ven-

Table 2 Basic Supplies and Equipment Recommended for Secondary Schools* (The quantities listed should be considered the minimum necessary for an adequate instructional program for a class of 35 students.)

Supplies & equipment	Quantity	Supplies & equipment	Quantity
Footballs	6	Uneven parallel bars	1
Soccerballs	8	Steeltape	
Basketballs	12	50 feet	2
Volleyballs	12	100 feet	2
Badminton rackets	30	High jump standards	1 set
Badminton birds (nylon)	1 gross	Pole vault pole	2
Archery standards and		Pole vault box	1
backstop	2 sets	Pole vault standard	1 set
Archery bows	12	Starting pistols and shells	
Archery arrows	4 doz	.22 caliber	2
Whistles	12	.32 caliber	2
Timer's clocks	2	Field hockey sticks	30
Pinnies (number 1–12)		Field hockey balls	15
Different colors	4 sets	Field hockey goalie pads	2 pairs
Medicine balls		Field hockey shin guards	30 pairs
6 pound	4	Tumbling mats	
9 pound	4	5′ × 10′ × 3″	20
Jump ropes	30	4′ × 16′ × 3″	8
Softballs	4 doz	Mat trucks	2
Softball bats	1 doz	Vaulting box	2
Softball gloves	24	Horizontal bar	1
Softball mask	4	Air pump	1
Chest protectors	2	Record player with	
Softball bases	4 sets	microphone and records	1
Home plates (rubber)	4	Stall bars	6 sets
Discus		Benches (stall bar)	4
men's	2	Standards (for nets)	8
women's	2	Volleyball nets (30 feet)	4
Shotput		Badminton nets	6
8 pound	2	First aid kit	1
12 pound	1	Climbing ropes	4
Discus circle	1	Traveling rings	10
Shotput circle	1	Pommel horse	1
Hurdles	20	Trampoline	2
Stop watches	4	Low parallel bars	1
Relay batons	20	Still rings (pair)	1
Balance beam	1	Swinging rings (pair)	1
Even parallel bars	1		

*Adapted from the *Physical Education Course of Study*, The Protestant School Board of Greater Montreal, Canada, 1966, pp. V7–V9.

tilation are important. The well-organized storeroom must have shelves and bins where material can be kept in an orderly manner. A counter window is necessary for the dispensing and receiving of equipment.

Clean towels, socks, shirts, and other washable articles which are issued frequently should be placed in bins near the issue window. Articles seldom issued and reserve supplies should be kept in more remote parts of the room. Equipment for sports which are not in season may be stored in less accessible areas.

A drying room is an important adjunct to the athletic equipment room. An accessible corner of the locker room or adjacent area can usually be found which will serve this purpose. When wet uniforms are placed in lockers they are likely to mildew and eventually to rot. Dryers are necessary when the school launders its own equipment.

Equipment room management. The physical education and/or athletic director is responsible for the efficient and successful management of the equipment room. But his or her duties and those of the physical education teachers and athletic coaches are so numerous that it is impossible for them to spend a great amount of time on the routine details that accompany management of the equipment room. If possible, full-time adult equipment custodians should be employed. If this is not feasible, students should be appointed to manage the equipment room. These students may be paid, but usually they are designated as student leaders or managers and are given an appropriate recognition for their services. Student leaders and managers must be carefully selected and trained for these positions of responsibility. Their honesty must be above reproach.

Issuing equipment. It is essential from the standpoint of economy and efficient management to account for every piece of equipment issued. An effective method of accounting for clothing and other athletic equipment is to number each item. Two systems of numbering are in general use. The first consists of numbering each article of equipment and then recording that number on an individual equipment record card as it is issued to the athlete. The other method is to assign each player an equipment number and stencil it on each article. The first system requires more bookkeeping but gives a better check on equipment issued.

Clothing which is laundered by the school and exchanged frequently by players, such as towels, quarter-sleeve shirts, socks, and athletic supporters, does not necessarily have to be numbered but should be stenciled with either the name of the school or its initials. Clean garments will be issued only when the players turn in articles with the stamp of the school on it. All equipment should be stamped exactly the same way, in indelible ink.

At the end of the season when equipment is returned, each item can be checked against the players' equipment cards.

Regardless of the system used for issuing equipment, the plan will not succeed unless the players are held responsible for equipment issued to them. The school should be reimbursed for all lost articles.

When equipment or supply items are issued to students in the physical education program, the intramural program, or for recreational play, the student should present proper identification to the equipment room manager. Some item of value may be retained by the equipment room manager to ensure the return of the items issued. Many public secondary schools now issue identification cards to students for a variety of uses in the school. The identification card should be surrendered to the equipment room manager at the time the items are checked out. When the equipment is returned, the identification card is returned to the student.

Cleaning equipment. Keeping garments clean is a cardinal principle in the care of physical education and athletic equipment. Cleaning not only preserves the garments but also protects the wearer's health.

Footballs, basketballs, shoes, and other leather goods should be cleaned frequently with saddle soap, since leather goods are easily damaged by moisture.

Woolen goods should be dry cleaned frequently. Cleaning prevents shrinkage and preserves color. Cotton equipment such as towels, shirts, and socks should be washed after each wearing. Some larger high schools have arrangements with commercial laundries to launder their cottons, but this is an expensive operation. Other schools have their own laundering equipment, in which case cottons can be laundered on the school premises. Managers or paid student help can handle the laundering service.

Storing equipment and supplies. At the end of the season equipment should be cleaned, repaired, and then stored. Following the check-in, the equipment should be carefully inventoried to determine what should be discarded, cleaned, repaired, and laundered. Cottons should be wrapped and stacked on shelves or in bins. Cases or racks should be provided for leather goods. Woolen goods should be stored in bins or trunks. Athletic supplies for each sport should also be stored in a safe place in racks or bins or on shelves for proper protection during that part of the year when the supplies are not in use. The same procedure is suggested for physical education supplies. All supplies should be stored in an orderly fashion for maximum protection.

Repairing equipment and supplies. Most schools make simple repairs to physical education and athletic equipment and supplies. Athletic uniform items that need extensive repairs are sent to reconditioning concerns. Generally speaking, the workmanship of these organizations is satisfactory and the school receives equivalent value for money expended. However, this type of reconditioning and repair work is too expensive for many secondary schools. Much more can be done by the schools themselves in repairing their athletic uniforms. Sewing classes of the home economics department may be used to repair athletic garments. Purchasing a sewing machine that can sew leather as well as textiles also saves the school many dollars.

CASE STUDY

The equipment and supplies budget of Whitehall High School was sufficient to permit the purchase of quality items in every activity. Mr. Jim Petty, the department head, had installed a pre- and postactivity inventory. At the end of the spring activity season he became alarmed at the shortages which were developing in several areas.

Under the present system either the instructor or one of the students would pick up the equipment and supplies for the class and return them at the end of the session. Although the preactivity inventory had shown an ample supply of tennis and golf balls, the postactivity inventory showed that the supply of these items was almost completely depleted. In addition, several golf clubs were missing. Several losses of this nature could cause a crippling situation in the budget of the department.

1. What issues are essential to this case?
2. What solutions or steps should be taken to resolve this dilemma?
3. Are there any budgeting principles involved in this case?

SELECTED REFERENCES

Bucher, Charles A. *Administration of Health and Physical Education Programs, Including Athletics* (5th rev. ed.). St. Louis, Mo.: C. V. Mosby, 1971.

Bylander, R. K. "Kid-Sized Hurdles," *Journal of Physical Education and Recreation,* **47** (May 1976): 46–47.

Collins, Don. "A Workable Athletic Equipment Inventory," *Athletic Journal,* **51** (April 1971): 64.

Corbin, D. E. "Using Tires in the Physical Education Program," *Physical Educator,* **30** (May 1973): 100–101.

Cowart, J. "Ball Retrieval Device for a Sedentary Table Tennis Player," *Journal of Physical Education and Recreation,* **47** (September 1976): 48.

Daughtrey, Greyson, and John B. Woods. *Physical Education Programs: Organization and Administration.* Philadelphia: W. B. Saunders, 1971.

———. *Physical Education and Intramural Programs: Organization and Administration.* Philadelphia: W. B. Saunders, 1976.

Diem, L. "Modern Apparatus for Elementary School Physical Education: Ideas from Germany," *Journal of Health Physical Education Recreation,* **41** (March 1970): 40–42.

Frederick, Bruce A. (ed.). *Two Hundred Twelve Ideas for Making Low-Cost Physical Education Equipment.* Danville, Ill.: School Aid Co., 1972.

Frost, Reuben B., and Stanley J. Marshall. *Administration of Physical Education and Athletics: Concepts and Practices.* Dubuque, Iowa: W. C. Brown, 1977.

Johnson, M. L. *Functional Administration in Physical and Health Education.* Boston: Houghton Mifflin, 1977.

"Quick! Tell Me How to Buy Athletic and Playground Equipment," *American School Board Journal,* **164** (February 1977): 11.

Scott, R. S., and W. B. Meiser. "Portable Climbing Apparatus," *Journal of Health Physical Education Recreation,* **44** (March 1973): 61.

Toman, T. G. "New Equipment Features Horizontal Ropes," *Journal of Health Physical Education Recreation,* **44** (March 1973): 61.

Watkins, S. M. "Apparel Design for Physical Activity," *Journal of Physical Education and Recreation,* **48** (February 1977): 40–41.

12

FACILITIES

STUDY STIMULATORS

1. From a physical educator's point of view, what factors are important in selecting a school site?
2. How is the number of physical education teaching stations determined for a secondary school?
3. What are some of the newer innovations in outdoor play space?
4. What factors should be considered in selecting the location of the locker and shower rooms?
5. What type of locker system is recommended for a large secondary school?
6. What are the advantages and disadvantages of the traditional rectangular pool?
7. What are the advantages and disadvantages of synthetic turf?

Three things are to be looked to in a building: that it stand on the right spot; that it be securely founded; that it be successfully executed.

JOHANN WOLFGANG VON GOETHE

The modern program of physical education, which includes interscholastic athletics, can be properly conducted only if adequate facilities, both indoor and outdoor, are available. While many programs are being carried on without suitable facilities, they are necessarily limited in scope. This chapter is divided into five major sections: (1) planning facilities for physical education, (2) outdoor physical education facilities, (3) indoor physical education facilities for elementary school physical education, (4) indoor facilities for secondary school physical education, and (5) swimming pool construction and administration.

PLANNING FACILITIES FOR PHYSICAL EDUCATION

With the rapid increase in school population that is being experienced in the United States, there is a need for long-range planning of school facilities to meet the educational needs of the students. Since physical education is considered an integral part of the educational program at all levels, the planning of facilities to conduct this program must be considered along with facilities for all other areas of the curriculum.

The acquisition of land and the planning of new school construction is a cooperative effort of many persons in a community.

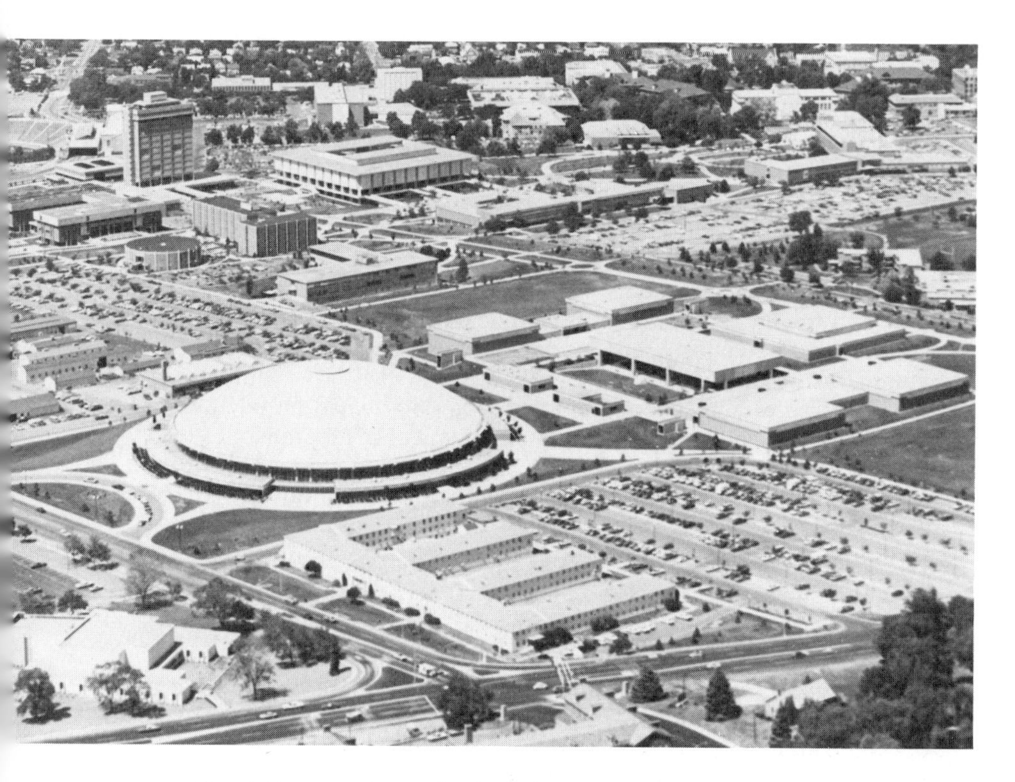

Fig. 1 Health, physical education, recreation, and athletic complex at the University of Utah, Salt Lake City. (Courtesy of the University of Utah.)

Leadership is provided by the board of education and the superintendent of schools. The need for land and a new school or schools for the community must be established first; then approval of a bond issue by vote of the people must be obtained to provide the necessary funds for planning and construction.

Every community sooner or later must face the problem of selecting a site or sites for public school buildings. This is a complex problem, since school location depends on many factors. Some factors which must be taken into consideration in the location of any school building are growth of population, direction of population growth in the community, cleanliness and safety of the environment (distance from traffic, noise, airport, railroad tracks, and industrial developments), adequate land for expansion of the school building and to meet recommended standards for play space, adequate water supply, and provisions for sewage disposal. In addition to the factors mentioned above, the city elementary school buildings should, ideally, be within walking distance of all children who attend the school. Buildings which service consolidated school districts should be within reasonable driving distance of all students' homes.

The *Guide for Planning School Plants* offers the following suggestions regarding the size of school sites:

> Experience has indicated that ultimate site requirements should be met with the initial site acquisition, because land adjacent to a new school soon becomes occupied with housing developments or commercial establishments.
>
> The size of any school site should be determined largely by the nature and scope of the contemplated educational program. . . . While it is recognized that for many schools much larger areas are preferred, the acceptance of the following suggestions will be an improvement:
>
> 1. For elementary schools, it is suggested that there be provided a minimum site of 10 acres plus an additional acre for each 100 pupils of predicted ultimate maximum enrollment. Thus an elementary school of 200 pupils would have a site of 12 acres.
>
> 2. For junior high schools, it is suggested that there be provided a minimum site of 25 acres plus an additional acre for each 100 pupils of predicted ultimate maximum enrollment. Thus a junior high school of 500 pupils would have a site of 30 acres.
>
> 3. For senior high schools, it is suggested that there be provided a minimum site of 35 acres plus an additional acre for each 100 pupils of predicted ultimate maximum enrollment. Thus a senior high school of 1,000 pupils would have a site of 45 acres.
>
> . . . The foregoing rules must be taken as minimums for which all should strive and which most should exceed.[1]

After the site or sites for the construction of a school or schools have been selected, an architect's firm must be employed to develop plans for the new construction. As plans develop, program specialists should provide the architect with necessary information as to the needs of the specific areas of the school. Program specialists include teachers in those subjects which require classrooms with special equipment as well as those teachers of subjects such as science, home economics, art, music, industrial arts, and physical

[1] National Council on School House Construction, *Guide for Planning School Plants* (1958 ed.): pp. 22–25. Reprinted by permission.

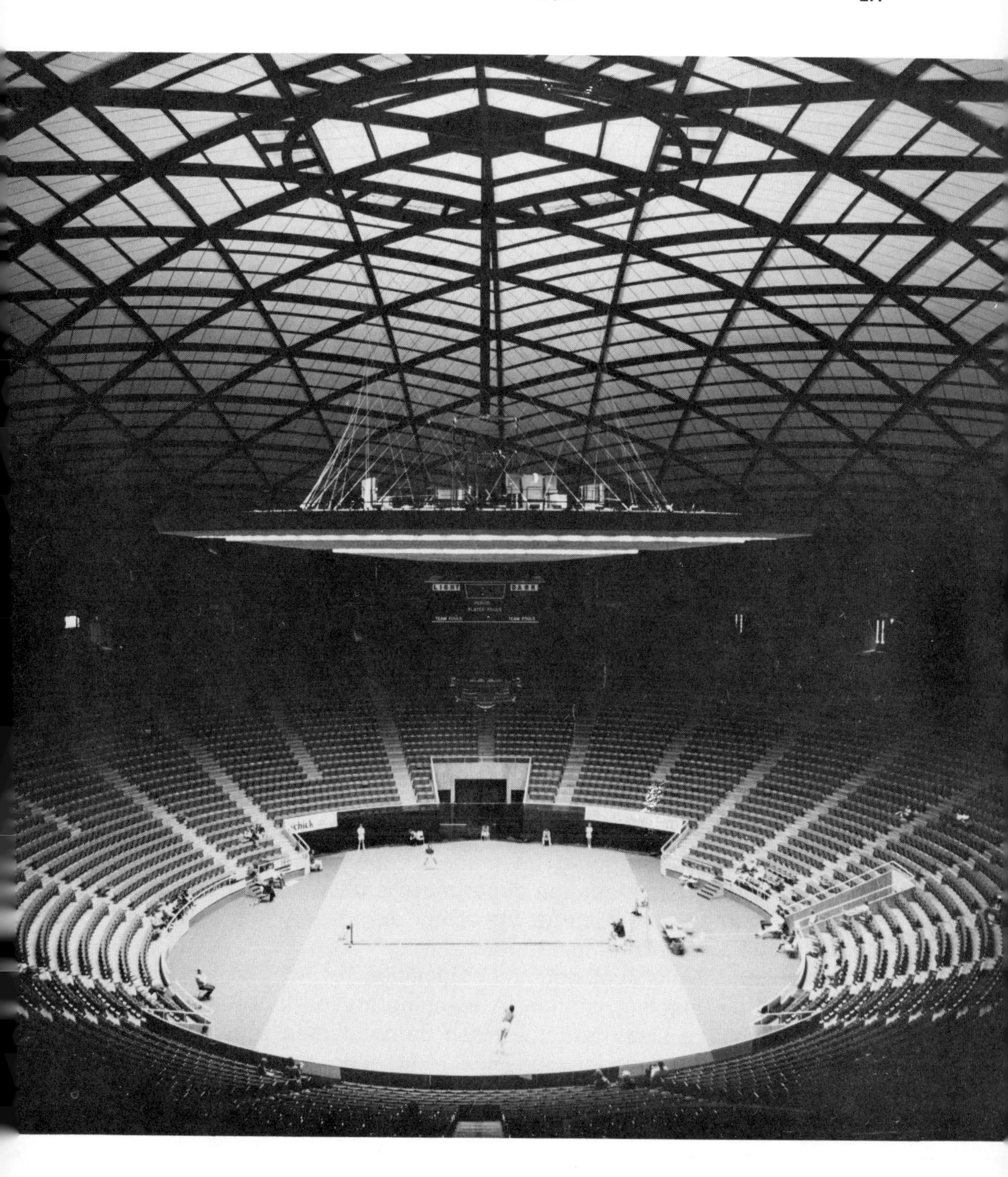

Fig. 2 Special events center at the University of Utah, Salt Lake City. (Courtesy of the University of Utah.)

education, where special facilities are needed. The school librarian, the nurse, and guidance counselors should also be consulted. Architects and program specialists should visit new schools in other communities to observe new facilities and discuss with the proper persons the advantages and disadvantages of specific facilities as they are related to the proposed new school. Scott sets forth the role of the program specialist in physical education in planning new facilities by listing the kinds of questions which that person should be able to answer:

1. For what purpose is the facility to be used?
2. What is the age range and sex of those who will use it?
3. How many will use it and under what conditions?
4. When and how often will it be used?
5. What special features will be required in design and construction to give it the maximum degree of usefulness?
6. What are the program trends and how could the facility be designed to allow for future program changes?
7. Where may the designer procure exact information regarding specifications for such matters as: dimensions of sports arenas, orientation of the facility, rules governing sports, and dimensions of equipment to be used.
8. What are the common errors of design and construction that need to be avoided, and where may examples of these be observed and studied?
9. Where may facilities be observed and studied that are reasonable examples of that which is desired? [2]

Special mention should be made of the fact that while the head of the physical education department is ultimately responsible for the planning of facilities for his or her area, every staff member should share in the planning.

Planning of physical education facilities revolves around the concept of the teaching station. A teaching station is an adequate facility in which a class or activity can be conducted without interference. Since the modern physical education program encompasses such a wide variety of activities, a variety of types of teaching stations are needed, including:

Indoor: gymnasiums, auxiliary gymnasium, gymnastic rooms, dance floor, classrooms, wrestling room, swimming pool, handball courts;

---

[2] Harry A. Scott, *Competitive Sports in Schools and Colleges* (New York: Harper and Bros., 1951): pp. 495–496. Reprinted by permission.

Outdoor: archery range, baseball fields, basketball courts, cross country course, field hockey fields, football field, one-wall handball courts, horseshoe courts, lacrosse fields, soccer fields, softball fields, and tennis courts.

Both indoor and outdoor facilities must be flexible for the department to obtain maximum use. Gymnasiums can be used for a wide variety of activities as can outdoor fields. For example, a football field can also be used for soccer, speedball, field hockey and lacrosse.

The National Facilities Conference Book, *Planning Areas and Facilities for Health, Physical Education, and Recreation gives a* formula for determining the number of teaching stations required to meet the needs of physical education programs at both the secondary and elementary levels, and illustrates this process with an example, as follows:[3]

Secondary

$$\text{Minimum number of teaching stations} = \frac{\text{Number of students}}{\text{Average number of students per instructor}} \times \frac{\text{Number of periods class meets each week}}{\text{Total number of class periods in school week}}$$

If a school with a projected enrollment of 700 students has six class periods a day with an average class size of 30 students, and physical education is required on a daily basis, the formula application is as follows:

$$\text{Minimum number of teaching stations} = \frac{\text{700 students}}{\text{30 per class}} \times \frac{\text{5 periods per week}}{\text{30 periods per week}}$$

$$= \frac{3500}{900} = \text{3.9 or 4 teaching stations}$$

Elementary

$$\text{Minimum number of teaching stations} = \text{Number of classrooms of students} \times \frac{\text{Number of physical education periods per week per class}}{\text{Total periods in school week}}$$

Thus, if an elementary school with six grades has three classes at each level (approximately 450 to 540 pupils) with ten 30-minute physical educa-

[3] *Planning Facilities for Athletics, Physical Education and Recreation* (Chicago: The Athletic Institute, 1974 rev.), pp. 11, 14. Reprinted with permission.

tion periods per day, since physical education is required on a daily basis, the number of teaching station needs can be calculated as follows:

$$\text{Minimum number of teaching stations} = 18 \text{ classroom units} \times \frac{5 \text{ periods per week}}{50 \text{ periods per week}}$$

$$= \frac{90}{50} = 1.8 \text{ or } 2 \text{ teaching stations}$$

Park-School Planning

While most school and park planners plan schools and parks as separate units, there is a trend toward planning the public school and city park as a single unit. This type of plan obviously necessitates close cooperation between the board of education and the city recreation commission. If this type of plan is adopted, it will provide facilities for indoor and outdoor physical education and athletics as well as indoor and outdoor recreation. Complete planning should include both an indoor and an outdoor swimming pool. Figure 3 illustrates this concept.

The park-school plan could be adopted at three levels of schools: elementary, junior high school, and senior high school. Each plan would be different to meet the needs of the students. Park-school planning provides maximum facilities for the most reasonable cost.

OUTDOOR FACILITIES FOR PHYSICAL EDUCATION

It is generally agreed by physical educators that when possible physical education activities should be conducted out-of-doors. The kinds of facilties used vary according to the level of the school. In this section, elementary and secondary school physical education facilities are discussed, together with general features common to both.

Elementary School

Authorities differ in their recommendations regarding the minimum size of elementary school playgrounds. However, the consensus is between five and ten acres, plus one additional acre for each 100 students. If the playground is to serve as both a school physical education facility and a community recreation facility, additional acreage is necessary.

The most important part of any playground should be its turfed area. This is the area where many games of low organization plus

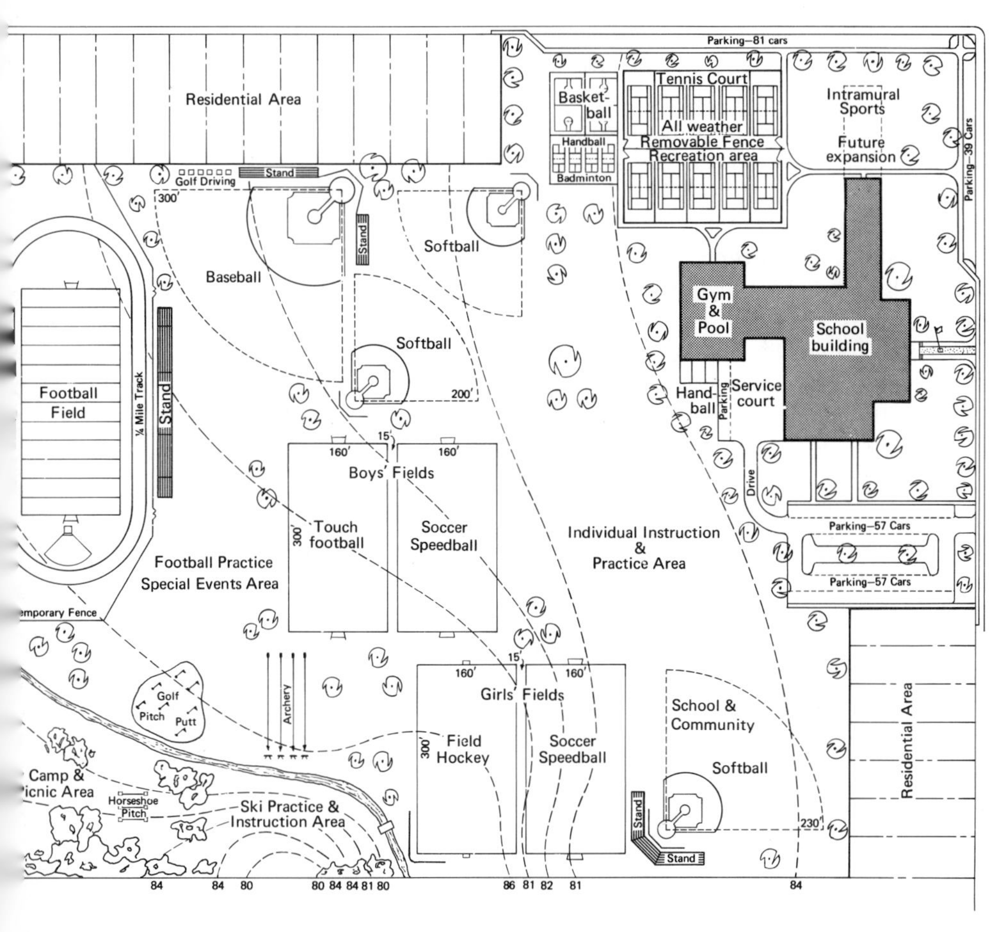

Fig. 3 Community park-school (senior high), one-building type. (Courtesy of the office of A. Carl Stelling, Consulting Landscape Architects and Site Planners.)

team games such as softball, touch football, and soccer are played. The grass should provide good cover and satisfactory wear tolerance. The variety of grass to plant varies with soil conditions and funds available. Also, new and better varieties are constantly being developed, so school authorities must keep informed if the best possible turfed area is to be provided for playgrounds.

Elementary school physical education facilities should include a hard-court area. The hard-court area is used for basketball, volleyball, hopscotch, shuffleboard, roller skating, dancing, games of low organization, and many other activities requiring a smooth surface. Scott states that the hard-court areas should be divided into two sections: one area for children in grades one through three, allowing 25 square feet per child, and a second area for children in grades four through six, allowing 50 square feet per child.[4] Both areas should be adjacent to the school.

The hard-court area should be surrounded by a chain link fence. Court lines using different colored paint for the various courts should be painted on the surface. Large circles should also be marked on the hard surface for group games and games of low organization.

The elementary school play area should also include a separate apparatus area. This area should include swings, seesaws, slides, jungle gyms, horizontal ladders and bars, climbing ropes, climbing mazes, balance beams, sandboxes, and merry-go-rounds. Good quality, rust-resistant apparatus which will give service for many years should be purchased. The apparatus should be located on either one end or one side of the playground relatively near the building. It, too, should be fenced off for safety.

Some elementary schools have supplemented their outdoor physical education facilities by erecting playsheds. These are roofed areas with either no sides or partial sides and with either a hard or grass surface. A playshed provides protection from inclement weather and also provides a shaded area for dance activities. The playshed could also include storage space for equipment and restroom facilities. The size of this facility will depend upon the size of the school and the funds available.

Secondary School

Secondary school outdoor physical education facilities must be planned to provide for the total needs of the program for both physical education and athletics. While in general the junior and senior high school outdoor facilities are similar, there is one basic difference. Junior high schools place less emphasis on facilities for spectators. The modern high school requires, as a minimum, a football stadium and a baseball field with bleachers for spectators. In some areas of the United States, provisions for spectators are also necessary on fields for soccer, lacrosse, and field hockey. In some of the larger cities, for reasons of economy, central football stadiums and baseball facilities have been developed for use by several schools.

As recommended by the National Council on School House

---

[4] Scott, *op. cit.,* p. 356.

Construction, total acreage for junior high schools should be 25 acres plus one additional acre for every 100 pupils of enrollment.

Senior high schools should have 35 acres plus one additional acre for every 100 pupils of estimated ultimate maximum enrollment. If this amount of land is available for the total school, there should be adequate outdoor space for physical education and athletic needs.[5]

Outdoor facilities should be provided for the following secondary school physical education and athletic activities: basketball, volleyball, tennis, field hockey, baseball, archery, softball, football, touch football, track and field, and soccer. Other outdoor activities for which facilities would be desirable include horseshoes, shuffleboard, handball, cross country, speedball, lacrosse, and golf. Recommended dimensions for outdoor game areas are given in Table 1.

General Features for Outdoor Facilities

When planning outdoor physical education and athletic facilities, administrators must consider certain general features. Some of these are drainage, surfacing, fencing, lighting, and orientation.

Drainage. To obtain maximum utilization of all unpaved physical education and athletic areas, adequate drainage (both surface and subsurface) of surface water must be provided. This is a job for the professional. The participants in the National Facilities Conference have the following to say about drainage:

> *Surface drainage.* Surface drainage on unpaved areas should be controlled by slope grading to natural or artificial surface. Water collectors, to carefully located surface inlets, or to catch basins connected to a storm water drainage system. In order to facilitate surface drainage of activity areas, a good general rule is to establish and maintain a minimum slope of one percent in noncompetitive sports areas. As a rule, the surface slope of paved areas should be a minimum of one percent except when used for competition. Exceptions to the above may be necessary. When certain soil and area use conditions exist, the degree of slope may lessen.
>
> *Subsurface drainage.* Subsurface drainage should be effected by using either porous subsoil foundations or perforated drain tile. In regions of severe frost, where surfaces are to be paved, natural or tile subsurface drainage is essential. All drainage tile should be installed after rough grading is completed.[6]

---

[5] National Counoil on Sohool Houco Conctruction, *op. cit.*, pp. 22–23.

[6] The Athletic Institute, *Planning Areas and Facilities for Health, Physical Education, and Recreation* (Chicago: The Athletic Institute. 1965): p. 18. Reprinted by permission.

Table 1 Recommended dimensions for game areas* †

Games	Elementary school	Junior high school	High school/ adults	Area size (including buffer space)
Basketball	40′ × 60′	50′ × 84′	50′ × 84′	7,200 sq ft
Basketball (college)			50′ × 94′	8,000 sq ft
Volleyball	25′ × 50′	25′ × 50′	30′ × 60′	2,800 sq ft
Badminton			20′ × 44′	1,800 sq ft
Paddle tennis			20′ × 44′	1,800 sq ft
Deck tennis			18′ × 40′	1,250 sq ft
Tennis		36′ × 78′	26′ × 78′	6,500 sq ft
Ice hockey			85′ × 200′	17,000 sq ft
Field hockey			180′ × 300′	64,000 sq ft
Horseshoes		10′ × 40′	10′ × 50′	1,000 sq ft
Shuffleboard			6′ × 52′	640 sq ft
Lawn bowling			14′ × 110′	1,800 sq ft
Boccie			15′ × 75′	1,950 sq ft
Tetherball	10′ circle	12′ circle	12′ circle	400 sq ft
Croquet	38′ × 60′	38′ × 60′	38′ × 60′	2,200 sq ft
Roque			30′ × 60′	2,400 sq ft
Handball (single-wall)	18′ × 26′	18′ × 26′	20′ × 40′	1,200 sq ft
Handball (four-wall)			23′ × 46′	1,058 sq ft
Baseball	210′ × 210′	300′ × 300′	400′ × 400′	160,000 sq ft
Archery		50′ × 150′	50′ × 300′	20,000 sq ft
Softball (12" ball)‡	150′ × 150′	200′ × 200′	275′ × 275′	75,000 sq ft
Football			160′ × 360′	80,000 sq ft
Touch football		120′ × 300′	160′ × 360′	80,000 sq ft
6-man football			120′ × 360′	54,000 sq ft
Soccer (men) minimum			165′ × 300′	65,000 sq ft
Soccer (men) maximum			240′ × 360′	105,000 sq ft
Soccer (women)			120′ × 240′	40,000 sq ft

* The Athletic Institute, *Planning Areas and Facilities for Health, Physical Education, and Recreation* (3rd ed.) (Chicago: The Athletic Institute, 1965): p. 18. Reprinted by permission.

† Table covers a single unit; many of above can be combined.

‡ Dimensions vary with size of ball used.

Surfacing. Outdoor physical education and athletic facilities require several kinds of surfaces, including grass, earth, concrete, bituminous, and synthetic. Many of the traditional outdoor activities (football, baseball (earth infield), soccer, lacrosse, golf, cross country, and some track and field events) are played on a grass surface. Turf has the advantage of being nonabrasive, durable, resilient, dustless, and relatively inexpensive to maintain.

The grass should be of a quality to provide good cover and satisfactory wear tolerance. Some of the best grasses are Bermuda, bent, fescue, and bluegrass. The types of grass used for outdoor activities areas depends on the climate of the area. For example, the Florida State Department of Education suggests that the best turf grasses for outdoor physical education activities in Florida are improved Bermuda varieties. Bohia grass is satisfactory but has the limitation of being fairly coarse.[7]

Both elementary and secondary schools are making extensive use of hard-surface areas as a part of outdoor physical education and athletic facilities. Outdoor hard-court surfaces are usually either concrete or bituminous. Concrete surfaces are expensive; however, they are very durable and require practically no maintenance. One major problem with concrete surfaces is its abrasiveness, which can result in injuries for participants.

The bituminous (black top) surface is initially expensive; however, the maintenance cost is low and there is excellent durability. As with the concrete surface, there is the problem of abrasiveness.

On hard surfaces, year-round participation is possible. Hard-court areas can be used for baseball, volleyball, tennis, handball, shuffleboard, roller skating, rhythms, dance, and games of low organization.

Several companies have developed new synthetic playing surfaces for outdoor sport and recreation areas such as basketball courts, tennis courts, running tracks, horseracing tracks, discus circles, long jump approaches, and pole vault runways. These surfaces are made of various materials such as compounded synthetic resin or polyvinyl chloride compound. Characteristics include resiliency, durability, uniformity, longevity, and ease of installation and maintenance.

Synthetic turf materials are rapidly emerging as a new material to replace grass and traditional hard-court surfaces for areas for physical education and sports activities. Many of the synthetics meet the criterion of durability. The synthetic turf substitutes are being used for baseball diamonds, football fields, running tracks, tennis courts, golf tees and putting greens, both indoors and out-of-doors. The synthetic turfs are basically made of nylon and vinyl. Time Magazine reported on synthetic turfs as follows:

---

[7] *Facilities for Physical Education* (Tallahassee, Florida: State Department of Education, 1954): p. 54.

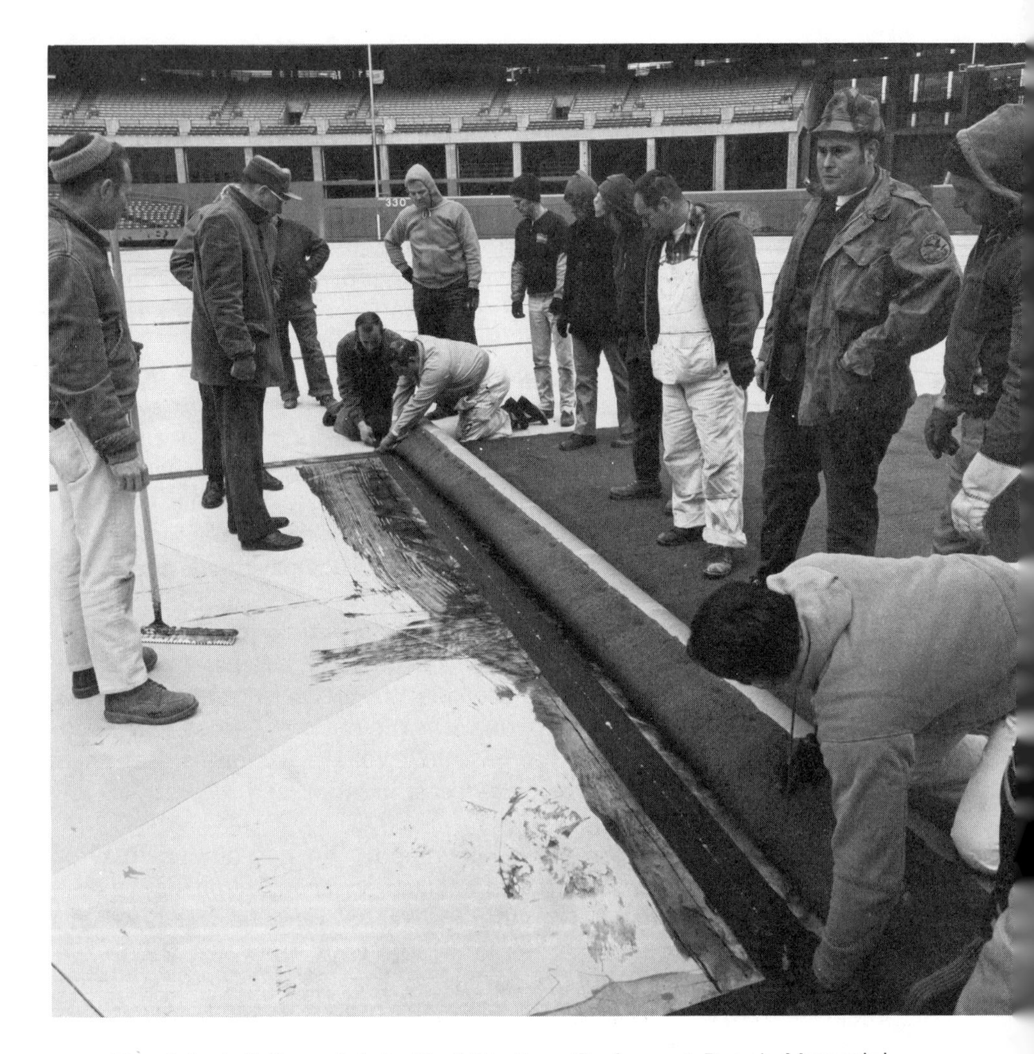

Fig. 4 Installation of AstroTurf Stadium Surface at Busch Memorial Stadium, St. Louis. (Courtesy of Monsanto.)

The newest look in grass is turf that never needs cutting, stays green all year, is maintained with a vacuum cleaner, cleaned by soap and water and dries in a trice. No fewer than 16 manufacturers are now turning out artificial turf—also called indoor-outdoor carpeting—for installation at . . . baseball diamonds, football fields and tennis courts.[8]

Research and development in synthetic turf began in the early 1960s; progress was rapid and by 1964 there were artificial turf

[8] *Time Magazine* (May 12, 1967): 57. Copyright Time Inc. 1967. Reprinted by permission.

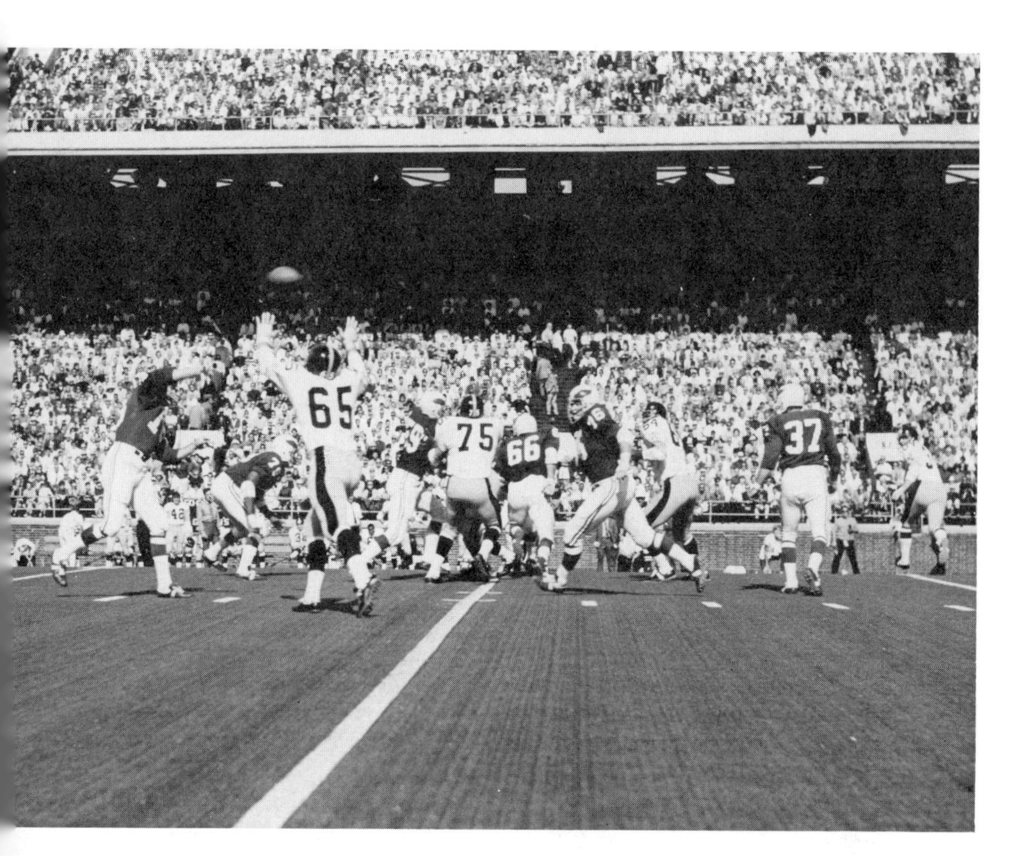

Fig. 5 AstroTurf in action at Busch Memorial Stadium, St. Louis. (Courtesy of Monsanto.)

fields in use in various parts of the United States. In 1966, synthetic turf was installed in the Astrodome in Houston, Texas because natural grass would not grow. The synthetic turf proved to be highly successful for baseball and football games as well as for a variety of other activities. The dramatic success of artificial turf in the Astrodome was the beginning of a new era in surfacing for both field-type sports (football, baseball, soccer, field hockey, lacrosse) and other types of sports, such as tennis and golf.

Installation of synthetic turf has greatly increased in the 1970s (see Figs. 4 and 5), and so has the variety of its use. Artificial turf is now installed for sports and recreational use at numerous colleges and universities, public schools, professional sports facilities, playgrounds, golf courses and motels, apartments, institutions, and homes.

Dick Adams, director of planning and construction at Oregon State University, made the following comments on the definition, component parts, and characteristics of synthetic turf.

> One definition (of synthetic turf), not too technical, might be a "man-made product for stadium use that simulates natural turf in color and playability, primarily for the sport of football, but also suitable for various other recreational uses such as, but not limited to: Soccer, Rugby, Lacrosse, Field Hockey, Baseball, Gymnastics, Wrestling, Physical Exercise, Jogging, Marching Band, Drill Team, miscellaneous physical education classes, and intramural sports." The Synthetic Turf shall consist of:
>
> 1. *Face Material:* A weather- and physical damage-resistant pile that simulates freshly mown natural turf, green pigmented and having a vertical pile height of not less than 1/2 of an inch.
> 2. *Face Material Backing:* Green pigmented, or dyed, to match Face Material.
> 3. *Backing Pad/Pads:* An energy absorbing cushion that shall provide a reasonable water-tight seal immediately beneath the face material backing. This backing pad shall retain its energy absorbing characteristics without damage to the Pad between 0°F. and 130°F. Minimum combined thickness of backing pad/pads shall be 9/16 inch.
> 4. *Adhesives:* As required for proper installation, shall be good for the useful life of the other materials making up the Synthetic Turf and shall provide positive adhesion for intended usage and for temperatures between 0°F. and 130°F. under both wet and dry conditions.
>
> *Characteristics of Synthetic Turf*
>
> 1. Resistant to deterioration and change in color from exposure to sunlight, weather, moisture and temperature range for this region.
> 2. Resists insects, rot, mildew or fungus growth.
> 3. All materials used shall be non-allergenic and non-toxic.
> 4. The face material and face material backing shall be highly abrasion resistant for the athletic uses described above.
> 5. The Synthetic Turf shall be shock resistant to falls and have good energy absorption characteristics.
> 6. The installed Synthetic Turf shall present a uniform playing surface and provide excellent traction under both wet and dry conditions with use of conventional sneaker type shoes, regular composition soled soccer shoes, or interchangeable traction cleats.
> 7. The Synthetic Turf shall drain water off the field reasonably well when installed according to the slopes and crown designed by the Engineer for these stadiums.

8. The Synthetic Turf shall be suitable for both temporary and permanent line markings providing good contrast for optimum visibility.
9. The Synthetic Turf must be composed of materials that can be easily cleaned of common stains and soiling. It shall not be damaged by the use of typical cleaning agents such as detergents or dry cleaning fluid.

From the layman's point of view it offers some tantalizing advantages. It doesn't, repeat, does not require mowing, watering, aerating or fertilizing. You don't have to replace the divots. A striping job may last for several games. And it's clean, man! No mud to mar the beauty of your favorite star in action. It does permit multiple use of the area and many more hours of use per day, thus reducing the number of fields which may be required for a physical education or intercollegiate athletic program. Some interesting surveys also indicate there are probably substantial reductions in knee and ankle injuries where these new turfs are used. And lastly, it appears the absence of mud-spattered gladiators aids the sale of tickets at the turnstiles.

On the other side of the coin, it will require periodic hosing and/or vacuuming. It is expected it may gradually fade or lose its color in part. It may gradually "flake" off due to the sun's rays and lose a part of the body of the fibers. It may cause some burns and abrasions to skin. The ball may bounce a bit funny. Special shoes for some sports are required. It doesn't drain near as well as good old grass, but aside from the hydroplaning effect, which intrigues but disturbs the audience, it provides an equally good footing, wet or dry. It cuts down on the laundry bills. It retains its color through the seasons, albeit it alters slowly through the years."[9]

Even though the cost of synthetic turf is relatively high, it appears that its use will continue to increase. The lifetime of synthetic-turf fields is unknown since most installations are only a few years old. However, available evidence indicates the longevity of synthetic fields should be sufficient to justify the cost.

Fencing. The enclosure of outdoor physical education and sports facilities with fencing enhances the utility of the areas. Appropriate fences aid in instructor supervision, provide protection for the participants, and serve to isolate the facility from spectators. The National Facilities Conference made the following suggestions regarding the fencing of outdoor facilities:

Some characteristics of good fencing are stability, durability, economy of maintenance, attractiveness and effectiveness. Among the many

---

[9] Dick Adams, "Synthetic Turf," adapted from a speech at the Facilities Clinic, New Orleans, Louisiana, conducted by the National Association of College Directors of Athletics, February, 1971. Reprinted by permission.

> types of suitable fencing available, woven-wire fencing of the chain-link type (minimum thickness—11 gauge) using H-type line posts or circular posts, has been found to meet requirements satisfactorily. All chain-link fencing should be installed so that the smooth edges are at the top and the sharp edges are at the bottom. . . . A hard surface strip about 12″ wide may be placed under the fence to facilitate maintenance.[10]

Lighting. Lighting facilities for physical education, recreation, intramural and interscholastic athletic competition areas greatly enhance the use of these facilities. Traditionally, at the secondary school level, the only outdoor facility to be lighted was the football field. As more and more public schools and municipal recreation programs coordinate facilities, many other types of outdoor facilities are lighted for school and community use, including baseball and softball diamonds, tennis courts, swimming pools, handball courts, shuffleboard courts, ice-skating areas, and golf driving ranges.

Proper lighting of facilities for sports and physical education activities can only be accomplished by consultation with experts in this area. Most local electric power companies can provide the necessary technical advice regarding cost, illumination intensity, and even distribution of light over playing surfaces.

According to the participants in the National Facilities Conference of 1965, the most complete source for sports-facility lighting is the Illuminating Engineering Society publication entitled *Current Recommended Practice for Sports Lighting.*[11]

Some errors that are often made in lighting outdoor physical education and sports facilities are poor quality of lighting installations, inadequate foot-candles of light intensity, failure to consult with experts on the technical aspects of lighting, inadequate housing of electrical controls, uneven distribution of light on playing area, inadequate protection of light units by nonbreakable guards, improper type of lighting fixtures, inadequate capacity of wiring systems, lack of automatic circuit breakers, and lack of spare circuits in panel to provide for future expansion.

Orientation. In planning outdoor fields and courts, the relationship of the facility to the sun's rays is a most important consideration. Proper orientation of the field or court is essential for the safety of participants and equitable playing conditions. Ideally,

---

[10] The Athletic Institute, *op. cit.*, p. 77. Reprinted by permission.

[11] *Ibid.*

fields and courts should be located so that the path of the sun is at right angles to the path of the ball. The final orientation of the facility is usually a compromise, with the determining factor being the time of day at which most contests are played. For games played on rectangular fields (football, soccer, lacrosse) the best orientation of the field is on a north-south axis, since the flight of the ball is parallel to the long axis of the field and the sun moves in an east-to-west direction. The north-south axis is also best for tennis, volleyball and track. Orientation of baseball and softball fields creates other problems. The nature of the baseball and softball fields and of the players' movement makes it impossible to prevent the sun's rays from shining in some participants' eyes. Therefore, the orientation must be such as to first protect the most vulnerable players, the batter and the catcher, and then as many other players as possible. Since most public schools have a limited number of diamonds, and since most of the baseball and softball activity is in the afternoon, a reasonable compromise of a southwest to northwest axis (home plate to third base) for the field layout is recommended.

INDOOR FACILITIES FOR PHYSICAL EDUCATION

Elementary School

Planning. The planning, construction, and utilization of the elementary school indoor physical education facilities should be based on goals which recognize that the total physical environment must be safe, attractive, comfortable, clean, practical, and adapted to the needs of the participants. Immediate and long-range planning should involve the efforts of the entire staff of the school. Planning, designing, and construction specialists should be utilized whenever necessary. Planning should always be done with the future in mind.

Choice of facilities. Elementary schools that serve only kindergarten and/or the primary grades (K through four) may find that a multipurpose room is sufficient to meet the needs of their physical education programs. It is recommended that elementary schools that serve grades one through six, grades one through eight, or any grade levels that may be classified as being intermediate, have a gymnasium. In the interest of economy of both finances and space, an elementary school gymnasium may be combined with the school auditorium but if at all possible it should be planned, constructed, and utilized as a separate unit.

Teaching stations. The elementary school gymnasium should provide the number of teaching stations as determined by the formula stated on page 279. This can often be facilitated by the use of a partition to divide the gymnasium.

Gymnasium location. The gymnasium should be located so that it is readily accessible from all other areas of the school plant. If properly planned, the gymnasium will be located in a separate wing of the school plant with access to the outside.

Size of the gymnasium. The recommended minimum overall length of the gymnasium is 86 feet and the minimum overall width is 54 feet. It is also recommended that there be a six-foot-wide safety zone at both ends and both sides of the gymnasium floor. This leaves a playing area that measures 74 feet in length and 42 feet in width. The size of the gymnasium may be modified according to the grade levels served, the anticipated community and spectator use, and/or the financial resources that are available.

Floor construction. The floor should have a concrete base that is covered with a high quality hardwood or linoleum tile. Linoleum tile can produce a floor that is warm, dry, nonglaring, easily cleaned, easily maintained, and nonabrasive. If a wooden floor is selected, hard northern maple is suggested. Wooden flooring should be tongue and groove at least $\frac{25}{32}$ inches thick.

Wall construction. All walls should have smooth nonabrasive surfaces, at least to the height of the doorways, and should be resistant to hard usage. All corners of all walls below this same height should be rounded. All equipment and apparatus that is attached to the walls should be completely recessed into the wall. The upper walls should be of a light color and should be adequately treated to prevent the undue transmission of sounds.

Ceiling construction. The ceiling of the elementary school physical education facility should be light in color, acoustically treated to prevent undue sound transmission, and at least 20 feet above the level of the playing surface.

Lighting. The lighting for the elementary school physical education facility should be provided from both natural and artificial sources. Windows that allow the natural light to enter should be on the east and west sides of the building and at least 12 feet above the playing surface. Directional glass blocks may be utilized. The artificial lighting that is used should be sufficient to maintain a lighting intensity of 20 foot-candles. All lights should be protected by screening, wire cages, and/or plastic shields.

Heating and ventilation. The heating and ventilation systems of the physical education facility should be based on economy of operation and the capacity to provide desirable atmospheric and thermal conditions. The heating and ventilation systems of the school plant will undoubtedly also be used in the physical education facilities.

Entrances and exits. There should be at least one exit that leads from the physical education facility directly to an outside area, and there should be at least one other exit that leads to the main school plant. Local and state fire codes and building regulations determine to some extent the number and location of the exits. It is also recommended that all entrances and exits be at least 40 inches wide and that all doors open outward into recesses.

Seating. No permanent seating should be provided in the physical education facility. If the area is also used as the school auditorium, roll-away bleachers may be provided. These bleachers should telescope to a depth of no more than two feet.

Drinking fountains. One drinking fountain should be installed at each end of the gymnasium, multi-purpose room, or other indoor play area. These fountains should be of vitreous china or stainless steel, and should be recessed in the walls to their full depth.

Electric service. The indoor physical education area should be equipped with a class signal bell, a fire alarm bell, exit illumination signs for all exits, several well-spaced wall outlets, and any other installations that are deemed necessary by school personnel. Included in this latter classification may be provisions for public address systems, intercommunication systems, and electrically powered maintenance equipment.

Storage space. A storage room or other storage space should be provided for all the equipment that is used for the physical education program of the school. This storage space should be directly accessible from the indoor physical education facility, should be adequately heated, lighted, and ventilated, and should be equipped with a doorway that will allow easy passage of the largest piece of apparatus that is to be stored in the room. It is desirable to have direct access to the storage area from the outdoor teaching stations.

Physical education office space. Physical education offices should be provided which are directly adjacent to the indoor physical education area. These offices should have at least 120 square feet of floor space per instructor and should include a toilet, lavatory, shower, ample space for dressing, desk, and storage space for necessary materials.

Dressing and shower rooms. Dressing and showering facilities should be provided by any school that serves any of the intermediate grade levels. Gang showers are recommended for installation in both boys' and girls' shower rooms, but at least one private cubicle should be provided in each area. This satisfies those parents who wish their children to shower in some degree of privacy as well as the occasional student who, at least in the beginning, is self-conscious. There should be eight to twelve square feet of floor space for each five individuals who will be using the facilities. Ample toilets, lavatories, and urinals should also be installed. Mirrors and lockers are also recommended. It is recommended that the above dressing, toilet, and shower facilities be grouped into one large room or area for the boys and one large room or area for the girls.

Secondary School

Planning. The planning of a gymnasium should be a cooperative effort of architects, administrators, boards of education, physical educators, coaches, and lay individuals. It is of utmost importance that the individuals using the facilities be consulted because of their awareness of the special needs in this area.

When planning new facilities, in many schools teachers are encouraged to make written recommendations for their areas of interest, as well as to meet with the architect and make recommendations on the proposed facility. Both of these methods can be utilized to increase staff morale and desirable teacher-administrator relationships.

The lay public can also be included in the planning by holding an "open" meeting and allowing the proposed plans for the facility to be seen. This offers an opportunity for the lay public to propose suggestions, and includes them in the planning procedures—a good public relations gesture.

Financing. The gymnasium will be financed as part of the total school building program. The two most common methods of financing school building programs are by tax levy and by bond issue.

Gymnasium location. Ideally, the gymnasium should be located in a separate wing of the building and serviced by a separate heating unit. The main advantages in locating the gymnasium as described are as follows: (1) to isolate the noise from physical education classes, (2) to eliminate having spectators travel through school corridors to reach the arena, and (3) to reduce or eliminate excessive hallway traffic of students, thereby decreasing the load for the custodial staff.

If there is not a separate heating unit for the gymnasium, the gymnasium should be located near the central heating plant to reduce the cost of heating.

Size of the gymnasium. The official secondary school dimensions for a basketball court and the recommended dimensions for end safety zones and side-court clearance areas should be adhered to by the planner of the facility. These dimensions are 84 feet by 50 feet, with provisions for at least six feet for safety zones and side-clearance areas.[12]

The amount of square footage available for activity should be at least 90 percent of the total square footage of the arena.

Mats should be provided on the end walls regardless of the size of the end safety zones.

Roll-away bleachers rather than permanent seating in balconies should be provided above and behind the arena floor seating. The bleachers should be properly lighted, ventilated, and provided with adequate entrance and exit areas.

Floor construction. One of the best materials for the construction of gymnasium floors is first- or second-quality, hard northern maple wood. This wood meets the criteria for acceptable gymnasium floors, which are that the floor should be resilient, light in color, nonglare, smooth, nonslippery, tight, dry, economical to install, easily maintained, easily cleaned, easily resurfaced, long-wearing, resistant to denting, and nonabrasive. In addition to hard northern maple, other woods that are acceptable for gymnasium floors are northern beech and birch.

> It is recommended that gymnasium floors placed on concrete have sleepers of 2″ × 3″ or 2″ × 4″, treated with a preservative, placed on a maximum of 16 inches on center, and anchored at not more than 24-inch intervals with floor clips set in the slab. The slab should be coated with one-fourth to one-half inch of hot asphalt pitch poured over membrane impervious to moisture. Subflooring of Douglas fir,

---

12 The Athletic Institute, 1965, *op. cit.*, p. 57.

> hemlock, pine, or spruce boards not wider than 6 inches should be placed on the sleepers at a diagonal and from one-eighth to one-fourth inch apart. A floor paper placed over the subflooring aids in the control of moisture. Maple flooring can then be laid at 90 degrees to the sleepers. Flooring should terminate 2 inches from the walls to allow for expansion. An angle-iron strip or shoe should cover the gap between the floor and the wall.[13]

The floor finish should be selected from a reputable manufacturer. A quality finish seals the grains of the wood and protects the wood from dirt and water, as well as making the floor nonslippery. Markings for all activities should be painted on the floor after the first sealer coat has been applied. Obviously, only official markings should be used. Colored tape is sometimes used as a substitute for painted lines on school gymnasium floors.

To make the playing floor more functional, floor plates should be used to support upright equipment. The floor can be marked for several activities including basketball, volleyball, shuffleboard, and badminton, and the lines for each activity should be a distinctive color and of varying widths.

Several companies have developed new synthetic playing surfaces for indoor sport and recreation use, made of the same materials as outdoor surfaces, that is, compounded synthetic resin or polyvinyl chloride compound. The characteristics are identical: resiliency, durability, uniformity, longevity, and ease of installation and maintenance. Some indoor facilities which are equipped with synthetic floor surfaces are basketball courts, field houses, indoor tennis courts, indoor tracks, locker rooms, roof decks, playgrounds and arena ramps.

Both hard wood and synthetic surfaces should be investigated for price and characteristics prior to selection of indoor playing surfaces.

Walls. The lower six and one-half feet of the gymnasium walls should be constructed of a material that will allow easy cleaning. Glazed ceramic tile is recommended because it is easy to clean and is rather decorative. The upper walls should be constructed of concrete blocks or other material which can easily be painted to aid illumination in the gymnasium. All projections or sharp edges should be eliminated; therefore, drinking fountains, fire extinguishers, and the like should be recessed in the walls.

---

13 The Athletic Institute, 1965, *op. cit.*, p. 164. Reprinted by permission.

Ceilings. The ceiling height should be at least 22 feet and it should be constructed of an acoustically treated material. The ceiling beams should be exposed to provide a place from which suspended equipment can be hung.

Lighting and electricity. Both natural and artificial lighting should be provided. The natural lighting should come from glazed window blocks or frosted window panes which prevent glare and at the same time provide direct lighting. Plain glass windows can be used in some cases and painted over to prevent glare; however, glazed windows are recommended.

In most arenas artificial lighting is provided by incandescent bulbs; however, fluorescent-type fixtures are increasing in popularity. Either type of artificial lighting is recommended for illumination in the gymnasium. The direct lighting should meet specified standards, cause no problem of glare and have proper brightness balance.

Scott and Westkaemper have made excellent suggestions concerning artificial illumination for indoor facilities for secondary school physical education. They state:

> A minimum of 30 foot-candles is recommended for illumination of gymnasiums. Artificial methods should ensure 30 foot-candles of light at all times and daylight would supplement the artificial source. . . . Direct lighting is used for most physical education activity areas. A shield is used to reflect the light in the desired direction. The shield also minimizes glare caused from having the source of light in the field of vision of the participants. . . . The functional use of lighting depends significantly upon the system of control. The cost of current required to provide adequate illumination can be held to a minimum by incorporation of a switch panel that permits control of lights individually, as units or in series. . . . All types of electric lamps have certain attributes and limitations, incandescent lamps have an average life of almost 1000 hours and are not significantly affected by the number of times the light is turned on or off. The lamps and fixture are not as expensive as the fluorescent types and require limited maintenance. The concentrated brightness represents the major disadvantage of the incandescent bulb. . . . Fluorescent tubes create little heat, have an effective life of about 2500 hours. . . . a fluorescent system is more difficult and expensive to clean and maintain than other types, but savings may accrue in wiring and costs of electricity. . . . The wiring of a building or a room must be of sufficient capacity to provide the necessary wattage for adequate illumination and operation of electrical equipment. . . . Wiring should exceed minimum needs. . . . Experts

should determine the type and number of fixtures essential to satisfy standards and calculate the wattage requirements.[14]

Scoreboards, public address systems, motion picture projectors, television cameras, cleaning equipment, class bells, and fire alarms should be positioned so that interference to the spectator is at a minimum.

Heating and ventilation. The type of heating system used should be the one most economical for that specific school. The most commonly used heating systems are steam, hot water, electric, oil, and gas. It is recommended that mechanical exhaust fans be provided for ventilation. If a louvered window is used, a combination of mechanical and natural ventilation should be used. The recommended temperatures for gymnasiums are 60 to 65 degrees Fahrenheit during periods of strenuous activities and 68 to 72 degrees Fahrenheit for mild activities.

Seating. The seating available should be adequate for all activities held in the gymnasium and should be constructed so as to allow for spectator and player safety. The seating should be readily accessible to drinking fountains, concessions, and restrooms.

Ideally, seating should be constructed so that spectator traffic on the arena floor is eliminated.

It is strongly recommended that roll-away bleachers be used since this prevents the seating from occupying otherwise usable space.

The seating capacity should be determined by the size of the school, the activities held in the arena, and the amount of spectator support of events. According to Taylor, the number of seats provided should be equal to one and one-half times the school enrollment.[15] It is recommended that more seats be provided than needed. There should be provisions for expansion of the seating facilities as the school enrollment increases.

Entrances and exits. The gymnasium wing should be provided with at least one main entrance, and the playing floor with at least two main entrances. The main entrance to the gymnasium should have a built-in ticket booth that is constructed in such a way that tickets may be dispensed from both sides of the booth.

---

14 Harry Scott and Richard B. Westkaemper. *From Program to Facilities in Physical Education.* (New York: Harper and Bros., 1958): pp. 303–305. Reprinted by permission.

15 James A. Taylor, "Planning the High School Gymnasium," *American School Board Journal,* **137** (October 1958): 44–48.

The number and size of the exit areas should meet with local and state regulations. All exit doors should open outward. If situated on the end walls of the playing floor, they should be located near the sidelines and not directly under the basket.

Uses. It is recommended that a stage not be constructed as part of the gymnasium area, due to conflicts in scheduling and damage to the gymnasium floor when school plays and other activities are held there.

The playing floor should be used exclusively for physical education classes and related activities, if possible.

Dressing and shower rooms. The dressing and shower rooms should be directly accessible to the playing floor, and there should also be a direct exit to the outdoor facilities.

The lockers should be raised above the floor level to facilitate cleaning. The floors in these areas should be constructed so that drainage is no problem. The dressing room floors should be constructed of cement which is sealed. Shower room floors should be constructed of a nonglazed ceramic tile, or of material that has been treated to prevent slipping. (See Fig. 6)

It is imperative that shower and dressing room space be adequate for any expansion in enrollment or additional teaching stations, since the cost of adding to this part of the facility is excessive and, therefore, prohibitive.

There are many different methods in use for the storing of clothing. Generally, the most satisfactory plan is to provide one full length locker for storage of street clothes to every six or eight small lockers. Each student is assigned a small locker for storage of the physical education uniform. The number of small lockers in each unit is dictated by the number of instructional periods in the school day. Another recommended method is the basket system (Fig. 7), in which numbered wire baskets are delivered to the locker room attendant, who stores them in tiers. Regardless of the system employed, provisions should be made for normal expansion of the school population.

The most satisfactory system for handling locks is to have students rent combination locks each semester. Such locks should be operable with a master key kept by the instructor.

The shower system in both the boys' and girls' locker rooms should be gang-type with at least one or two individual shower stalls. The showering facilities should meet recommended standards for handling peak loads.

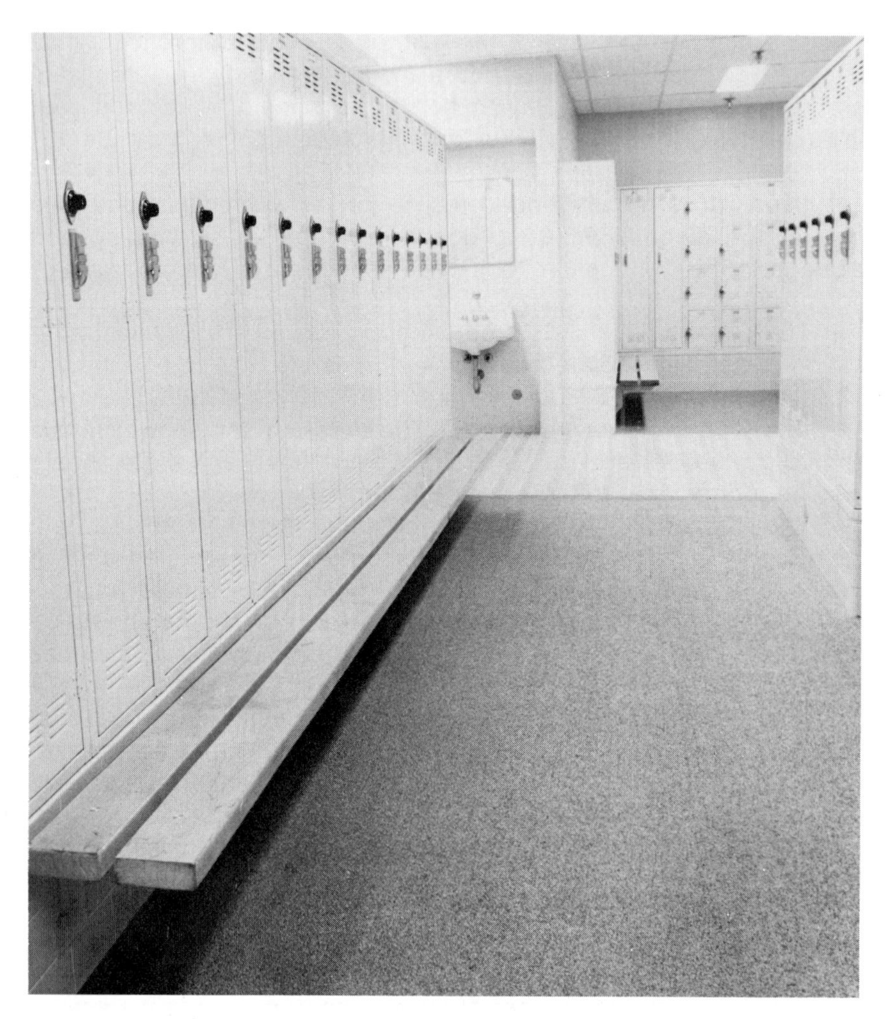

Fig. 6 Women's locker room at the University of Utah, Salt Lake City. (Courtesy of the University of Utah.)

Ventilation in the locker room should be primarily mechanical in nature with supplementary aid from natural ventilation.

It is strongly recommended that a drying area be provided in which students can dry themselves before entering the dressing room, since this prevents excess water from being tracked into the dressing room.

The recommended number of lavatories, urinals, toilets, mirrors, and drinking fountains should be provided in the locker rooms.

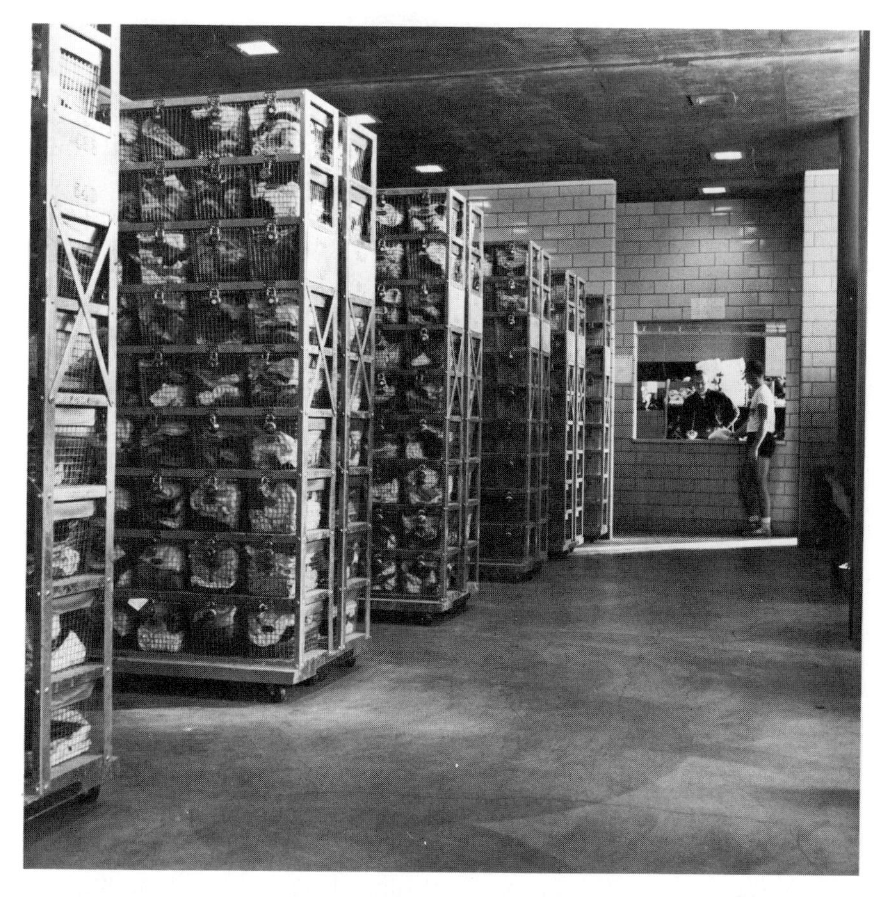

Fig. 7 Basket system of storage. (Courtesy Department of Physical Education, Ohio University.)

Spectator restrooms. These restrooms should be accessibly located for the spectator and should be properly heated, lighted, and ventilated. The number of lavatories, urinals, and toilets will vary according to the school; however, recommended standards should be followed. Scott recommends that toilet facilities for public accommodations be as follows: one urinal for each 40 individuals, and one lavatory for each 75 individuals.[16] Other recommendations are that there be at least two restrooms each for men and women. The men's and women's restrooms should each have at least three lavatories. The men's restroom should have at least three toilets,

[16] Scott and Westkaemper, *op. cit.,* p. 329.

while the women's restroom should have at least four toilets. The men's restroom should be provided with at least four urinals.

Offices. The instructors' office should be located in the locker room and should provide private dressing, showering, and toilet facilities. The office should be constructed to allow for visual supervision of the locker room. There should be separate offices provided for both the men and women instructors, and they should be large enough to accommodate the entire staff. Offices should also be provided with adequate storage space.

Team rooms. In addition to the physical education locker rooms, separate locker rooms should be provided for both the home team and the visiting team. The team rooms should be connected by a passageway that can be securely locked if desired. The construction should be such that these rooms can be used by the physical education classes if necessary. The team rooms should be adequate in size to provide facilities for the largest athletic squad.

These rooms should be adequately heated, lighted, and ventilated, as well as provided with a separate shower room and full-length lockers.

Training room. A training room or area should be provided not only for athletic use, but also for general school use. This room should be connected to the boys' locker room and the team room and should naturally be properly lighted, heated, and ventilated.

Drying room. A room at least eight feet wide and twelve feet long should be provided for the drying of athletic equipment. It is important that this room be properly heated and ventilated.

Accessory activity room. A room that can provide an additional teaching station should be included as part of the total gymnasium. This room allows for activities such as handball, dancing, gymnastics, wrestling, individual exercises, and weight training. It is recommended that this room be at least 30 feet wide and 50 feet long.

Equipment room. Well-planned and organized equipment rooms of sufficient size for the storing, issuing, collecting, and repairing of physical education and athletic equipment are most important in the conduct of the secondary school physical education program.

For the storage of large pieces of equipment, such as net standards, mats, trampolines, parallel bars, and other pieces of apparatus, at least one large room with double doors adjacent to the main gymnasium should be provided. Obviously, the double doors should be of sufficient size to permit easy passage of the largest pieces of equipment.

Equipment, supplies, and uniforms for physical education, athletics, and recreation activities should be stored in a room adjacent to each locker room for maximum accessibility to instructors and students. This room should be well ventilated, well lighted, and sufficiently large to store those pieces of equipment and the uniforms which are unique to the boys' or girls' program.

Such equipment storage areas should have at least one dispensing window with a metal covered counter for the issue and return of equipment and supplies. The equipment room should be separated from the locker room by a metal mesh grill for equipment security as well as for locker room supervision.

The number and types of shelves, drawers, bins, and cupboards that should be built in the equipment room depend on the purposes for which the room is to be used, the number of students and instructors to be served, and the curricular offerings. If the room is used to service physical education, athletic, and recreation programs, shelves should be built to store all types of sports equipment. Some shelves should be used to store equipment in current use, while others should be available for equipment that is seasonal and not in current use. Large bins or drawers should be provided for storing a wide variety of small items of sports equipment and clothing. If towels are dispensed to physical education classes, or if towels, athletic supporters, T-shirts, and socks are provided for athletic teams, bins or drawers for these items should be built beneath the dispensing counter to implement their issue. Cupboards should be built in which athletic team uniforms can be stored. At the end of the season, the uniforms should be cleaned and mothproofed before storing. If possible, a separate cupboard should be available for uniform storage for each sport. Racks for storing such items as golf clubs, golf bags, baseball bats, lacrosse sticks, and tennis rackets should also be available. A work area in the form of counter space or a large table is a valuable asset to the equipment room for the inspecting and marking of uniforms and equipment and the handling of towels and uniforms. A sewing machine and leather-stitching machine are valuable aids in repairing uniforms and leather items.

Classrooms. It is recommended that a classroom be a part of the gymnasium. It should be large enough to handle the largest physical education class or athletic squad, and should be properly heated, lighted, and ventilated.

NEW IDEAS IN THE DEVELOPMENT OF FACILITIES

In recent years, many new and creative ideas have evolved in the development of facilities for physical education, athletics, and recreation.

In addition to traditional outdoor physical education and athletic facilities (football, baseball, soccer and field-hockey fields, tennis courts, and track and field facilities), new facilities have been developed for colleges, universities, and public schools, that have enlarged the scope of program offerings. Some of these new facilities are: field-archery areas, paddle-tennis courts, marinas (for canoeing, boating, and sailing), roller-skating rinks, angling and casting areas, bicycle paths, bridle paths, ice-skating rinks, ski areas, rifle ranges, outdoor education laboratories, school camps, and one of the newest outdoor facilities parcour (jogging exercise trail).

A variety of new indoor facilities have been added to the traditional basketball arena for college, university, and public school gymnasiums, thus enabling the range of course-offerings and recreation play activities to be increased. These facilities include fencing areas, rifle ranges, tennis courts, handball-racketball courts, deck- and paddle-tennis courts, street-shoes-usage rooms, indoor archery ranges, personal-defense rooms, weight/exercise rooms, golf practice areas, bowling lanes, diving pools, ice-skating rinks, and curling ice-sheets (see Fig. 8).

Following are some new ideas developed to enhance the use of existing facilities in physical education, athletics and recreation: improved lighting of indoor facilities, both in quality and quantity of light; lighting of outdoor facilities for competitive sports, physical education, and recreation; air-conditioned gymnasiums and field houses; electric-powered equipment for moving partitions and telescopic bleachers; improved acoustics; synthetic surfaces for gymnasium floors, indoor/outdoor carpeting for locker rooms; tennis courts, running tracks, field-events facilities; synthetic turf for football, baseball, soccer, and lacrosse fields; conversion of football stadiums to multipurpose use; conversion of swimming pools for use in both warm and cold weather by mechanically moving the

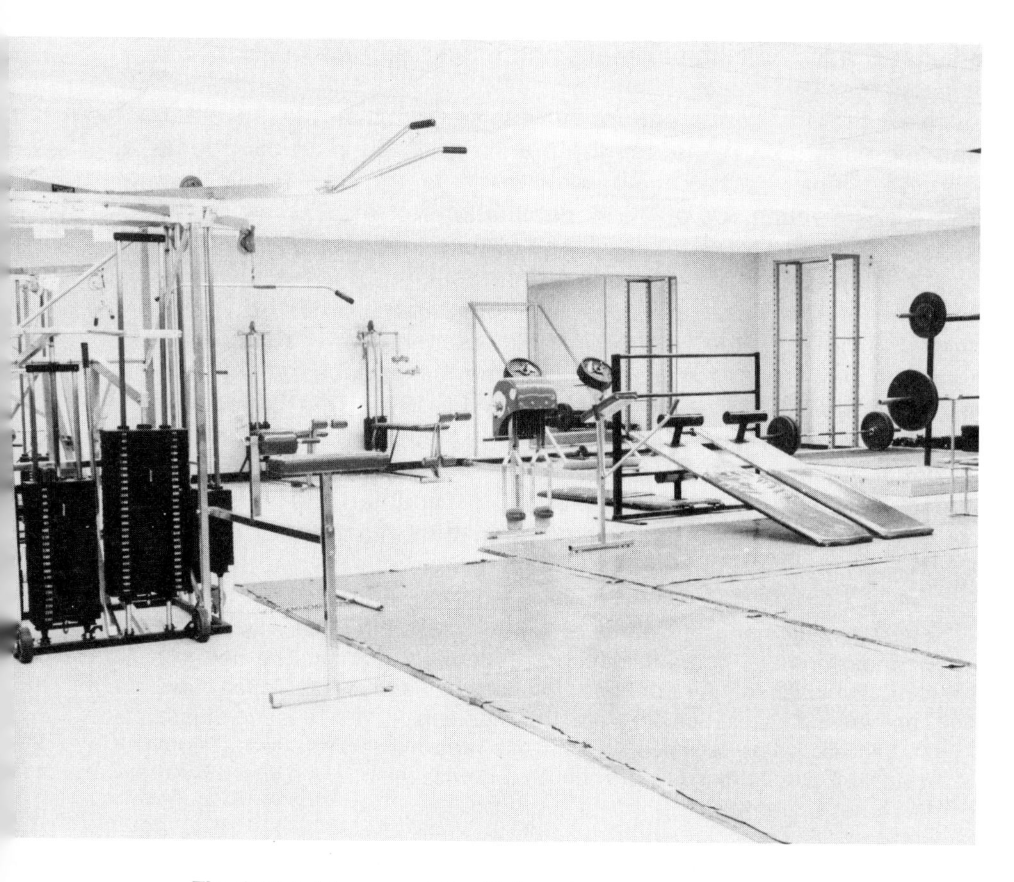

Fig. 8 Weight room at the University of Utah, Salt Lake City. (Courtesy of the University of Utah.)

pool enclosure on a sliding track; conversion of outdoor football stadiums to indoor multiuse stadiums for such activities as indoor track and field, basketball, soccer, festivals, and concerts.

New concepts in facilities construction include: covering sports facilities with air structures; field houses adjacent to secondary schools; Quonset-type gymnasiums; "play sheds" consisting of a roof and steel supports for elementary school physical education programs; circular-shaped gymnasium providing better spectator viewing; geodesic-domed field houses; arched and gabled roofs for sports arenas (see Fig. 9 (a), (b), (c), (d); and stacking facilities, for a school district, by placing a complete sports facility in a few locations and minimal facilities in the remainder of the district to reduce costs. More economical building materials such as cement block, laminated wood for structural members, and corrugated steel are being increasingly used.

New factors in our culture have emerged that will have far-reaching effects on the future, the planning of new physical education and athletic facilities. Some of these factors are Public Law 94–142 and Section 504 of the Rehabilitation Act of 1973, which became effective on October 1, 1977, and require that public school, college, and university physical education facilities be constructed to meet the needs of all students, including those who are handicapped; Title IX of the Educational Amendment Act of 1972 is designed to end sex discrimination in American education. All provisions of the act had to be met by July 21, 1978. Title IX requires that physical education facilities meet the needs of all students on an equal basis and that all physical education classes except contact sports must be coeducational. In addition, conversion to the metric system is gradually emerging; thus planners of new in-

Fig. 9 (a) Eight thousand yards of Teflon-coated Fiberglas stretch over one and one-half acres at LaVerne College, California. The new student activities center, dubbed "Supertent" and "The Tepee," will combine a physical activities area for men and women, athletic offices, student activities facilities, classrooms, and a fine arts area. (Photograph by Sid Fridkin. Reprinted by permission of the University of LaVerne, California.)

Fig. 9 (b) "Supertent's" physical activities center is equipped with up-to-date moveable facilities, lockers for every student, and training rooms for men and women. Women are invited to try out for all sports at LaVerne. (Photograph by Sid Fridkin. Reprinted by permission of the University of LaVerne, California.)

Fig. 9 (c) Student activities facilities at LaVerne include socializing areas mixed among pool tables, student organization offices, book store, radio station, photographic darkroom, small cinema, post office, and a soon-to-be-built snack bar. (Photograph by Sid Fridkin. Reprinted by permission of the University of LaVerne, California.)

Fig. 9 (d) Two levels compose "Supertent's" unique structure. The first level has four main interest areas, each of which is completely flexible as to its use. The physical activities area is equipped with a variety of weight-lifting and exercise devices including a trampoline, parallel bars, horizontal bars, gymnastic rings, and side horses. (Photograph by Sid Fridkin. Reprinted by permission of the University of LaVerne, California.)

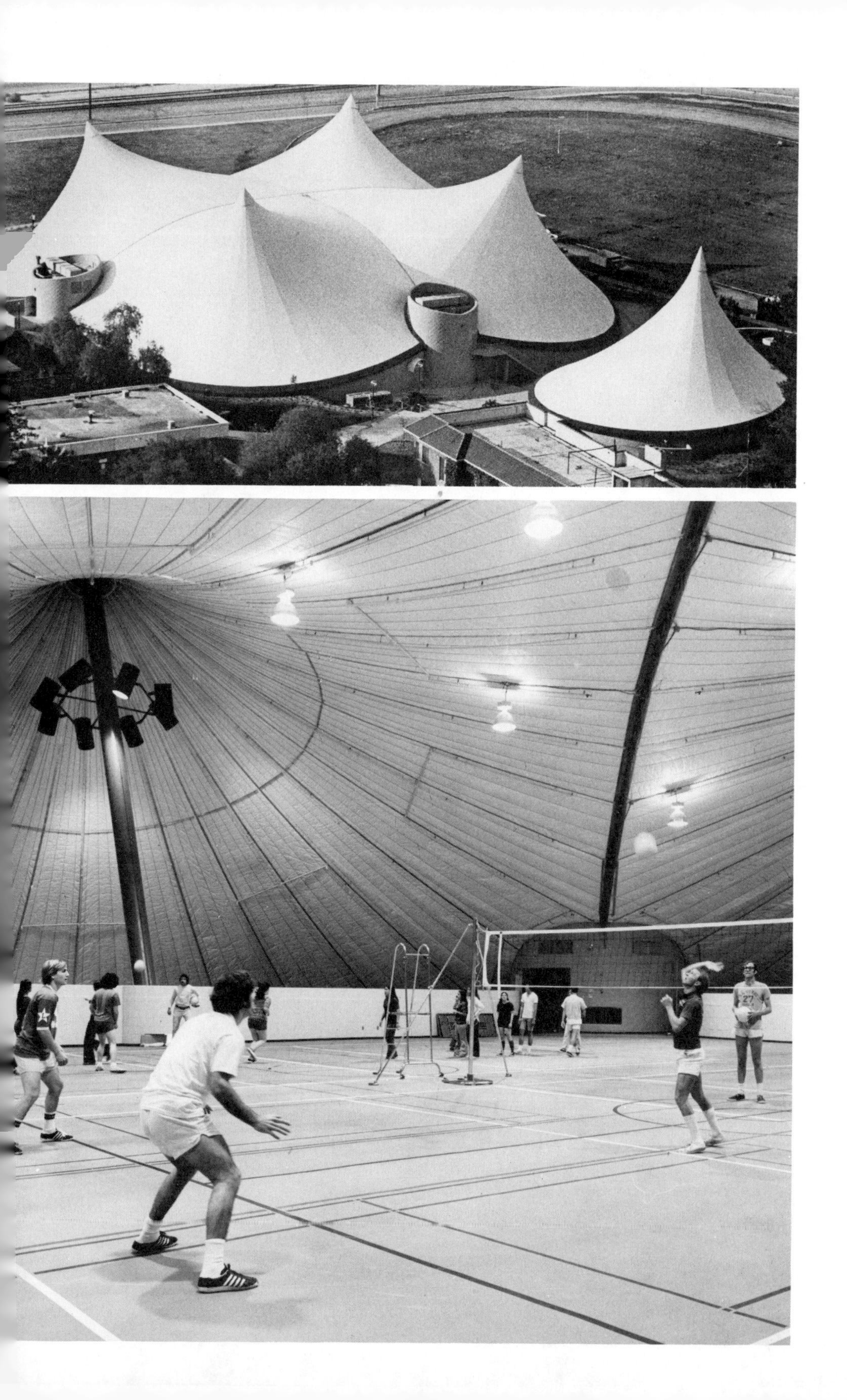

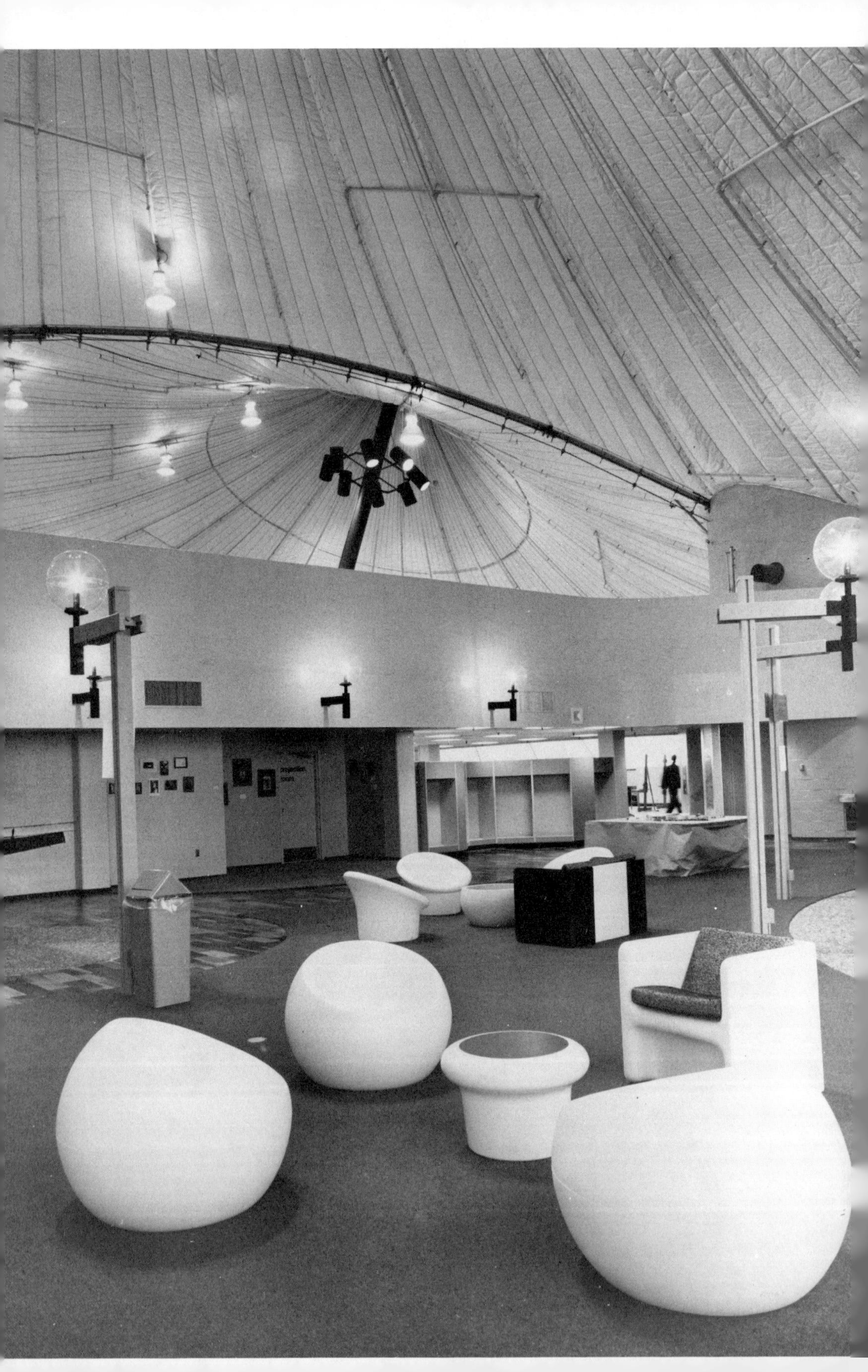

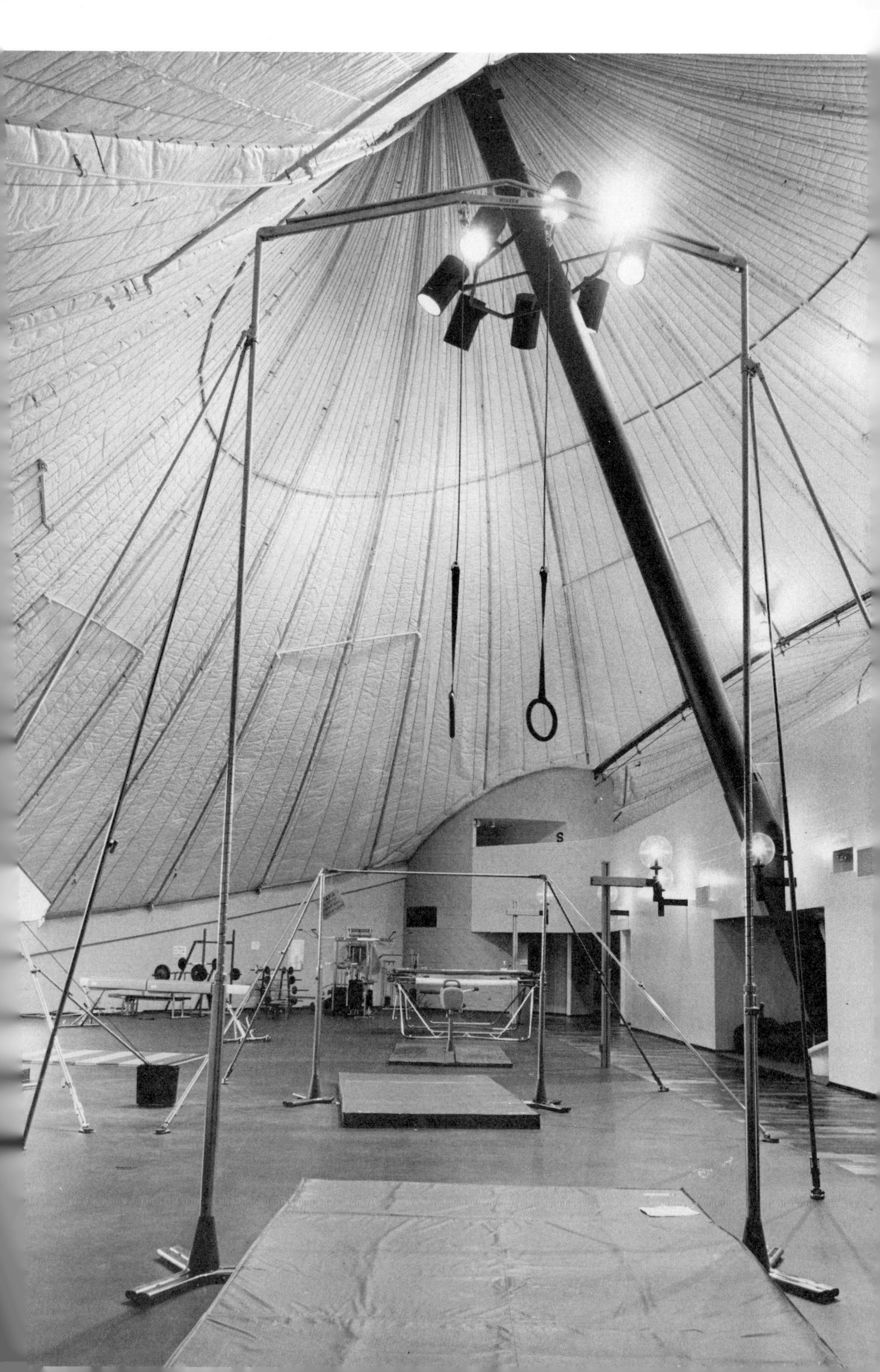

door and outdoor facilities must consider the use of the metric system for their fields, courts, and swimming pools. The energy crisis and the rising cost of utilities (heat, electricity, air conditioning, telephones) will be major items of concern in facility planning. Solar energy is one possible answer to the heating problem in the future.

Additional innovations in physical education and athletic facilities are: development of neighborhood and community school–parks used for both public school physical education and athletic programs and community recreation; rooftop tennis courts and rooftop playing fields (with artificial turf); portable swimming pools; surfing pools with wave-generating machinery; and audiovisual centers in gymnasiums at the secondary school and college level. It appears the revolution in facilities development for physical education, athletics, and sport will continue into the foreseeable future.

PUBLIC SCHOOL SWIMMING POOLS

A complete discussion of the swimming pool as a school physical education facility is beyond the scope of this book; however, the basic elements of planning size, shape, construction, and administration are presented.

In the United States there has been an increase in water activities of all types. The number of public school swimming pools at both the elementary and secondary level is rapidly increasing, although a majority of public schools still lack this important facility. Obviously, the major deterrent is cost. Therefore, when a school system is able to finance a swimming pool, it is most important that maximum value be received for each dollar spent. This means careful planning, excellent design and construction, proper maintenance and supervision, and a well-rounded aquatic program providing maximum pool use.

Many communities have justified the construction of a public school swimming pool on the basis of total community use. This means that adults, as well as school-age children, have access to the pool. Since the public schools belong to all citizens in the community, total community use of the pool is justified.

When a choice is available between building an indoor or an outdoor pool, the indoor pool is recommended. In most areas of the United States, use of an outdoor pool is restricted to a few months of the year. The indoor pool is more expensive to build, but the cost can be justified in terms of year-round use.

Planning the Swimming Pool

Because of the technical nature of swimming pool construction, it is imperative that a competent pool architect or engineer be employed. Planning decisions can only be made by those who are knowledgeable about locations, construction costs, plumbing, acoustics, wiring, size and shape of pools, construction materials, state and local building codes, water sanitation, and filtration systems. As in the construction of all physical education facilities, the physical education aquatic specialist should consult with the architect regarding the kinds of activities to be conducted in the pool, as well as the type and number of persons expected to use the pool. School swimming pools should be planned for multiple use including instruction, recreation, and competition.

Size and Shape of the Swimming Pool

In determining the size and shape of the swimming pool, the program specialists and architect must work cooperatively, since the pool, to be functional, must meet the needs of the aquatic program. Funds available for pool construction are always the limiting factor in pool design.

The most common design for public school swimming pools is the rectangular shape. With careful planning, the rectangular pool can provide for all the needs of the program. This shape pool is the most economical to construct, maintain, and supervise. The recommended length is 75 feet, one inch; the recommended width, is 36 or 42 feet. With varying water depths, the needs of all areas of the instructional program can be met. The following are guidelines for water depths as suggested by the participants in the National Facilities Conference. "For educational purposes, a pool should be divided with lifelines, or moveable bulkheads, separating the water areas into deep (over 5′0″), intermediate (3′9″ to 5′0″), and shallow (2′10″ to 3′9″)." [17] One problem with the rectangle-shaped pool is that diving, when it is a part of the aquatic program, interferes with swimming.

There are numerous other swimming pool shapes that can be used; the value of each depends on aquatic program needs, emphasis, and funds available. Included among them are the L-shape, T-shape, Z-shape, V-shape, and W-shape (see Fig. 10). The L- and T-shaped pools are modifications of the rectangle which provide

---

[17] National Facilities Conference, *op. cit.*, p. 174.

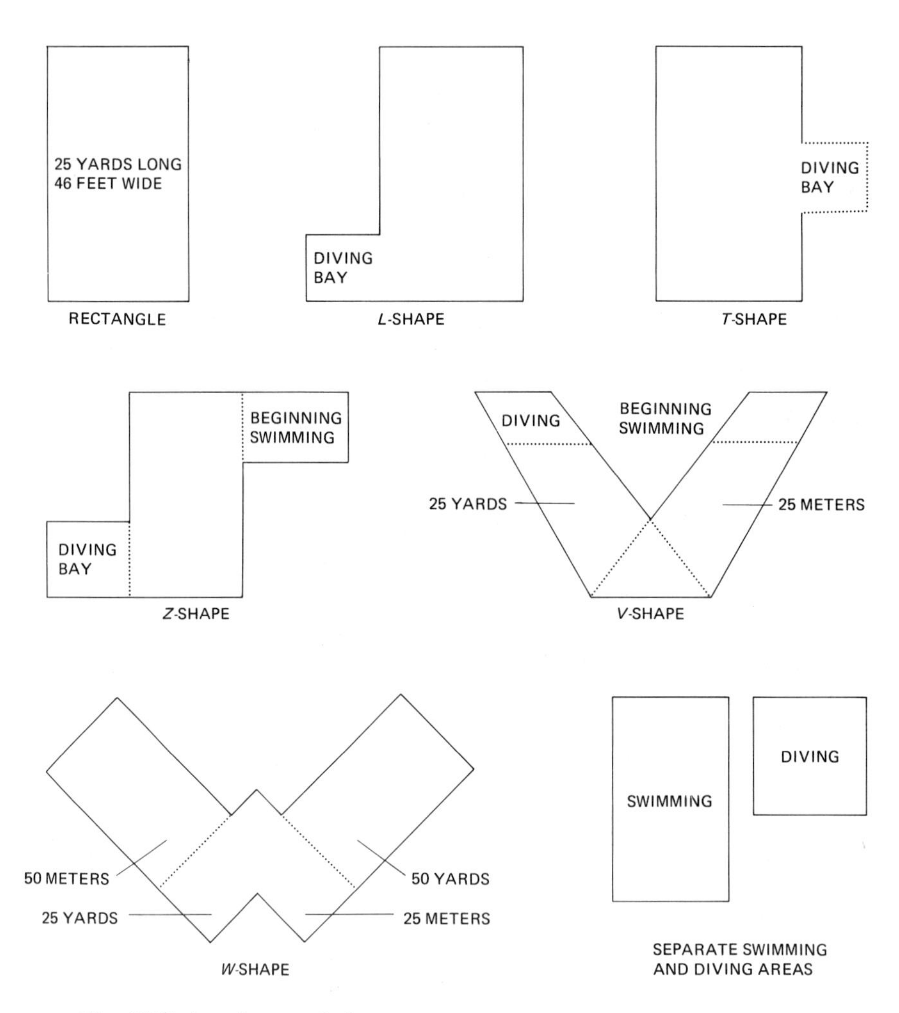

Fig. 10 Swimming pool shapes.

diving bays so that swimming and diving activities can be conducted simultaneously. The Z-shaped pool is designed to provide for diving and the teaching of beginning swimming, in addition to the rectangular area for instruction and competition. The V-shaped pool provides for diving and beginning swimming at the 25-yard and 25-meter distances for competition and instruction. The W-shaped pool is designed to provide all the competitive distances, the 25-yard and 25-meter distance (short course) as well as the 50-yard and 50-meter distances (long course). Another design that should be mentioned is that of separate swimming and diving pools.

This is probably the most desirable, but also the most expensive.

The participants in the National Facilities Conference suggest the following dimensions for public school swimming pools:

The elementary school pool

Minimum width: 16′
Desirable widths: 20′, 25′, or 30′
Minimum length: 36′
Desirable lengths: 50′, 60′, or 75′

The junior-high school pool

Minimum width: 25′
Desirable widths: 30′, 36′, or 42′
Minimum length: 60′
Desirable length: 75′

The high school pool

Minimum width: 36′
Desirable width: 45′
Minimum and desirable length: 75′ and 1″ [18]

Construction of Swimming Pools

Much of the information in this section is adapted from John J. Krumb's article "How to Plan the School and/or Community Pool." [19] Most of the concepts presented apply to both outdoor and indoor pools.

After being presented with certain preliminary facts, such as general location of the pool, pool uses, and estimated size and shape, the architect reacts to these preliminary specifics and renders judgments as a technical expert. After the site has been selected, the architect requires a survey which must include topography, sewer lines, water availability, and any other details which might affect the design of the pool. The indoor school swimming pool should be planned as a part of the total physical education facility and should be adjacent to the boys' and girls' locker and shower rooms.

Pool shell. A decision must be made regarding the pool shell structure. Form-poured concrete basins have proven to be excellent for construction. Also gunite (premixed concrete "shot" under pressure from a nozzled flexible hose) is considered one of the better methods of constructing the pool shell. Other materials include cement block, brick, steel, and aluminum.

---

[18] *Ibid.*, p. 181. Reprinted by permission.

[19] John J. Krumb, "How to Plan the School and/or Community Pool," *Swimming Pool Data and Reference Annual* (Fort Lauderdale, Florida: Hoffman Publications, 1964): p. 24.

Pool shell finish. For maximum satisfaction, well-chosen quality paints for the interior finish of the shell will prove to be the most economical in terms of continued use. In selecting colors for paints, light colors should be selected, since they improve the appearance of the water and thus add to the overall aesthetic effect. Also, light-colored paint of good quality tends to be more permanent, since it resists the influence of the sun and the chemicals in the water.

The top 12 inches of the pool side should be finished in tile to facilitate the removal of the body oils from the walls. The finish of pool surfaces (pool wall and floor finish) should be reasonably smooth, enduring nontoxic, inert and impervious material. Available finishes are plaster (preferably a white cement plaster of marble aggregate), ceramic tile, paint on concrete, or the plastered surface. Gunite pool surfaces must be plastered in order to be reasonably smooth. In recent years, many pool shells have been treated with epoxy, a plastic paint substance. Epoxy surfaces are glossy in appearance, easy to clean, and have no joints.

For indoor pools a white finish should be applied to the bottom and sides of the pool, to provide the clearest vision; for outdoor pools light blue is generally recommended. Dark contrasting material should be used for swimming lane markers that are painted on the pool bottom.

Copings and gutters. The deck coping above the gutters should extend completely around the pool, so as to separate decks from the basin edges and to prevent a flow of deck water into the pool. The edges of the gutter and coping should be finished in a color different from that used on the basin sides.

Steps and ladders. Recessed steps built into the pool sides are recommended. If ladders are used, they should also be recessed, and the tread of the ladders should be painted in a dark color. All rough edges and sharp corners in the pool should be rounded and smooth, with a minimum of a one-half-inch radius.

Underwater viewing room. An underwater viewing room is desirable as a teaching aid. However, the expense of such a room generally precludes its construction in the public schools.

Pool markings. Permanent pool markings are necessary to indicate pool depths, various distances along the sides, finishes for competitive races, swimming lanes, and water polo areas. These markings should be of a color that is in contrast to the color of the surface finish.

Numbers or letters indicating depths or finish marks should be four inches to six inches high. Depth markings should indicate depths in feet, and they should be placed on the deck and the side of the pool above the water level. For competitive swimming, lanes must be provided. The lanes should be seven feet wide and marked by either eight- or ten-inch-wide lines of a dark color extending along the bottom the length of the pool, but terminating five feet from each end and marked with a short perpendicular line.

Pool decks. Deck area width depends on usage and local conditions. The total deck distributed around the pool should be adequately drained with a slope of one and one-half inches in the first foot from the pool edge to the deck area. The surface should be a nonslip material. Decks should slope away from the pool and/or in the direction of drain points at the rate of one-fourth inch to the foot, with the exception of the first foot. Bleacher space for spectators is not included as deck space. The only public entrance to the pool deck should be directly from the shower room and should be used only by swimmers. A service entrance, ten feet wide with eight feet of overhead clearance, should also be provided.

Diving facilities. Public school pools should include facilities and equipment for diving. Diving is a popular activity and facilities should be provided for instruction, competition, and recreation. Minimum water depths necessary for diving are 10 feet of water for a one-meter springboard, 11.5 feet of water for a three-meter springboard.

The National Collegiate Athletic Association requires 12 feet of depth below diving equipment for one-meter through five-meter competitions.

Other space requirements for diving are as follows: the diving board should extend five feet over the edge of the pool; the indoor pool ceiling height should be 15 feet above the water level for one-meter boards and 25 feet above the water level for three-meter boards; and the minimum distance between two diving boards (center to center) or from the center of one diving board to the side of the pool should be ten feet.

The required depths of the pool below diving equipment should be maintained five feet beyond the end of the one- and three-meter springboards. This depth should be continued to a distance of five feet on either side of a one-meter board and ten feet on either side of a three-meter board. The rise of the pool beyond this point should not be greater than six inches per five feet for the following distances from the board: one-meter board, fifteen feet; three-meter board, 20 feet. In diving pools, the wall opposite the boards should be a minimum of 25 feet from one-meter boards and 33 feet from three-meter boards.

Spectator area. The amount of space provided for spectators depends on the interest in the competitive program and on funds available. Balconies, permanent bleachers, and roll-away bleachers are available options. In most cases, roll-away bleachers are suggested, since this provides additional deck space for instruction when the bleachers are rolled flush with the wall.

Other Construction Features

In planning the indoor school swimming pool, other construction features that must be considered are heating, ventilation, humidity control, acoustics, lighting, service tunnel, and storage area.

Heating, ventilation, and humidity control. Heating, ventilation, and humidity control are most important considerations when planning the indoor swimming pool, and thus the services of a heating engineer are required. Scott makes the following suggestions regarding these areas:

> The heating system should permit constant and automatic control of water temperature in the pool. The locations of tank inlets should distribute warmed water evenly throughout the pool so that a uniform temperature is maintained. The recommended temperature of 83 degrees Fahrenheit for the pool area should be maintained for all seasons. Humidity control is necessary for comfort and elimination of condensation. A humidity of 40 to 60 per cent is desired in most instances. The ventilation system should recirculate air rapidly, but without creating a draft effect in the area occupied by swimmers. In some instances dehumidifiers are placed near the ceilings or in the ventilation system serving the area. The heating and ventilation systems for natatoriums should operate separately from those systems for other sections of the physical education building.[20]

Acoustics. Effective acoustical control is necessary in an indoor swimming pool. High ceilings create problems, and therefore the ceiling and walls should be acoustically treated to control noise and sound distortion. An acoustical engineer should be consulted.

Lighting. Considerable thought should be given to the electrical work in the pool area, since the attractiveness and safety of the pool will depend on the placement of the lights. Scott suggests a

---

[20] Scott and Westkaemper, *op. cit.*, pp. 201–203.

minimum of 30 foot-candles of artificial illumination at water level.[21] Underwater lighting is essential to the indoor swimming pool to facilitate instruction and competition; it is also valuable for recreational swimming and all special aquatic events. Illumination engineers should be consulted.

Service tunnel. A service tunnel, located around the perimeter of the pool shell, is essential for the modern indoor swimming pool, since it facilitates the repair of the pool shell, lights, pipe lines, valves, and windows.

Storage area. A storage area is necessary at pool deck level for storage of the many pieces of equipment that are necessary for the conduct of the aquatic program. The largest individual pieces of equipment are diving boards and canoes. Therefore, according to Scott and Westkaemper, the area should be at least 20 feet long with a total area of 140 square feet and an opening five to six feet wide; it should also have an elevated threshold to prevent water from the pool deck from entering the storage area.[22]

CASE STUDY

The population of East High School had tripled in the past five years. Its gymnasium at that time had been more than adequate, but now several serious problems were developing. One problem in particular was causing the department head to reevaluate his space and facilities. Up to the present year, each male student was assigned a full-length locker for the entire year for physical education classes. The head of the department was informed by the principal that in the coming year the increase in male students would approach 20 percent. The present locker room was completely full and there was no hope for any type of expansion. Mr. Wells sent a memo to his staff asking for suggestions.

1. What are the issues in this case?
2. What are the possible solutions for this situation?
3. Are there any guidelines or principles which evolve from this problem?

SELECTED REFERENCES

"Alternative Athletics: Planning Facilities for Lifetime Sports," *College and University Business,* **55** (September 1973): 51–58.

---

[21] *Ibid.,* p. 203.

[22] *Ibid.,* p. 197.

American Association for Health, Physical Education and Recreation. *College and University Facilities Guide for Health, Physical Education, Recreation and Athletics.* Washington, D.C.: The Association, 1968.

———. *Planning Areas and Facilities for Health, Physical Education and Recreation.* Washington, D.C.: The Association, 1966.

Browne, R. L. "Innovations in Sports Facilities," *American School and University,* **44** (November 1971): 24.

———. "Multi-Purpose Facilities: More Use Per Inch, Per Hour, Per Student," *American School and University,* **47** (November 1974): 23–27.

Bryant, J. E. "Don't Knock Your Facilities!" *Physical Educator,* **28** (May 1971): 74–75.

"Bubble, Bubble: Less Cost, Minimum Trouble," *Nation's Schools,* **85** (February 1970): 76–78.

Budd, B. "Lacking Facilities? Improvise!" *Instructor,* **82** (January 1973): 52–53.

Buskirk, E. R., et al. "Microclimate Over Artificial Turf," *Journal of Health Physical Education* Recreation, **42** (November 1971): 29–30.

"Campus Climate Limits All Outdoor Activity Except Skiing and Skating So Other Sports Have an Indoor Center," *College Management,* **6** (May 1971): 40–41.

Chung, T. B. "Building Coverage: A Typical Assignment of Physical Directors," *Journal of Physical Education,* **74** (March 1977): 48.

Coates, E. "Role of the Physical Educator in Facility Planning," *Physical Educator,* **28** (May 1971): 88–91.

Crudo, A., and K. Reed. "No! You Can't Have the Gym," *Journal of Health Physical Education Recreation,* **44** (September 1973): 73–74.

Daughtrey, Greyson, and John B. Woods. *Physical Education Programs, Organization and Administration.* Philadelphia: W. B. Saunders, 1971.

———. *Physical Education and Intramural Programs: Organization and Administration.* Philadelphia: W. B. Saunders, 1976.

David, W. E. "Stadium for All Seasons: Idaho State University's New Minidome," *College Management,* **7** (February 1972): 21–24.

Day, C. W. "Field Turf System Has Irrigation Down PAT: Prescription Athletic Turf System," *Nation's Schools,* **92** (November 1973): 28.

Englehart, N. *Complete Guide for Planning New Schools.* Englewood Cliffs, N.J.: Prentice-Hall, 1970.

Ezersky, E., and P. R. Theibert. "City Schools Without Gyms," *Journal of Health Physical Education Recreation,* **41** (April 1970): 26–29.

"Facilities for Lifetime Sports," *The Ohio High School Athlete* (November 1973): 79–92.

"Focus on Facilities in Public Schools," *Journal of Physical Education and Recreation,* **47** (September 1976): 15–21.

"Four Thousand Tires Died for This: New Track Surface Made of Tires Mixed with Asphalt," *Nation's Schools and Colleges,* **1** (October 1974): 68.

Frost, Reuben B., and Stanley J. Marshall. *Administration of Physical Education and Athletics: Concepts and Practices.* Dubuque, Iowa: W. C. Brown, 1977.

Gabrielsen, M. Alexander. *Swimming Pools. A Guide to Their Planning, Design and Operation.* Fort Lauderdale, Florida: Hoffman, 1969.

"Geodesic Dome Shipped 3,000 Miles to Construction Site," *School Management,* **15** (September 1971): 45.

"Gigantic Gym; Remodeled Stadium at University of Minnesota," *Nation's Schools and Colleges,* **2** (February 1975): 23.

Glenesk E., and F. Cords. "There'll Be Some Changes Made! Survey About Physical Education Programs and Building Design," *Journal of Physical Education,* **72** (September 1974): 4–7.

Grieve, A. "Safety of Facilities," *Journal of Health Physical Education Recreation,* **45** (October 1974): 24–25.

"Gym Floor in Perfect Condition for 18 Years," *School Management,* **15** (May 1971): 43.

"Gymnasiums in the Round: Huron High School, Ann Arbor, Mich.," *American School and University,* **43** (June 1971): 24.

Johnson, M. L. *Functional Administration in Physical and Health Education.* Boston: Houghton Mifflin, 1977.

Karabetos, J. "Facilities for the 70's," *Physical Educator,* **27** (December 1970): 171–172.

Keene, C. "Using Balconies in Physical Education Programs," *Journal of Physical Education and Recreation,* **48** (April 1977): 64.

Keller, R. J. "Making the Most of Your Old Facilities," *Journal of Health Physical Education Recreation,* **42** (June 1971): 26–28.

Kelsey, F. L. "Sports Facilities: The New Breed," *Phi Delta Kappan,* **56** (January 1975): 321–325.

Levenson, S. "Now Is the Time to Build That Pool," *Times Educational Supplement,* **3000** (November 24, 1972): 15.

Mittelstaedt, A. H. "Preparing Health, Physical Education and Recreation Professionals to Deal With Facilities and Equipment," *Journal of Health Physical Education Recreation,* **45** (October 1974): 22–23.

Meditch, C. "Physical Educators Plan Facilities," *Journal of Health Physical Education Recreation,* **45** (January 1974): 32–33.

"Multi-Purpose Mammoths," *College Management,* **5** (August 1970): 18–21.

"OSU Puts Sports Where the Students Are," *American School and University,* **49** (December 1976): 32–33.

"Pavilion Built for Basketball: Stanford University," *College and University Business,* **49** (July 1970): 46–48.

Penman, K. A. "Let's Build Useful Gyms," *American School and University,* **42** (August 1970): 14–15.

———. *Planning Physical Education and Athletic Facilities in Schools.* New York: Wiley, 1977.

———. "Sports and Noise: How Much Is too Much?" *American School and University,* **49** (March 1977): 23.

Pettine, A. M. "Planning a Gymnasium," *Journal of Health Physical Education Recreation,* **44** (October 1973): 58.

"Physical Education Center Built Underground; Columbia University, New York," *American School and University,* **47** (March 1975): 15–17.

"Physical Education Center: More Facility for the Money; Merrimack College, Andover, Mass.," *American School and University,* **47** (October 1974): 441–444.

Piper, J. E. "Painting Plastic Turf; Painting Lines on the Field," *American School and University,* **49** (March 1977): 36.

"Pool Maintenance Costs Plunge with Automatic Controls," *American School and University,* **44** (December 1971): 20–22.

"Primer on Synthetic Surfaces," *American School and University,* **43** (August 1971): 44–45.

Puckett, J. R. "Planning Educational Specifications for Health and Physical Education," *Physical Educator,* **30** (December 1973): 203–204.

———. "Two Promising Innovations in Physical Education Facilities," *Journal of Health Physical Education Recreation,* **43** (January 1972): 40–41.

"Raising the Roof on Inflation; Air-Supported Activities Center at the University of Santa Clara," *Nation's Schools and Colleges,* **2** (May 1975): 23.

"Remodel the Armory or Build a New Gym?" *American School and University,* **43** (December 1970): 20–24.

Ridini, L. "Suggestions for Effective and Efficient Utilization of Space for Large Student Enrollments," *Journal of Physical Education,* **71** (May 1974): 130.

"Sampling the New Sports, Surfaces and Services," *College and University Business,* **55** (September 1973): 59–60.

Seaborne, Malcolm. *Primary School Design.* Boston: Routledge and Kegan Paul, 1971.

Sliger, I. T. "Student Aquatic Center Recreation Complex at the University of Tennessee," *Journal of Health Physical Education Recreation,* **41** (February 1970): 42–43.

"Sports Dome Offers Something for Everybody; University of Northern Iowa," *American School and University,* **49** (December 1976): 30–31.

"Synthetic Covering for College Field House," *American School and University,* **42** (August 1970): 18.

"Texas District Finds Success with Synthetic Playing Fields," *American School and University,* **45** (June 1973): 30.

Theibert, P. R. "P. Richard Theibert on Facilities for Lifetime Sports: Interview," *American School and University,* **44** (November 1971): 14–18.

"Two-Story Gym Solves Traffic Problem: Wisconsin State University, Eau Claire," *American School and University,* **43** (June 1971): 22–23.

Watson, J. R. "Care and Feeding of Athletic Fields," *American School and University,* **43** (May 1971): 46–47.

Woods, H. W. "Vinyl Flooring the Surfacing of the Future," *Athletic Journal,* **53** (December 1972): 16.

Zingale, D. P. "Skiing Facility for the College Physical Education Program," *Physical Educator,* **29** (March 1972): 3–5.

PART III

INTRAMURAL AND INTERSCHOOL SPORT

13

THE INTRAMURAL AND EXTRAMURAL PROGRAMS

STUDY STIMULATORS

1. What purpose(s) justifies the time and efforts involved in administering a program of intramural activities?
2. How can an administrator involve students in the administration and management of the intramural program?
3. What basic units for competition can be utilized in setting up a program of intramurals?
4. What are the advantages and disadvantages of different types of tournaments used in intramurals?
5. What is the case for awards in the program? How many, and on what basis?
6. Should there be eligibility rules for intramural competition?
7. Is it necessary to have structured, organized programs? Is there merit in simply opening the facilities for "free play"?

Play up! Play up! And play the game.

SIR HENRY NEWBOLDT

The purpose of intramural programs in schools and colleges is to offer an opportunity for voluntary participation in a population not skilled enough for or not sufficiently interested in a varsity-type program.

Quite sophisticated programs of intramural activities are in existence today in many school systems. These programs are the result of several contributory factors which are briefly traced below.

HISTORY

Intramurals began in a rather haphazard manner during the decade from 1850–1860 when male students at some of the eastern universities formed club teams in various athletic activities and challenged each other to matches. In spite of the somewhat poor, unorganized planning for these activities under student leadership, the programs flourished and participation increased to the point where faculties decried the emphasis placed on such "frivolous, ungentlemanly" contests. Nevertheless, student interest increased and challenging units became associated with classes, clubs, and Greek societies. Such competition then spread to extramural proportions and thus became the forerunner of the modern-day intercollegiate program. In the early 1900's, the intramural program for men had expanded to such an extent that colleges saw the need for some form of faculty supervision and control, although student leadership was still fundamental. As a result, in 1913 the University of Michigan and Ohio State University established Departments of Intramurals and each named one man to direct the entire program. In 1917 an

Intramural Sports Section was established as a part of the Research Section of the organization known today as AAHPER (American Alliance for Health, Physical Education, and Recreation). Intramurals for women were introduced into the colleges in 1923, and since then the operation of women's programs has remained largely in the hands of students.

By 1925, the intramural program was extended into the secondary schools. The National Intramural Association was established in 1950, and this organization continues to exert strong leadership in the intramural area. Although its primary concern is the promotion of intramurals on the college level, its influence is felt throughout the entire educational spectrum. An Intramural Advisory Committee, organized through the AAHPER in 1964, has as one of its purposes to encourage the formulation of intramural programs within each state of the union.

There is a trend today, particularly at the college level, to move the responsibility for the intramural program from a department of physical education or athletics to an office of student affairs. Such an organizational structure makes possible the scheduling of all student activities in one office and thus tends to overcome the problem of conflicting events (see Fig. 4). Regardless of where the intramural program is officially housed, the director of the program needs to be educated specifically for the assignment, as discussed below.

CURRENT TRENDS

Perhaps three factors can be cited as being significant today. The first is the public's increased awareness of the importance of physical fitness and the attendant recognition that a good intramural program in which every boy and girl can participate will help meet this goal. The second, particularly apropos at the college level, is an increased awareness of the many ramifications of the concept of leisure, in part advanced by the behavioral scientists, and the congruent need for recreational facilities where less structured programs can be conducted. The third is the increasing number of professional preparation programs in intramural administration. Preo[1] believes that we "need to adopt a more sound process of preparing individuals to become intramural administrators," and he proposes the model shown in Fig. 1 as the basis for such a process.[2] Whereas

---

[1] L. S. Preo, "Professional Preparation of Administrators of Intramural and Physical Recreation Programs," in J. A. Peterson (ed.), *Intramural Administration: Theory and Practice* (Englewood Cliffs, N.J.: Prentice-Hall, 1976), pp. 12–19.

[2] *Ibid.*, p. 15.

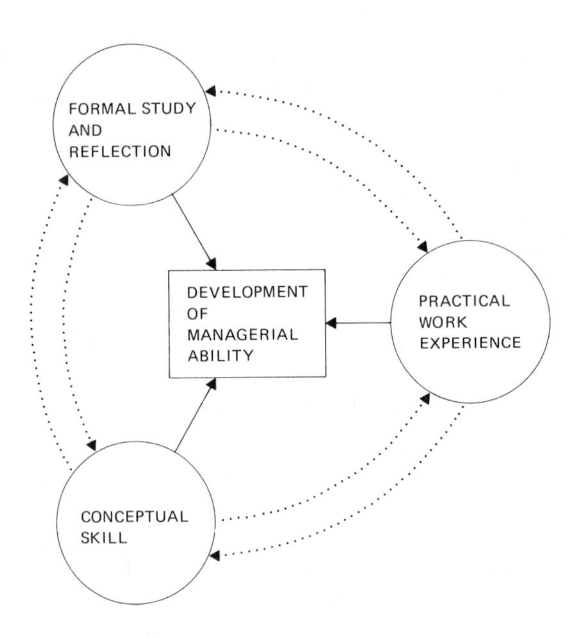

Fig. 1 Proposed model for the professional preparation of intramural administrators. (James A. Peterson, *Intramural Administration: Theory and Practice,* © 1976, p. 15. Reprinted by permission of Prentice-Hall, Inc., Englewood Cliffs, New Jersey.)

an apprenticeship used to be the primary, if not the only, prerequisite for securing a position as a director of intramurals, this model clearly depicts that practical work experience is but one of three areas of skills and knowledges which together comprise a concept of managerial ability. Each of these is examined briefly below.

The intramural program in the public schools is gradually increasing in stature, size, and scope. The problem of heavy demand on inadequate facilities, which in the past has allowed for little or no intramural offerings, is now being handled more intelligently as administrators become more cognizant of their responsibility to provide cocurricular activities for *all.* More and more, the people who must conduct activities in these facilities are meeting together with building principals and cooperatively coming up with ways of sharing facilities. Very important, too, is the recognition that less desirable times must be shared. For example, a typical high school with one divided gymnasium (Gym A and Gym B) has the following cocurricular activities to schedule into this gymnasium: boys' varsity basketball, girls' varsity basketball, boys' reserve basketball, and boys' and girls' intramurals. Cooperative planning on the part of all the advisers concerned resulted in the following schedule.

Day and time	Gym A	Gym B
Monday		
3:15–4:00	Boys' varsity basketball	Boys' intramurals
4:00–4:45	Boys' varsity basketball	Boys' varsity basketball
4:45–5:30	Boys' reserve basketball	Girls' varsity basketball
Tuesday		
3:15–4:00	Boys' varsity basketball	Girls' intramurals
4:00–4:45	Boys' varsity basketball	
4:45–5:30	Boys' reserve basketball	Girls' varsity basketball
Wednesday		
3:15–4:00	Boys' varsity basketball	Boys' intramurals
4:00–4:45	Boys' varsity basketball	
4:45–5:30	Boys' reserve basketball	Girls' varsity basketball
Thursday		
3:15–4:00	Boys' varsity basketball	Girls' intramurals
4:00–4:45	Boys' varsity basketball	
4:45–5:30	Boys' reserve basketball	Girls' varsity basketball
Friday		
3:15–4:00	Boys' intramurals	Girls' intramurals
4:00–5:30	Girls' varsity basketball game	
6:30–9:30	Boys' reserve & varsity basketball games	

Admittedly, it is fairly easy to schedule just these four activities. In case other groups, such as the wrestling team, cheerleaders, and boys' and girls' leaders' clubs, also need to be scheduled into these facilities, additional time periods such as 7:00 to 8:00 in the morning and 6:30 to 9:00 in the evening can be used on some days. The concept of sharing undesirable times is a significant one. Although it is ideal to schedule one activity (for example, boys' varsity basketball) at the same time every day, it is educationally unjustifiable always to schedule another activity (for example, the wrestling team or girls' varsity basketball) at a less desirable time, such as 7:00 a. m.

The second trend, which is particularly noticeable at the college level, is the demand for facilities where less structured programs can be carried on. As a result, more and more recreational facilities are being built in and around residence hall complexes. Modern complexes of this type often have hard-surfaced, multipurpose play areas adjacent to the buildings for such activities as basketball, volleyball, tennis, and badminton. In addition, bowling lanes, game rooms for billiards, table tennis and the like, and even swimming pools are often found inside the buildings.

Many colleges and universities now have gymnasium-type buildings which are specifically set aside for intramural activities. Less structured, informal recreational programs as well as the traditionally organized competitive intramural programs are carried out in buildings of this type. This trend is perhaps indicative of a new "philosophy" of intramurals, as formulated by Jones,[3] in which each of four related areas is shown as a functioning entity with its own unique identity. A horizontal model, then, is necessary to show that no program is seen as more important than any other (Fig. 2), although the solid line between athletics and intramurals connotes a closer relationship than that which exists between instruction and recreation. This is in marked contrast to the traditional vertical model, which places intramurals at the midpoint of a hierarchy between the programs of instruction and varsity athletics (Fig. 3).

The third trend, that toward specialized professional preparation programs in intramural administration, encompasses a concurrent concept of extending campus recreational programs to include not only physical recreation activities, but also such other leisure-time pursuits as arts and crafts, music, and theater, all under the guidance of a single administrative unit. Stevenson proposes an organizational model for an endeavor of this type (Fig. 4), which he believes will ensure proper coordination of all types of recreational activities.

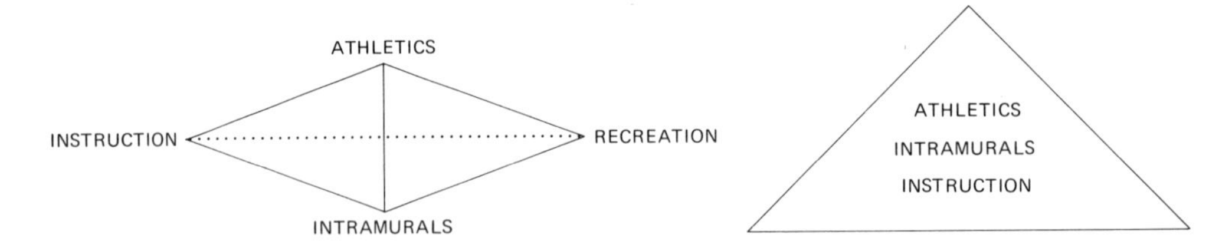

Fig. 2 Horizontal model.

Fig. 3 Vertical model.

---

[3] Tom R. Jones, "Needed: A New Philosophical Model for Intramurals," *Journal of Health, Physical Education and Recreation,* **42** (November–December 1971): 34.

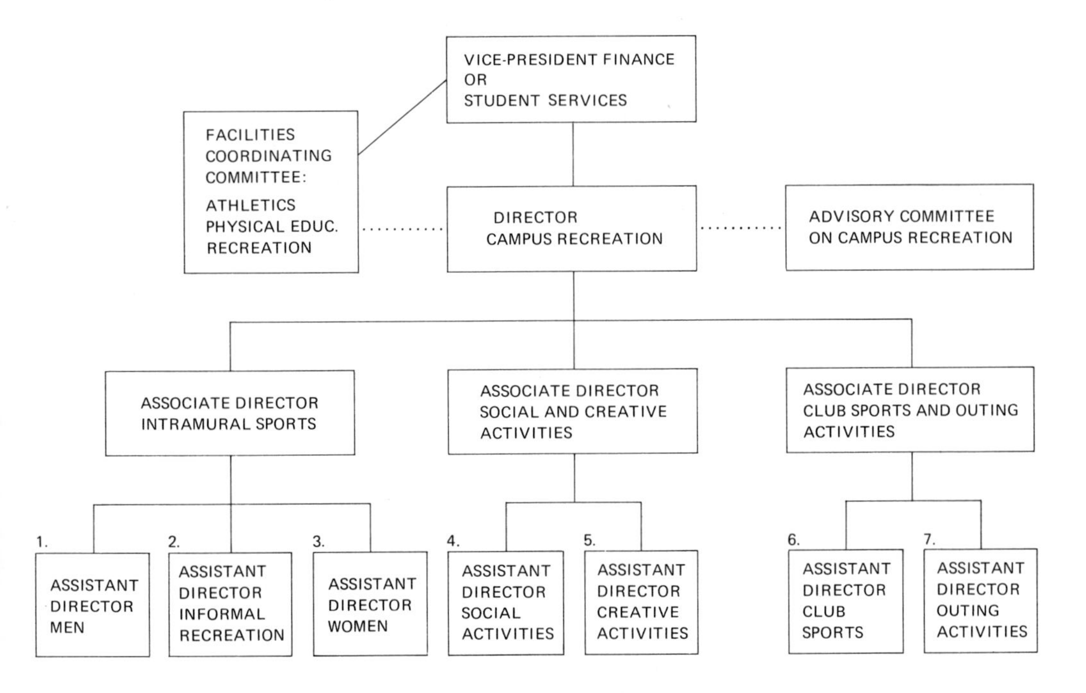

LEGEND FOR MODEL

(1) = Responsible for team, dual, and individual competitive intramural programs for men.

(2) = Responsible for informal/ "free-play" activities program.

(3) = Responsible for team, dual, and individual competitive intramural programs for women, and for competitive co-recreational intramural program.

(4) = Responsible for social activities such as nonphysical recreation, dances, parties, and so forth.

(5) = Responsible for music, dance, drama, lectures, and so on.

(6) = Responsible for organization and administration of physical recreation-oriented sports clubs.

(7) = Responsible for orienteering, hunting, fishing, sailing, skating, skiing, and similar activities.

Fig. 4 Model for structuring a division of campus sports and recreation. (James A. Peterson, *Intramural Administration: Theory and Practice,* © 1976, p. 27. Reprinted by permission of Prentice-Hall Inc., Englewood Cliffs, New Jersey.)

INTRAMURAL TERMINOLOGY

As with all other programs, certain terms are important in any discussion of intramurals and therefore should be defined.

Intramurals is a term which in modern usage designates the entire spectrum of the program whose offerings range from tournaments in basketball, badminton, bridge, chess, and other activities to interest clubs in such diversified activities as dance, weight-lifting and SCUBA. "Intramural" literally means "within the walls" and this meaning still applies. In other words, an intramural program is one that is carried on within the confines of a school or institution. Chronologically, the term applied to the entire program has gone from "intramural athletics" to "intramural sports" to "intramural activities" to the present somewhat standard, all-inclusive "intramurals."

Extramurals implies a program which is an outgrowth of the intramural program, but which is not confined to a single institution. For example, in a city school system the intramural winners in a particular activity from all junior high schools compete against each other for the city junior high school intramural championship. The term has been used, too, to designate the very informal competitive program for girls which some schools sponsor. This concept is explored further in Chapter 15.

Play day is a day in which representatives from two or more schools engage in one or more competitive activities, but the identities of the schools are not retained. Instead, the contestants are mixed on teams according to some prearranged system.

Sports day is a day in which two or more schools compete in one or more activities and the identities of the schools are maintained.

The faculty person in charge of the program is known as the *director of intramurals* or the *intramural adviser.*

The *activity adviser* or *club adviser* is a person other than the intramural director who is in charge of a specific activity. This could conceivably be a student.

The *intramural board* is composed of representatives from the various participating units. It serves as a liaison between the students and the director and, in many cases, it formulates policies and regulations.

A *managerial system* is advisable in a well-run program of intramurals. *Managers* are students who handle the routine details of a particular activity. Such details may include, for example, securing officials, scheduling games, and distributing equipment. In addition to activity managers, a *managerial board* may be incorporated into a large program. This board is composed of one or two representatives from each class who handle less routine details, such as publicity and point records and under whose guidance the activity managers operate.

A *protest board* is probably a necessity in a flourishing program, particularly one which is at least partially student run. It is the duty of this board to adjudicate all protests submitted to it.

THE PLACE OF INTRAMURALS IN THE SCHOOL PROGRAM

As was noted, intramurals developed in a random manner and within a framework which was almost entirely outside the province of the school. From this beginning, intramurals have evolved into a program which today is considered by most educators a vital part of the school's cocurricular offerings. Never before in the history of the world has there been such a need for recreation. Modern-day pressures permeate even the field of education, and therefore most people recognize the need for everyone, including the young, to be provided with outlets through which tensions can be released. Only in this way can people recreate themselves, becoming lost momentarily in some form of play. Although recreation does not have to be of a physical nature, it is doubly beneficial if it is, since physical activity simultaneously releases tension and exercises the body.

Objectives

Many objectives can be legitimately advanced for an intramural program. The degree to which each is met depends, of course, on a variety of factors, such as the activity, the educational level of the participants, and the leadership.

Recreation ("*re*-creation") is probably the paramount objective. If one can become lost in play and thus forget pressures and tensions, one will be more productive upon returning to the task at hand, whether one is a student, a laborer, or an executive. An intramural program is educationally justifiable in an age in which more and more children join the ranks of the mentally ill, commit suicide, or become deviants from society. The time-honored motto of "A sport for everyone and everyone in a sport" is still apropos today, although the concept has broadened to include more than "sports" activities.

Group loyalty is a worthy objective in modern America. Societal mores, especially at the senior high school and college level, seem to protest vigorously against this concept and to label persons who embrace such values as being "square." Nevertheless, education professes a belief in this value and can foster it by providing a well-run intramural program.

The objective which encompasses the *wise use of leisure time* can well be achieved through a diversified program of intramurals.

Sports skills learned in the physical education class can be refined in the intramural program. Since ability in an activity is an important factor in one's interest and participation in that activity, the student needs the opportunity to develop a skill to the point where it will somewhat guarantee participation for the rest of one's life. Especially important here are the so-called "lifetime sports."

Interest in *physical fitness* has never been greater in our society. Many of the activities within an intramural program are conducive to the development of this attribute. Since most intramural participation is limited to once or twice per week, it must be recognized that some activities contribute much more to this objective than do others.

The ramifications of the term *social skills* are many and varied. Not only can the student become more competent in certain activity skills through which one can gain psychologically necessary social contacts, but he or she can learn concomitant skills such as cooperation, respect, and fair play which make these contacts more pleasurable and thus help develop self-confidence.

These are only the most important objectives of intramurals; many others could be listed which no doubt are capable of being met to some degree. If the above aims are met to the fullest extent, the program needs no other justification!

Principles

If an intramural program is to meet the above objectives and if, indeed, it is to be educationally sound, certain principles must underlie the program.

The welfare of the participant must be a paramount consideration. Physical welfare is but one aspect of this picture. It is also necessary to consider such things as the *time* when activities are scheduled and the *stress* placed upon them.

The "sports for all" idiom dictates that another prime *principle* shall be that of *nonexclusion.* There must be an opportunity for everyone to participate—regardless of skill level, regardless of physical or mental handicap, and regardless of scholastic achievement. If the objectives for the program are good ones, they are good for everyone! It is important to recognize that participation can and must, in a democratic society, be extended beyond the playing of a game. It includes as well such aspects as managing an activity or a team, officiating, and keeping the point records up-to-date.

The program must be voluntary. In spite of the fact that many fine outcomes are possible, cocurricular activities should not be mandatory.

The objectives of the program must not be stressed to the point where undesirable aspects also develop. For example, under the guise of group loyalty, rivalry might develop to the extreme that too often characterizes the interscholastic athletic program. Likewise, even though group loyalty is significant, the concept of individuality should not be lost.

The old adage of "change occurs slowly" dictates that *organizational alterations should be made only after thorough evaluation of existing policy.* Such changes should come about as a result of democratic interchange of ideas between the director and the participants or their representatives. Above all, if a change is made which later seems to be productive of no or poor results, the change should be rescinded. A word of caution is necessary here: The results of an alteration in policy or procedure should not be evaluated too quickly. It takes time for results to become apparent.

Administration of the Program

A sound program of intramurals is impossible without wise, responsible leadership. The authority for developing the program should be invested in a faculty member who is generally called the intramural director. Ideally, the director should be a professionally trained physical educator who has time to devote to the program, who is genuinely interested in it, and who has no other cocurricular assignments. However, since in many physical education departments all staff members not only teach but also coach one or more varsity teams, it becomes necessary to change the intramural director as the athletic season changes. For example, the football coach can direct intramurals during the basketball season, and the basketball coach can take over during the baseball season.

The role of students in the administration of the program is a vital one. As explained earlier, at the beginning intramurals were entirely student conducted, and even though the program flourished to the extent that faculty supervision became imperative, student involvement is still desirable. The framework within which students operate is largely the managerial system as set up by the Intramural board. In the sample administrative line chart (Fig. 5), the Intramural Board has divided the managerial system into two main components: (1) activity managers, and (2) class managers.

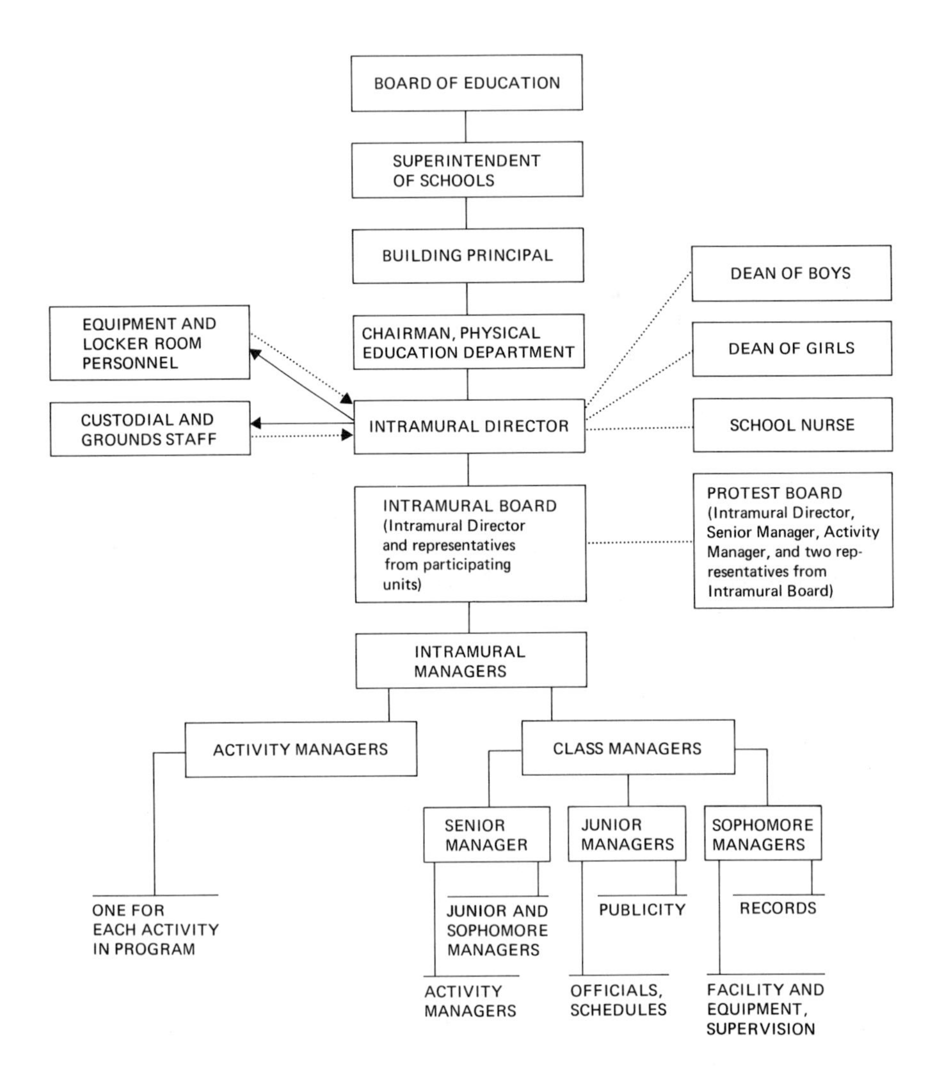

Fig. 5 Sample administrative line chart (for senior high schools).

Each activity has its own student manager. Generally this is someone particularly interested in the activity and, in the case of club activities, someone who can instruct or assist in the instruction. The point system may be so arranged that activity managers receive points for their services.

The class manager system, if well organized, can relieve the director of much of the necessary routine work. In the example in Fig. 5, there are two managers from both the sophomore and the junior class, and one senior manager. Since this is not a seasonal responsibility (as in the case of activity managers), it is perhaps well to award points for these duties. The managerial system is an apprenticeship system in which the senior manager might even be a paid position (particularly at the college level).

As the line chart (Fig. 5) suggests, several of the school's personnel used in advisory capacities by the intramural director who, in turn, shares this advice with the Intramural Board or the advisory personnel can report directly to the Board. In any event, if the intramural director believes in the democratic process, he or she will allow the program to be largely prescribed by students.

Program of Activities

Just as the name of the subject has evolved from "intramural athletics" through "intramural activities" to "intramurals," so too has the program of activities undergone a change from a strictly athletic type of offering to a program which offers individual sports as well as activities such as chess, frisbee, wrist-wrestling, checkers, and bridge. Several factors underlie the selection of activities to offer in the program. Time, facilities, equipment, and finances are usually problems to one degree or another. Therefore, in view of the philosophy of an activity for everyone, it is advisable to offer a few well-conducted activities which service the majority of students. Generally speaking, very vigorous activities should be offered only if there is the opportunity to require a training period of some kind. Most activities, especially sports activities, are more or less seasonal; therefore, they should be offered during the season when interest is highest. Also, if it is at all possible, approximately the same number of activities should be offered each season.

Types of Activities

Team sports continue to be very popular and are probably the backbone of the intramural program, especially at the secondary level. Such activities can be conducted within a framework of tournament competition.

Individual sports are also very popular and are largely conducted within a tournament framework. If the recreation objective is to be achieved to its fullest, the program in individual sports must be broad.

Meets are usually "one shot" affairs such as a swimming meet or a track-and-field meet. However, since such meets are quite vigorous, it is recommended that some kind of premeet practice and training be required.

Interest clubs are comprised of individuals who have a great interest in a particular activity. Usually, one of the prime objectives of an interest club is the refinement of skill. Clubs which are popular in intramurals encompass such diverse activities as dance, gymnastics, chess, and weightlifting.

Corecreational activities are becoming more and more popular in the intramural program. Various activities in each of the types above are conducive to corecreational participation. Any superiority that either sex may have in a specific activity can be counterbalanced if care is taken when organizing the competition. Thus even a highly competitive situation can be challenging, stimulating, and interesting to both sexes. Some universities even offer very successful coed tournaments in ice hockey.

Mini-tournaments, which extend over a very brief time period such as a holiday or a weekend, can be conducted in almost any activity. Many persons who might not ordinarily participate are attracted by mini-tournaments since the time needed to determine a final winner is short.

Special activities such as faculty play nights, or parents' nights when students invite either or both parents to participate with them, have a definite place in the program, especially as an effort to foster better public relations. Various activities for handicapped persons, such as wheelchair basketball, are gaining in popularity.

Time and Place

As described earlier, all groups should have equal opportunity to use school facilities at times which are conducive to maximum participation. The most popular, and probably the most desirable, time is immediately after classes are over in the afternoon. Other possible times are before school starts in the morning, during the lunch hour, in the evening after dinner, on Saturdays, and even during the summer recess. Each of these times has advantages and disadvantages, depending on such factors as availability of students, transportation, health considerations, and availability of adequate faculty supervision.

PARTICIPATING UNITS

The intramural director must be thoroughly acquainted with the school and its administrative organization as well as the social climate of the times before he or she can identify the various competing units intelligently. Some of the more popular units are classes, home rooms, geographical areas, and independent groups.

Class units are particularly desirable in very small schools and at the elementary school level. Usually there is a feeling of cohesion among class members that makes for spirited competition. However, in the average secondary school, unless several teams can be entered from the same grade level, the use of the class unit is a delimiting participation factor.

Homeroom units are probably the best all-around units for competition in the typical secondary school today. This is particularly true if the administrative setup is such that a student's homeroom, first assigned when he or she enters the school, remains fixed throughout the school years. In this case, pupils get to know one another well, and a feeling of loyalty to the homeroom usually exists.

Geographical or neighborhood units are increasing in popularity, and the intramural director should explore all facets of this possibility. Facilities are often the limiting factor in a secondary school program. Most elementary schools, however, have gymnasiums and often they are not used to capacity. Therefore, scheduling participation in these facilities according to neighborhood units solves several problems, not the least of which is transportation. Generally, the elementary school is within walking distance of the students' homes. It is a simple matter, then, to transport secondary school pupils to the elementary school, so that after the activities are finished, the participants can walk home.

Independent or "pick-up" or arbitrary units are often used. However, generally speaking, their use can be questioned on at least two counts. First, since such groupings may constantly change, the achievement of objectives such as group loyalty is difficult. On the other hand, a group of skilled players can get together, enter a team in nearly every activity, and therefore monopolize the program. This can be circumvented if the director, with student help, assigns to teams all individuals who desire to participate in a certain activity.

Other possible units are the clubs such as the Science Club, F. T. A., Hi-Y, and the like.

Some activities are more conducive to a particular form of competing unit than others. The intramural director needs to consider all ramifications of the program in order to ensure maximum participation.

In general, the larger the unit, the more difficult it is to organize, but intelligent preplanning should overcome the built-in problems.

TYPES AND SELECTIONS OF TOURNAMENTS

The success of any kind of tournament depends on careful advanced planning. Too often intramural programs seem to get in a rut in that every tournament is organized as the previous one was. Variety in the types of tournaments should help to maintain interest in the program. Tournaments can be divided into basically three types: elimination, round-robin, and extended.

Elimination tournaments are used to a greater extent in the intramural program than any other type. This is understandable since time and facilities are usually at a premium and this type of tournament determines a winner in the shortest possible time.

An elimination tournament is based on the elimination of one-half of the contestants in each round. After a match, the winner advances to the next round, and the loser is either eliminated completely or dropped to some form of a losers' bracket. The original placement of entries on the tournament draw chart can be either by chance or according to seeds. The use of seeds (an attempt to rate the players' abilities and place them so that the two best contestants or teams meet in the final round) is questionable in the intramural program. If seeds are used, however, a general rule-of-thumb is to award no more than two seeded places for every eight contestants. The drawing of an elimination tournament chart must be governed by certain rules. If the number of entries is a power of two, no problem arises, since each round will automatically follow the same pattern. However, if the original number of entries is not a power of two, byes must be inserted. A bye is simply a free ticket to the second round. *All byes should be eliminated in the first round.* The number of byes necessary is determined by subtracting the number of entries from the next higher power of two. For example, is the number of entries is 9 ($2^3 + 1$), the number of necessary byes is 7, since the next higher power of two above 9 is 16 (2^4), and sixteen minus nine is seven. In this example, since the number of byes is nearly equal to the number of entries, the draw sheet usually *implies* the byes. Byes and/or seeds should be placed on the draw sheet according to the following scheme: number one at the top of the top bracket, number two at the bottom of the bottom bracket, number three at the bottom of the top bracket, number four at the top of the bottom bracket. Continue to alternate in this way until all are placed. Figures 6 and 7 illustrate these principles. Note that contestants are shown by capital italic letters, rounds are shown by Roman numerals, the order in which games are played is designated by Arabic numerals and seeds—in this case the theoretical maximum, four—are shown parenthetically.

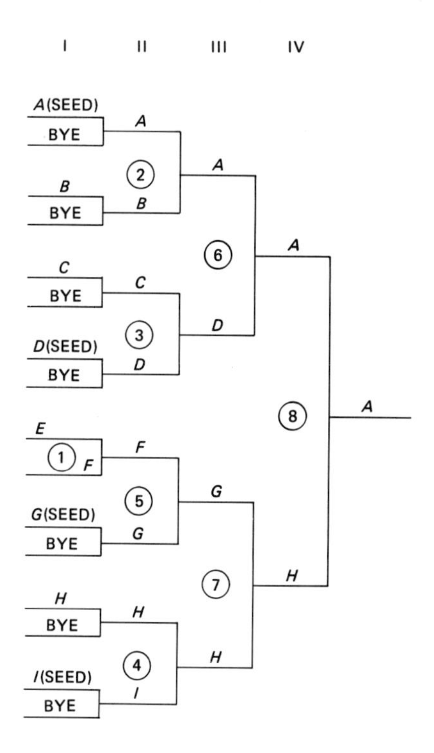

Fig. 6 Nine-team single elimination, byes and seeds shown.

The most popular types of elimination tournaments are the single elimination, the double elimination, and the consolation. It is important to remember that arbitrary decisions about any of these types can be made so long as they are made *and publicized* before the tournament begins. For example, in a single elmination tournament (see Fig. 6), A is obviously the champion and H (the entry which upset seeded I) is the runner-up. An arbitrary decision about third and fourth place can be made. It can be decided that the loser in round III to the ultimate champion is the third-place winner, or it can be decided that the losers in round III must play-off for third and fourth place. In either event, the decision should be made ahead of time.

In *single elimination* tournaments, certain formulas based on the number of competitors are used to determine how long it will take to finish the tournament. To determine the *number of matches* required to select first and second place, subtract one from the total number of entries (9 entries, 8 matches). If a play-off is to be held for third and fourth place, one additional match is necessary,

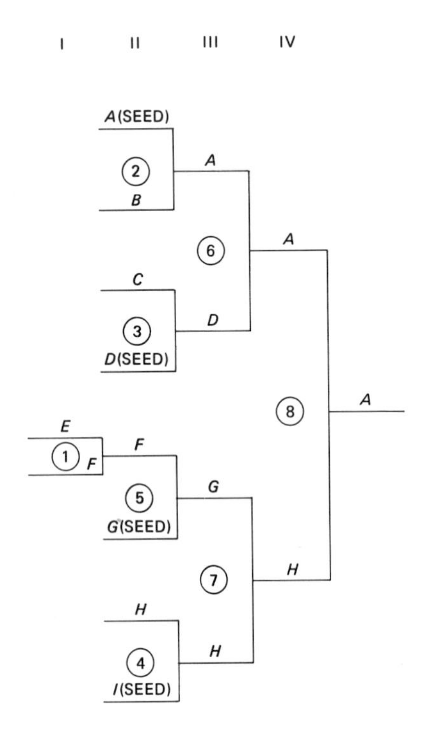

Fig. 7 Nine-team single elimination, byes implied.

and thus the formula becomes: the number of matches is equal to the total number of entries. To determine the *number of rounds* necessary to determine first and second place, determine the number of times two has to be multiplied by itself (that is, the power of two) to equal or exceed the number of entries. For example, with 9 entries 2 must be raised to the fourth power, or 16, to equal or exceed the number of entries. Therefore, four rounds are necessary.

A *double elimination* tournament is one of the fairest types since each entry must be defeated twice before being eliminated. This is one of the more complicated tournaments to show graphically, since the losers' rounds keep adding new contestants as entries drop out of the winners' rounds. The losers' rounds can be drawn to the left of the initial first round, with the winners' rounds going to the right (Fig. 8); or the losers' rounds can be drawn as a separate tournament (Fig. 9). The formula for determining the *number of matches* is $(N \times 2) - 2$, where N is the number of entries. If there are 12 entries (N), 22 or 23 matches are required. (If the win-

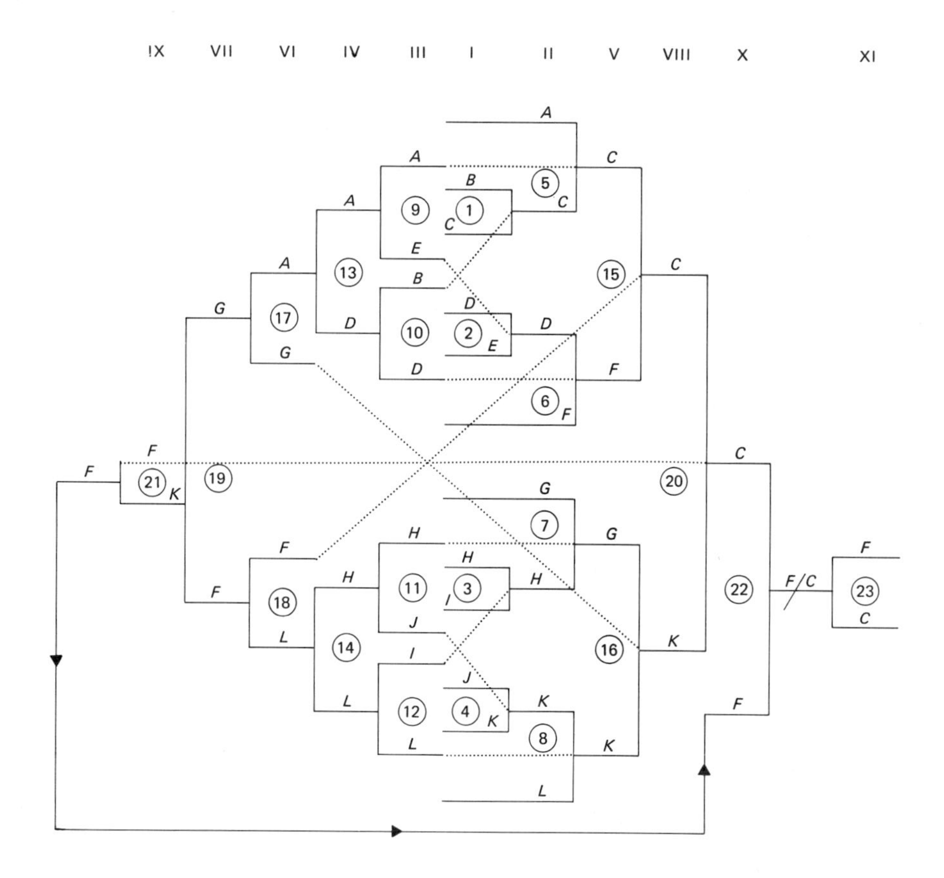

Fig. 8 Twelve-team double elimination, byes implied (side by side).

ner of the losers' rounds defeats the winner of the winners' rounds, one additional match is necessary.)

In order to ensure that losers do not meet the same contestant twice, or to postpone their meeting as long as possible, brackets should be crossed as the loser's are dropped down. (This is indicated by dashed lines in Fig. 8.)

Consolation tournaments are used when there is time to allow *first* round losers (or second round losers who drew byes the first round) to play again. The draw sheets can be drawn with losers to the left and winners to the right or as separate tournaments. Usually in a consolation tournament the winner of the losers' bracket is allowed to challenge the winner of the winners' bracket. This arbitrary decision should be made, however, before the tournament

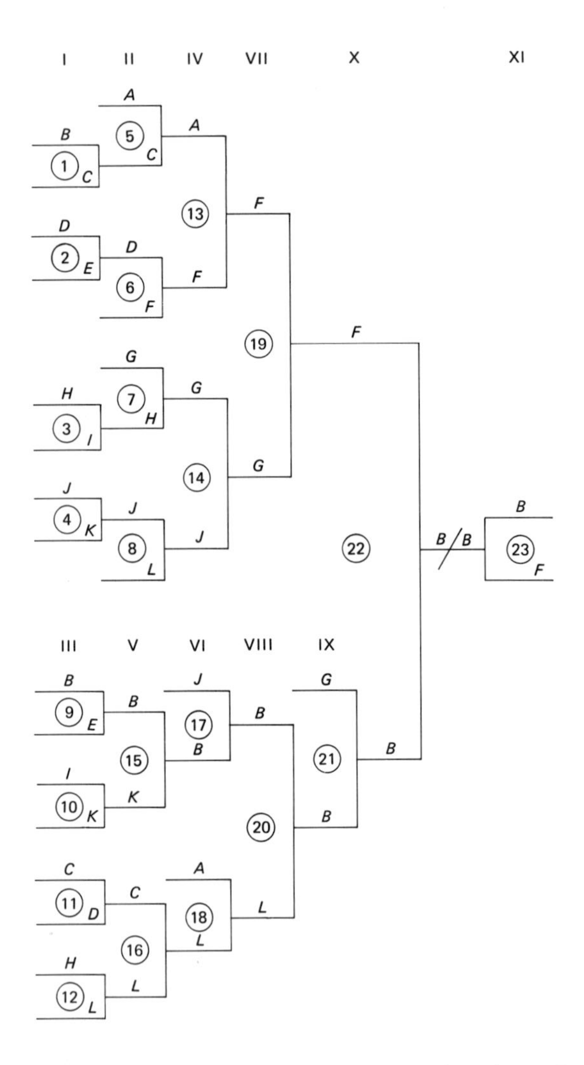

Fig. 9 Twelve-team double elimination, byes implied (separate tournament for losers).

commences (Fig. 10). Note in the example that *A* and *L*, who drew first-round byes, won the first time they played. However, *F* and *G*, who also drew first-round byes, were defeated the first time they played; therefore, even though their losses occurred in the second round, they are entered on the losers' side.

Another type of consolation tournament, one which selects winners through fourth-place, is popularly referred to as the "wrestling-

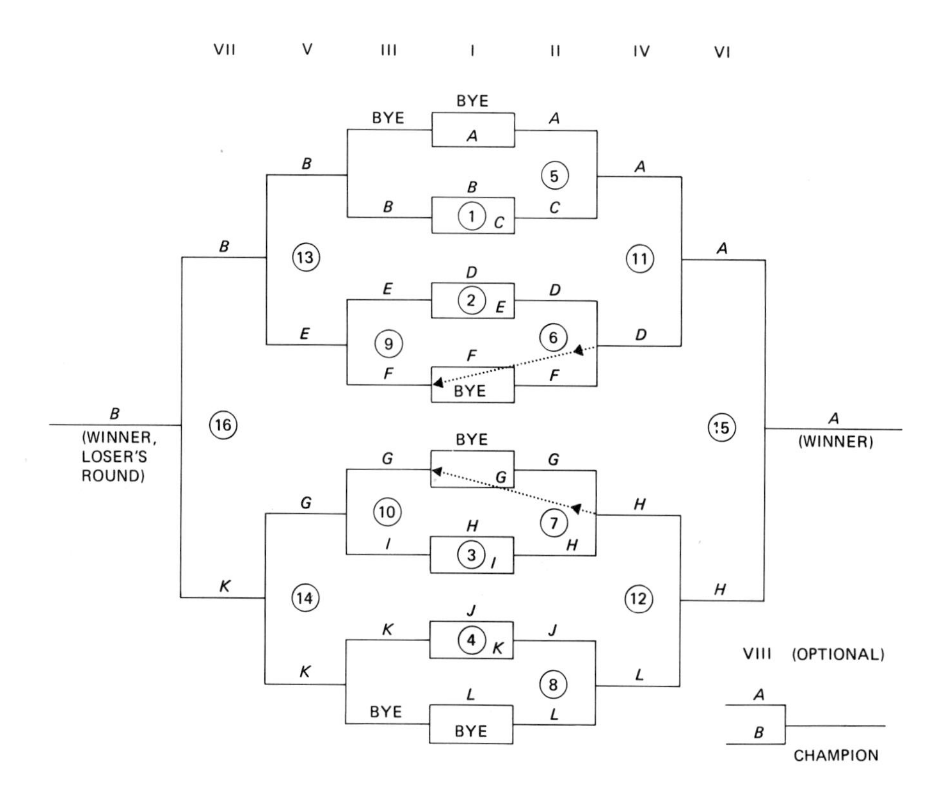

Fig. 10 Twelve-team consolation tournament, byes shown.

type" tournament. Here, all losers to the ultimate first- and second-place winners compete again for third and fourth place (Fig. 11).

Round-Robin Tournaments

Round-robin tournaments, in which each contestant plays every other contestant, are recommended if sufficient time is available. This is one of the fairest types of tournaments, since each contestant competes against the total entry. It also has the advantage of allowing contestants to become better acquainted.

In order to keep a running account of where each entry stands, points can be awarded as follows: win, 3; tie, 2; loss, 1; and forfeit, 0. This scheme is recommended because it gives some credit to the teams which show up to play and are defeated as opposed to those teams which forfeit.

The formula for determining the number of games *per round* is $\frac{1}{2}N$ when N (the number of entries) is even, and $(N - 1)/2$ when N

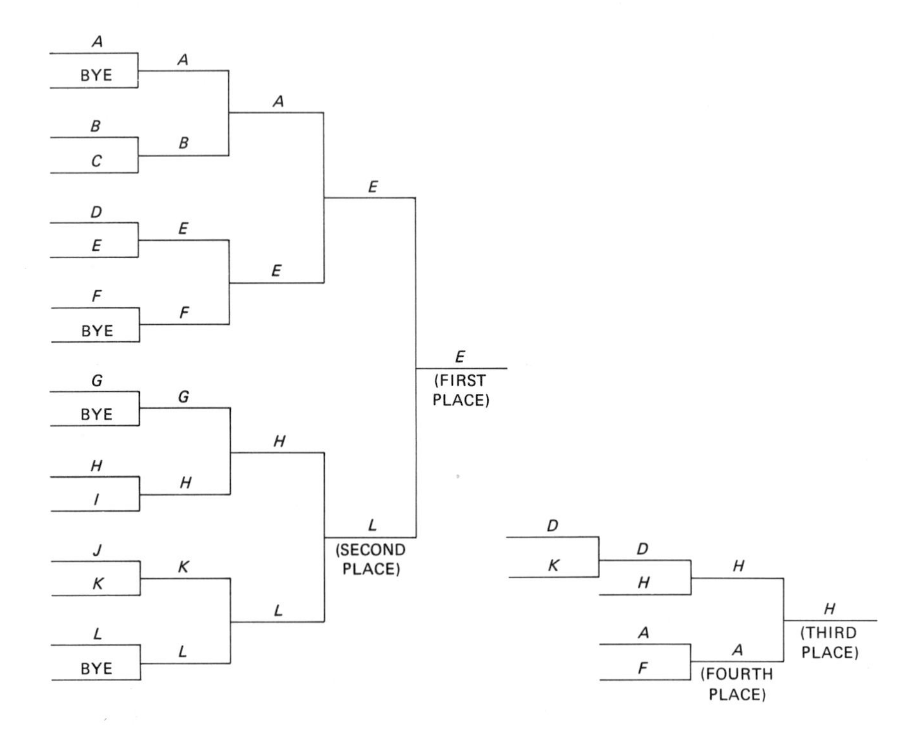

Fig. 11 "Wrestling-type" tournament, twelve entries, byes shown.

is odd. (For instance, for 8 entries there must be 4 games; for 11 entries, 5 games.) The number of rounds is equal to the number of entries if *N* is odd, and to the number of entries minus one if *N* is even.

The formula for determining the *total number of games* necessary to complete a single round-robin is $N (N - 1)/2$.

If time is a factor, one can reduce the total number of games required by breaking down the total entry into leagues. For example, 8 entries can be divided into two leagues of 4 entries each, thus reducing the total number of games required from 28 to 12—a significant difference! Regardless of the number of leagues, some arbitrary decision must be made on what method to use to determine ultimate winners. A popular method is to place the first- and second-place winners from each league in a single elimination play-off.

Drawing the schedule is facilitated by giving each team a number, and then rotating the numbers around a "pivot point" for each round (see Fig. 12). If the number of teams is an odd one, designate the bye with a zero.

Round I	Round II	Round III	Round IV	Round V
0–9	0–8	0–7	0–6	0–5
1–8	9–7	8–6	7–5	6–4
2–7	1–6	9–5	8–4	7–3
3–6	2–5	1–4	9–3	8–2
4–5	3–4	2–3	1–2	9–1
Round VI	**Round VII**	**Round VIII**	**Round IX**	
0–4	0–3	0–2	0–1	
5–3	4–2	3–1	2–9	
6–2	5–1	4–9	3–8	
7–1	6–9	5–8	4–7	
8–9	7–8	6–7	5–6	

Fig. 12 Round-robin schedule, nine teams.

A simple way to keep the participants informed of the progress of the tournament is shown in Fig. 13. The numbers assigned to the teams are listed at both the top and side of the chart. (A list of the teams and their assigned numbers should be posted nearby.) The date, time, and playing area for all games can be recorded in advance. As soon as a game is completed, the score should also be posted in the square across and below the competing numbers. In order that all may understand who the winner is, always record the score of the left-hand team first. (For example, in the figure the entry in the square below team 5 and opposite team 4 indicates that team 5 was scheduled to play team 4 on September 21 at 4:30 on field II, and that team 4 forfeited the game.) Assuming that the first activity in the fall is a soccer tournament and that two fields are available at two different times, two days a week, Fig. 13 shows that the first round has already been played. It also shows that team 1 defeated team 8, 2–0; team 7 defeated team 2, 3–1; teams 3 and 6 tied; and team 4 forfeited (therefore, team 5 won, 1–0). It is well to post accumulative scores nearby also. If this is done, the totals to date would show teams 1, 5, and 7 tied with 3 points; teams 3 and 6 with 2 points each; teams 2 and 8 with 1 point each; and team 4 with no points. (See our earlier discussion for a recommended scoring system.)

Extended Tournaments

Tournaments of this type are conducted over a period of weeks or months. Since contestants usually schedule their own matches, an

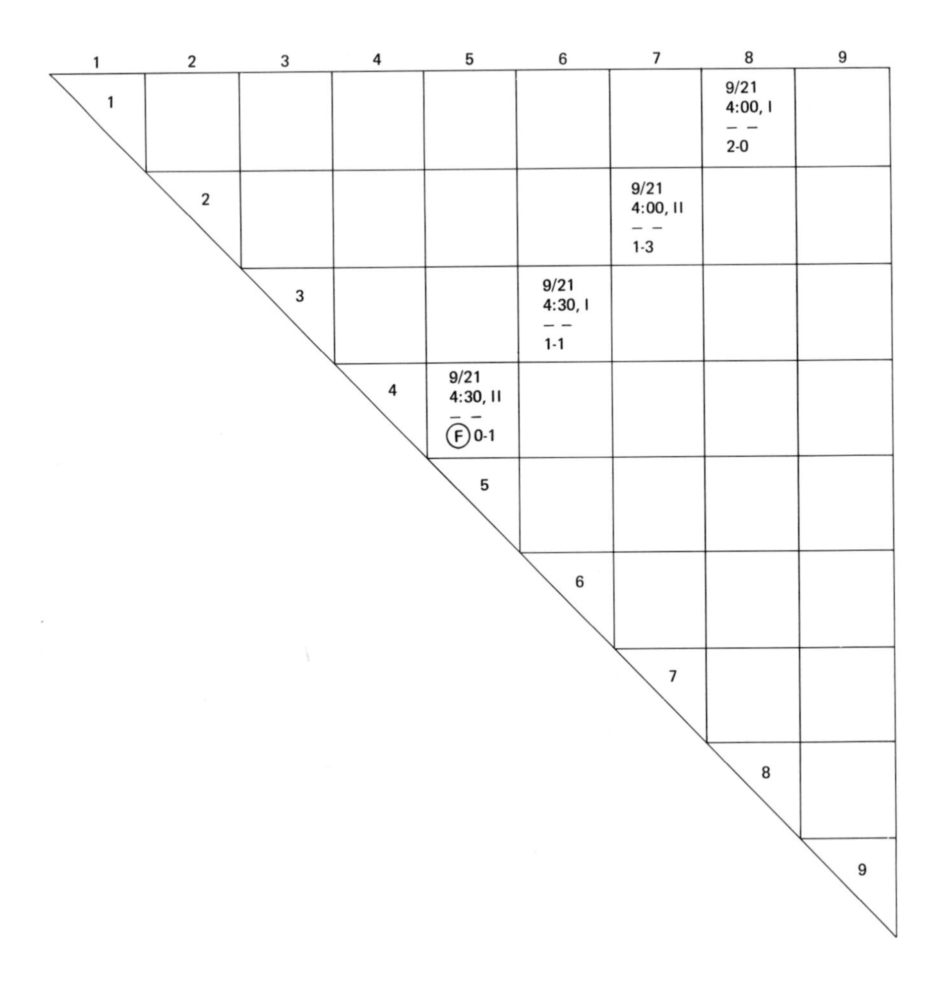

Fig. 13 Sample round-robin record sheet.

extended tournament is fairly easy to organize and requires little supervision. Probably the most popular types are the ladder, the pyramid, and the accumulated.

The *ladder tournament* is undoubtedly the best known and most used of the extended type. It is particularly appropriate for individual competition. The objective in a ladder tournament is to work one's way to the top and remain there. Advances to the top are gained by challenging someone on a higher rung and defeating him or her. Initial spots on the ladder usually are determined by chance. If seeding is used, all entries are listed in order of ability and the list is then inverted; in other words, the best player starts on the

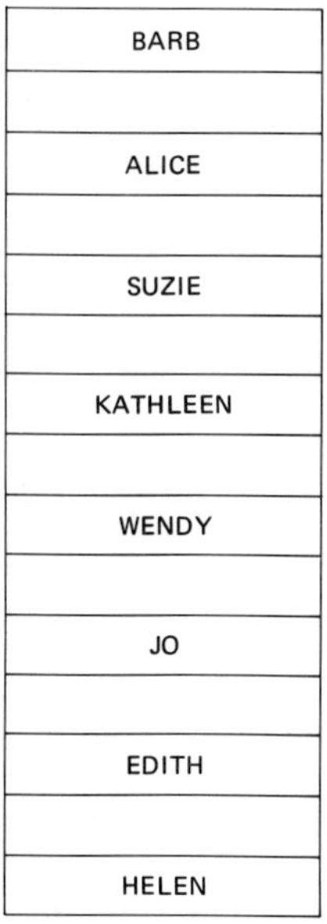

BARB
ALICE
SUZIE
KATHLEEN
WENDY
JO
EDITH
HELEN

Fig. 14 Sample ladder tournament.

bottom rung. Some of the arbitrary decisions which need to be made are (1) how many rungs above his or her own the contestant can challenge (usually only one or two), (2) what the position of the challenger will be if he or she wins (usually he or she exchanges spots with the defeated person), (3) the final date of the tournament, (4) the minimum and maximum number of matches that can be played in a certain time period (for example, at least one but not more than two per week), and (5) which challenge must be accepted (usually the first one offered). Figure 14 shows an example of a diagram of a ladder tournament.

There are several types of *pyramid tournaments* and each has differing regulations. The most popular, and also the simplest, is the so-called "standard" type in which all the spaces in the pyramid are filled, by lot, before the activity starts. Any player may challenge any other player in the same horizontal row (see Fig. 15). The winner may then challenge anyone in the row above. Upon winning, he or she changes places with the defeated contestant. Other general hints and rules are the same as for a ladder tournament.

An *accumulation tournament* is suited to either individual or team competition. Since the object is to reach some goal which has been preset, this type of tournament can be used to develop ability as well as interest and participation. An example might be to run to New York City and back. Assuming that this distance is 1000 miles

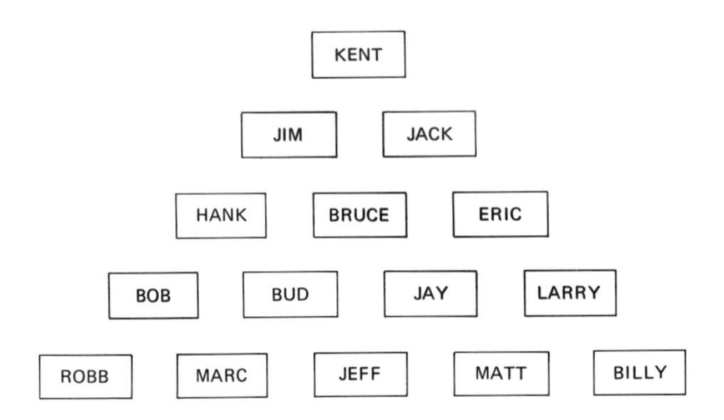

Fig. 15 Sample pyramid tournament (standard type).

and that the distance around the track is one-quarter mile, then it takes 4000 laps around the track to achieve the goal. It can arbitrarily be decided that a team consists of five runners, each runner may run no more than sixteen laps per day, and the laps run by an individual must be consecutive ones. At this rate it will take between two and three months to achieve the goal, assuming that at the start the contestants are not capable of running sixteen consecutive laps.

POINT SYSTEMS AND AWARDS

Whether or not point systems and awards are necessary in a program in intramurals remains a debatable subject. Theoretically, participation in an activity is its own reward and extrinsic motivating devices are not needed. This ideal may be approached in a college program, but most other educational levels seem to need some kind of award system. Awards do not dictate point systems, however, since awards often go only to winners.

Those in charge of an intramural program probably need to wrestle with the philosophic question of whether participation or achievement (winning) is more important. A rationale can be developed for both concepts and quite often, particularly at the secondary level, each is assigned equal importance. In this case a point system is necessary if awards are to be given also for participation.

Point systems can be kept for individuals, for groups, or for both. For example, Homeroom 202 may enter a basketball team which wins second place in the tournament. This homeroom, then, can obtain so many points for entering a team and completing its schedule without default and so many extra points for winning second place. The team can also receive a trophy, a banner or the like for receiving second-place honors. In addition, each team member can receive so many points for fullfilling his or her obligation to the team. At the end of the year, the homeroom with the highest total number of points may receive an All-Sports Trophy, while individuals who accumulate a designated number of points may win a school letter, a tie-tack (boys), a bracelet charm (girls), or some other kind of individual award.

It is obvious that point systems, if used, must be simple; otherwise, the keeping of necessary records becomes an insurmountable task in terms of time and effort involved.

When awards are given, they should be simple and inexpensive. In the case of an accumulative year-to-year individual point system, awards should increase in value to the participant, but they should remain of little monetary value.

SPECIAL PROBLEMS

Many of the problems which are unique to intramurals require regulations to govern them. Regulations, however, should be kept as minimal as possible in order not to overstructure the program.

Eligibility

Problems of eligibility revolve around factors such as scholarship, participation by varsity players, and participation by professionals. As indicated previously, there should be no scholarship barriers. The argument advanced about requiring certain scholastic standards for varsity participation because players will have less time for study cannot be justified for intramurals, since the average participant in this program spends perhaps one, or at the most, two hours per week in the program. In general, varsity, reserve, and professional players are not allowed to compete in intramurals in the same activity.

If classes are used as the participating units, the number of credits or hours which constitute each class must be clearly defined.

In the college program, a decision must be made concerning the status of fraternity (sorority) pledges. Generally, they are not allowed to play for the fraternity or sorority.

Finances

Theoretically, the money necessary to run any cocurricular program should come from the board of education. If this occurs, the program director must assess cost-benefit analyses realistically and well. Existing or increased financial support cannot be justified if it cannot be conclusively shown that program objectives are attainable. When board of education funds are not available, other frequently used sources are the physical education budget, athletic receipts, student activity fees, dues, and various money-making projects such as concession stands at athletic contests, paper drives, and car washes.

Forfeits

The problem of forfeits is a constant one in spite of determined efforts to avoid them. Certainly any forfeiting team or individual should not receive points. The intramural director needs constantly to conduct educational campaigns against forfeits—campaigns based on a plea for responsibility to carry out the commitment made on entrance into the activity. The director's efforts to schedule events well in advance and to publicize all details generally pay dividends.

Protests

Protests should be avoided whenever possible. If regulations such as the filing of a thorough written protest within a minimal time limit and one based only on such factors as the use of ineligible players or other violations of regulations are adhered to strictly, the number of protests will be small. It is doubtful that any protest against the judgment of an official should be honored. All protests should be handled quickly and objectively by whatever group is designated to consider them.

Insurance and Legal Liability

Most school insurance covers injuries which occur in an intramural program. However, legal liability (see Chapter 4) is still a factor in any school sponsored activity. Therefore, the director should make sure that all activities are thoroughly supervised and that all equipment and facilities are safe. It is perhaps well to demand parental permission forms from all participants. Although such forms are technically meaningless, they do place a moral responsibility on the parent to accept certain results which might accrue, such as an injury in an activity such as touch football where an assumption of risk is involved.

Moral and Ethical Values

The attainment of moral and ethical values is sometimes listed as an objective for the program. In this instance, the values are primarily those which revolve around a concept of sportsmanship, such as accepting officials' decisions without complaining, winning fairly and humbly, and losing graciously. One way of working toward this objective is to use a system whereby the officials rate the teams on sportsmanship items immediately after the conclusion of a game and, conversely, the captains of the teams rate the officials on competency, fairness, and the like.

Moral and ethical values are perhaps more easily achieved, at least outwardly, in individual sports, which are generally officiated by the contestants themselves.

Officiating

Since officials play such an important role in an intramural program, it is imperative that every possible step be taken to ensure quality. Since few programs at the secondary level pay officials, most directors must depend on volunteers. These volunteers must be trained to officiate as well as possible. Participants in the program must be educated to realize that their peers who officiate are, at best, neophytes and that mistakes—which are bound to occur—usually penalize both teams equally. The sex of the official is perhaps irrelevant; in fact, it is rather common practice today to assign officials only on the basis of competency and availability.

EVALUATION

There are many ways to evaluate a program of intramurals. Simple numerical statistics such as the number of participants and participations, the number of activities offered, and the number of forfeits will tell whether the program has grown and to what extent. School administrators are always interested in securing this kind of information and annual reports should be submitted to them. (Figure 16 shows a sample annual report.)

Certain evaluative check lists such as that developed by the Washington Conference[4] can be employed. Outside study groups,

---

[4] American Association of Health, Physical Education, and Recreation, *Intramural Sports for College Men and Women: Washington Conference Report.* (Washington, D.C.: The Association, 1956.)

Activity	No. of Teams	No. of Individuals	No. of Participations	Forfeits	Injuries	Personnel Needed		Cost		Winners	Comments
						No.	Type	Amount	Item		
Volleyball	15	135	705	3	1-Sprained ankle	12 6 6	Umps Scorers Timers	$10.95	New time clock	1. Homeroom 102 2. Homeroom 305	Interest high. Try coed tour next year.
Chess Club	–	11	–	–	–	Mr. Smith, Math., Adviser		–	–	1. Robb Moses 2. Suzy Smith	New activity this year. Good reception.
Track and Field Meet	10	327	549	–	–	1 1 10	Starter Judge Timers	$5.00	Ribbon for awards	1. Dandy Dudes 2. Beatles	Required 4 practice sessions prior to meet
Totals											

Fig. 16. Sample annual report (summary).

such as a visiting team of experts from the state physical education association, can be invited to visit the program and evaluate it. Intramural directors can visit well-known schools to observe their programs in action.

Since the program is for students, they should not be overlooked as a potentially valuable source of evaluation. Techniques for getting students' responses are suggestion boxes, discussion groups, and brainstorming sessions.

Last, but not least, the director should become acquainted with the professional research and literature in the field. The annual *Proceedings of the National Intramural Association* is an invaluable resource for information on what's happening in the field throughout the United States.

CASE STUDY

Among the regulations for intramurals at Wilson High School is one which forbids any member of a varsity squad to compete in the same sport in intramurals. This is not a problem in most sports, since the intramural competition begins well into the sport in season. Since scheduling events in the pool had always been a problem, George Wyatt, the Intramural Director, decided to conduct the swimming intramural competition in the fall season. As soon as the announcement of sign-ups was posted, he was besieged by many complaints that almost the entire swimming team had entered the intramural competition. Wyatt called several of these participants for conferences and explained the purposes of the program to them. Most of them remarked that since the season had not yet begun, they were not members of any squad and furthermore they were not assured of making the varsity swim squad. They refused to withdraw.

Mr. Wyatt convened the Intramural Council to consider this problem.

1. What are the issues?
2. What solutions are possible?
3. What policies or principles evolve from the considerations in this case?

SELECTED REFERENCES

American Association for Health, Physical Education, and Recreation. *Intramural Sports for College Men and Women: Washington Conference Report.* Washington, D.C.: The Association, 1956.

———. *Intramurals for the Elementary School.* Chicago: Athletic Institute, 1964.

———. *Intramurals for the Junior High School.* Chicago: Athletic Institute, 1964.

———. *Intramurals for the Senior High School.* Chicago: Athletic Institute, 1964.

Beeman, Harris F., Carol A. Harding, and James H. Humphrey. *Intramural Sports: A Text and Study Guide.* Dubuque: W. C. Brown, 1974.

Boyden, E. Douglas, and Roger Burton. *Staging Successful Tournaments.* New York: Association Press, 1957.

Hyatt, R. W. *Intramural Sports: Organization and Administration.* St. Louis, Mo.: C. V. Mosby, 1977.

Hyatt, Ronald (ed.). "The Intramural Story." *Journal of Health Physical Education Recreation.* **45**: 3 (March 1974): 39–54.

Jones, Tom R. "Needed: A New Philosophical Model for Intramurals," *Journal of Health, Physical Education and Recreation,* **42**: (November-December 1971): 34.

Kleindienst, Viola, and Arthur Weston. *Intramural and Recreation Programs for Schools and Colleges.* New York: Appleton-Century-Crofts, 1964.

Leavitt, Norma, and Hartley Price. *Intramural and Recreational Sports for High School and College.* New York: Ronald Press, 1958.

Means, Louis E. *Intramurals.* Englewood Cliffs, N. J.: Prentice-Hall, 1973.

Mueller, Pat. *Intramurals: Programming and Administration.* New York: Ronald Press, 1971.

National Intramural Sports Council. "Financing Intramurals," *Journal of Physical Education and Recreation,* **46** (January 1975): 22–25.

Peterson, James A. *Intramural Administration: Theory and Practice.* Englewood Cliffs, N.J.: Prentice-Hall, 1976.

Preo, L. S., "Professional Preparation of Administrators of Intramural and Physical Recreation Programs," in J. A. Peterson (ed.) *Intramural Administration: Theory and Practice,* Englewood Cliffs, N.J.: Prentice-Hall, 1976.

Rokosz, Francis M. "Student Relations in the Intramural Program." *Journal of Health Physical Education Recreation.* **45**: 3 (March 1974): 59–60.

14

INTERSCHOLASTIC ATHLETIC ADMINISTRATION

STUDY STIMULATORS

1. Are interscholastic athletics a part of education? of physical education?
2. Who is responsible for the conduct of the participants? of the spectators?
3. What are the functions of a state high school athletic association?
4. What are the most relevant problems concerning eligibility which confront the administrator?
5. What are the minimum safety and health regulations essential for the welfare of the participant?
6. What are valid criteria for athletic awards?

The battle of Waterloo was won on the playing fields of Eton.

DUKE OF WELLINGTON

Interscholastic athletics are an important part of the educational program of our American high schools. With each passing year, the significance of interschool competitive sport becomes greater, not only to the schools but to the local communities as well. Secondary school administrators are becoming increasingly concerned about how best to conduct their interscholastic athletic programs on a sound educational basis in light of the ever increasing student and community interest.

Interscholastic athletics are one of the most engrossing parts of the school curriculum; they are important to the vitality and morale of the school, and contain implications for the total community. High school administrators, however, have quite often chosen not to administer the school athletic program on the same basis as the rest of the curriculum.

Secondary school administrators conduct most of their school program with a thorough regard for educational principles and procedures. Interscholastic athletics should be conducted in the same manner. In dealing with the interscholastic athletic problems, school administrators often forsake educational policies and standards, and they are inconsistent in their attitude toward athletics in relation to the rest of the school program and sound educational policy. Administrators often allow interference from alumni and downtown coaches.

Because of the tremendous popularity of interscholastic athletics, a great deal of responsibility rests on those who administer the program. Though ultimately all responsibility is placed on the school principal, the athletic director and teachers of sports have as great an obligation as the principal to conduct a sound program of athletics. By virtue of their professional preparation and experience these people are experts on athletic matters, and the chief school officer must depend on them for guidance and advice.

It is possible to eliminate the ills and evil influences of interscholastic athletics when administrators are willing to recognize these activities as one part of the physical education program. It is necessary, however, for these administrators to have a thorough knowledge of the many facets of the interscholastic program.

The educational values of interscholastic athletics have been the subject of many periodical articles in the past; they have also been discussed by many authors of books on physical education and athletics. Most authors agree that interscholastic athletics are a part of the physical education program and as such make a definite contribution to the student, school, and community.

Athletic programs in high schools were at first opposed, later tolerated as a necessary evil, and then recognized as an integral part of the educational program. Interinstitutional athletics developed rapidly as the high schools followed the lead of the colleges. Originally most of the management and coaching was done by students, since the attitude of the school officials was one of indifference. The last two decades of the nineteenth century were marked by an expansion and elaboration of athletics. Interschool competition developed out of undirected play and intramural sports. In colleges undergraduate leadership was soon replaced by voluntary supervision by graduates and finally by salaried managers and coaches. As expenditures for interinstitutional sports mounted, the practice of charging admission at the gate was introduced. During these last two decades of the nineteenth century, most of the evils of interschool athletics took root. This happened because faculties had ignored interschool athletics in one of its most critical periods, its period of greatest growth. Then school officials took a position of vigorous opposition to athletics, but much of the damage had already been done. School administrators, realizing it was inadvisable to abolish interschool sports, made an effort to control them. The widening conception of education as concerned with more than mental growth made it logical to put this branch of school life under the supervision of school administration.

THE PERSONNEL OF LOCAL INTERSCHOLASTIC ATHLETIC PROGRAMS

In discussing the role of athletic administration in the modern high school, it must be emphasized that there is a variety of organizational patterns for the conduct of the interscholastic programs. The organizational pattern selected depends on the size of the school district, the number and sizes of the schools, the extent of the interscholastic athletic program, and the number of athletic staff members.

The local interscholastic athletic program is only as good as the persons who administer it. The program can be evaluated in terms of how well those responsible for the conduct of the program have attained the aims and objectives established for that program. The successful high school athletic program requires that administrators display team work and cooperation, as well as an understanding of the educational implication of athletics and of each person's role in the program. These include the superintendent of schools, the school principal, athletic director, and the athletic coaches.

The role of the superintendent of schools. In the final analysis, the superintendent of schools, as the chief executive officer, is responsible for the athletic program of a school. In many of the smaller schools one person, designated as superintendent, performs all the duties of both superintendent of schools and principal.

The superintendent has several important functions to perform with regard to the athletic program. The superintendent keeps the board of education informed of the athletic program and policy of the school or schools, is instrumental in forming school athletic policy, informs the community at every opportunity that athletics are a part of the educational program and must be conducted as any other part of the school curriculum, and, in cooperation with the school principal, has the duty of selecting the athletic coaches, who are key persons in the interscholastic athletic program.

The role of the principal. The high school principal has immediate authority and responsibility for the conduct of the interscholastic athletic program. Usually the principal's relationship to the athletic program is more definite and detailed than that of the superintendent of schools. The principal is responsible for planning interschool athletics as part of the curriculum and as part of the physical education program. The wise principal adopts the philosophy that athletics are subjects to be taught, subjects from which both participants and spectators derive educational values. He or she thoroughly understands the school athletic policy, and if the school is in a city or league system of several schools, the athletic program is conducted in accordance with the policies, rules, and regulations pertaining to all the schools in that system. The principal keeps the superintendent of schools informed about the school athletic program.

In smaller schools the principal will necessarily handle many details of the program alone. In larger institutions responsibility and authority may be delegated to an athletic director, a faculty manager, or athletic coaches.

It is good administrative practice for the principal to meet early in the year with those persons to whom responsibilities are delegated and to make sure that they understand their individual duties. The principal works in close cooperation with the athletic director or faculty manager. Usually it is the principal's responsibility to apportion existing facilties to the physical education, intramural, and interscholastic athletic programs for both boys and girls. It is essential that consideration be given to all parts of the program and to all students in order to equitably distribute available facilities.

The thoughtful principal strives for friendly relationships, attends as many contests as possible, and sets an example for the students and adults in good sportsmanship. The principal seizes every opportunity to inform the student body and the adults of the place interschool athletics maintains in the balanced physical education program.

It is apparent that the role of the principal is a varied and important one. The fact that the principal is the person immediately responsible for the interschool athletic program must always be kept in mind.

The role of the athletic director. Regardless of the organizational pattern, responsibility and authority for the conduct of the interscholastic athletic program should be centered in one person. This person, titled the athletic director, usually combines the athletic directorship with teaching and coaching duties. In some large school districts, one person may have a full-time position as director of athletics or director of physical education and athletics for the school district whose job is to coordinate the programs of the directors in each of the high schools in the school district. Some schools designate a faculty member, other than an athletic coach, as faculty manager of athletics.

A member of the athletic coaching staff is usually given the position of director of athletics as an additional duty. That person is responsible for administering the total athletic program and should be given the necessary authority commensurate with the many duties of the position.

This person should be an experienced coach and should possess the ability to organize and direct the program. This requires leadership qualities of the highest order including the ability to maintain harmony among all members of the athletic staff.

With the aid of the coaching staff, the superintendent, and the principal, the athletic director should establish the philosophy for the program. The athletic director should be a member of the school Athletic Council and should present important items pertinent to the conduct of the athletic program to the Council for policy decisions. Once the policies are adopted by the Council, the athletic director must conduct the athletic program within the framework of the established policies. It is important that all policies be written down, preferably in the form of a policy book. In addition, the athletic director must keep abreast of new ideas, new concepts, and changes that occur in the area of interscholastic athletics.

In conducting the interscholastic athletic program, the athletic director must devote attention to numerous duties. Among these are to supervise all areas of the program; to conduct the program according to the policies, rules, and regulations established by the Athletic Council, the department, the conference, the State Association, and the National Federation of State High School Athletic Associations; to organize the staff for the most effective results; to make staff assignments; to recommend staff promotions and changes; to supervise all business matters; to prepare the budget; to supervise the expenditure of all department funds; to establish bookkeeping and accounting procedures; to handle the administration of tickets; to purchase all equipment and supplies; to serve as a consultant in the planning and building of facilities; to provide proper health and medical services; to represent the department in dealing with all agencies outside the department; to develop an effective public relations program; to prepare contest schedules and game contracts; to make all home contest arrangements; to hire game officials; to prepare eligibility lists; to make all away contest arrangements; to prepare all written reports for specific contests, for the school administration, the conference, and state athletic association; to continuously evaluate the program; to make emergency decisions when necessary.

The role of the faculty manager of athletics. In some high schools the position of faculty manager of athletics, as well as that of athletic director, is included in the administrative arrangement. While the athletic director is usually one of the athletic coaches, the faculty manager of athletics is normally not a coach, but an interested faculty member. It is advantageous for this person to have had business training. The duties of the faculty manager of athletics vary from handling all the administration of the interscholastic athletic program to having a few specific responsibilities usually in the areas of finance and ticket administration. The extent of the duties depends on the duties assigned to the coaches and the extent of the program. Whatever duties are assigned the person in this position, they should be clear and in writing, to avoid any misunderstanding. The advantage of having a faculty manager of athletics is that this person is not encumbered with coaching duties and thus can concentrate on the administration of the interscholastic athletic program. One disadvantage is that without direct contact with the teams a manager may not be in a position to know the needs of the coaches and their teams; therefore, there must be a close liaison between the coaches and the faculty manager of athletics if this administrative plan for the conduct of the interscholastic athletic program is to be successful.

The role of the athletic coach. The athletic coach is the key figure in the local interscholastic athletic program whose principal athletic duty is to teach sports activities to the members of the squad; however, a position in athletic coaching involves much more. Besides doing the best teaching job possible, the athletic coach must set an example of good personal living in both the school and the community. The athletic coach must work closely with the school administration in carrying out the school athletic policy and must be fair and honest in the relationship with team members, assistants, colleagues, fellow coaches, the alumni, press, and general public. He or she needs such personal qualifications as enjoyment of working with adolescents, irreproachable character, leadership ability and enthusiasm, knowledge of techniques and ability to impart such knowledge to others, and good common sense. The coach must also understand the place of athletics in the total school curriculum.

Since the athletic coach holds such a prominent place in the secondary school, and thus can be such a tremendous influence for good or ill on not only the members of the team but the rest of the student body and community, selection must be made with great care. The principal and superintendent must employ only those who can meet the stringent qualifications that the modern athletic coaching position requires.

ORGANIZATION OF LOCAL INTERSCHOLASTIC ATHLETIC PROGRAMS

In high schools the organization of the interscholastic athletic program varies according to the size of the schools.

The interscholastic athletic program should be organized as one part of the total physical education program. Although interscholastic athletic programs have certain common characteristics, it is obvious that the organization of the program in a high school of 300 students and that in a high school of 5000 students will differ. However, the chief difference in organization is in the number of athletic coaches, rather than in the number of students, after a certain minimum has been reached. After a school has reached the size at which the personnel of the interscholastic athletic program is composed of an athletic director, a faculty manager, and athletic coaches, the number of students in the school has little bearing on the organization of the program.

The board of education is the policy-making group for the local school system. The superintendent of schools is charged with the responsibility of carrying out the policies established by this board. The superintendent initiates procedures to aid in carrying out this responsibility and also delegates responsibility and authority to the school principals to further assist in complying with the policies of the board of education. School principals in turn develop procedures to fulfill their responsibilities, including procedures for interscholastic athletics. School boards through high school principals delegate to the school athletic council the authority to determine policy and procedure for the interscholastic athletic program. As a member of the athletic council, the principal helps to determine these policies and procedures.

An athletic council is a must, regardless of the size of the school or the extent of the interschool sports program. Interscholastic athletics command wide student and adult interest, which sometimes leads to overzealous feelings that can cause the destruction of an otherwise rational program. Therefore, a representative group of school personnel is essential to aid the principal in controlling and administering the program of interscholastics. The athletic council is the "board of trustees" for the athletics of the school; it counsels on athletic matters. The council must be a well-informed group.

The personnel and functions of the athletic council vary from school to school. The members of this group may include any or all of the following: a member of the board of education, the superintendent of schools, the principal, the athletic director, the faculty manager, the athletic coaches, other members of the faculty, the director or a supervisor of health and physical education, and students. The functions of the council include any or all of the following: to determine policy procedure and program; to control the administrative aspects of the program; to consider schedules, game contracts, equipment, awards, finances, budgets, player eligibility; and to prevent athletic excesses.

Interscholastic Athletic Program Offerings

Table 1 shows activities suitable for the interscholastic program according to season. It is difficult for any high school to offer all of them, but the school administrator and athletic director should be able to select a suitable program including a good portion of carry-over activities.

Selecting the activities for the school interscholastic athletic program is a very important task and requires the consideration of

Table 1 A Suggested Program of Interscholastic Athletics

Season	Individual and dual sports	Team games
Fall	Golf Archery Tennis Cross country	Football Speedball Soccer Lacrosse
Winter	Fencing Wrestling Bowling Table tennis Badminton Handball Swimming	Ice hockey Basketball Volleyball
Spring	Archery Golf Tennis	Baseball Softball Track and field Lacrosse

many factors including student interest, finances, staff, facilities, and equipment. Meyers developed criteria which serve as a guide in the proper selection of activities to include in the program of interscholastic athletics:

1. The practice should be safe and contribute to the attainment of the objectives of general education.

2. The practice should be safe and contribute to the total physical and organic development of the individual and to the attainment of maximum health and physical efficiency.

3. The practice should foster development of desirable social and moral qualities.

4. The practice should contribute to development of sound mental and emotional attitudes concerning physical activities.

5. The practice should contribute to development of desirable psychological qualities.

6. The practice should meet student needs.

7. The practice should be of interest to students.

8. The practice should be commensurate with the abilities of the students.

9. The practice should provide opportunities for the student to evaluate himself.

10. The practice should possess carry-over value.

11. The practice should contribute to the development of a high degree of skill in one of a variety of physical activities.

12. The practice should contribute to the development of general and specific skills valuable in self protection and in the protection of others.

13. The practice should be administratively feasible in an educational situation.[1]

The School as a Member of the State High School Athletic Association

Most state high school athletic associations were organized just prior to, or shortly after, 1900. Among the first associations were those in Wisconsin, Michigan, Illinois, and Indiana. By 1925 there were associations in all states. These associations were designed by school officials of the high schools in the various states because it became apparent that as interscholastic athletics grew in scope

---

[1] Carlton R. Meyers, "An Evaluation of Boxing as a Sports Activity in Institutions of Higher Learning" (Ed.D. project, Teachers College, Columbia University, 1949): pp. 20–28. Cited by Harry A. Scott, *Competitive Sports in Schools and Colleges* (New York: Harper and Bros., 1951): pp. 359–360. Reprinted by permission.

and importance, better administrative regulations than those provided by local leagues and conferences were necessary to ensure uniformity and equality of competition.

Today there are three types of state associations: those affiliated with the state department of education, those under the supervision of a state university, and those that are of a strictly voluntary nature. Most of the associations are of a voluntary nature. In states in which the association is affiliated with the state department of education, or a state university, all public, private, and parochial schools are automatically members of the state athletic association. In states in which membership is voluntary, no high school is required to join the association. However, in these states a vast majority of the high schools belong to the association because of the many advantages of membership.

Association membership includes both advantages and obligations. Some of the functions of state associations that are advantageous to member schools are

1. establishment and enforcement of regulations for the conduct of contests,
2. maintenance of athletic accident or insurance plans,
3. registration and classification of athletic officials,
4. publication of magazines and bulletins,
5. establishment of athletic standards,
6. acting as a final authority to whom questions may be addressed, controversies presented, and appeals made.

The obligations of membership include compliance with all rules and regulations of the association, cooperation and loyalty, and support of those undertakings of the group which are in the interest of better interscholastic athletics.

Eligibility Requirements for School and Participants

The state high school athletic associations in the various states assume the duty of making and enforcing eligibility rules for their member schools. In fact, the necessity for eligibility standards was one of the original reasons for establishing these associations. The secondary school administrator must understand that these regulations are designed as guides by which the administrator may plan local policy for the conduct of the athletic program. These regulations are for the protection of the school administration and the participants against those schools which would voluntarlly take advantage of opponents to gain athletic supremacy.

Eligibility requirements are divided into two categories: those pertaining to schools and those pertaining to individual participants. Eligibility requirements pertaining to schools that are common to most state high school athletic associations are:

1. Play only member schools.
2. Limit the value of awards.
3. Use official contracts.
4. Exchange eligibility lists.
5. Prohibit postseason games.
6. Limit the length of seasons.
7. Limit the number of games.
8. Certify coaches as teachers.
9. Prohibit spring practice of football.
10. Require a specified number of days of practice prior to the first game.

Eligibility requirements for players, like those for schools, should be regarded from a positive point of view. They are established to protect the students who are good school citizens, not to place unwarranted restrictions upon them. Since participation in interscholastic athletics is regarded as a privilege, the student in turn must undertake certain responsibilities. Certain eligibility requirements which are common to most state high school athletic associations are given below. Players must:

1. Have reached a certain age.
2. Have taken a certain number of subjects and attained a certain average in the previous semester.
3. Be currently taking a certain number of credits and maintaining a certain average.
4. Pass a physical examination.
5. Obtain parental permission.
6. Be an amateur.
7. Participate a given number of semesters, or years.
8. Abstain from play on nonschool teams.
9. Be currently enrolled in the school.
10. Observe transfer rule. Student eligible only if parents transfer to a new school district and student resides with parents.

The School as a Member of an Athletic Conference

Interscholastic athletic conferences are patterned after college conferences. They perform similar functions except in the matter of setting up and enforcing eligibility rules; this function is performed by the state high school athletic association.

Within every state there are many secondary high school athletic conferences composed of schools in close proximity to one another. Usually the schools are of approximately the same size. The chief purposes of these conferences are to assign athletic officials, to keep records, to declare league champions, and to arrange schedules.

When a school maintains membership in an interscholastic athletic conference, the school is obligated to fulfill all requirements and abide by all rules of that conference. Much has been done by high school conferences to place athletics on an educational basis; hence administrators, athletic directors, and athletic coaches would be wise to investigate the possibilities of joining an athletic conference if they are unaffiliated.

The most practical size league is composed of from six to eight schools. Fewer schools provide inadequate competition while more prove to be cumbersome. A six- seven- eight-team league in football allows a one-round schedule, with time for several games outside the organization. In basketball a home-and-home program may be scheduled and teams will still have time for several nonleague games. In other sports such as track, golf, tennis, baseball, and swimming, this size league makes for interesting as well as efficient competition.

SCHEDULING INTERSCHOLASTIC ATHLETIC CONTESTS

The arrangement of varsity athletic schedules is a major facet of interscholastic athletic administration. Obtaining opponents of equal or nearly equal ability within a reasonable traveling distance is often a difficult task. When a school is a member of an athletic conference, its schedule-making problem is simplified by its obligation to play other conference schools.

The basic criterion in scheduling secondary school interscholastic athletic contests is the health and welfare of the participants. Schedules should be made by one person, usually the athletic director, subject to the approval of the athletic council, the superintendent, the principal, or the school board. The key point is that interscholastic athletic schedules should be reviewed by responsible persons or by a duly authorized group.

Interscholastic athletic schedule making is affected by national, state, league, and local policies and regulations. For example, at the national level the National Federation of State High School Athletic Associations, along with the concerned state associations, must sanction any game which requires a team to travel more than 600 miles round trip.

State high school athletic associations place restrictions on local interscholastic athletic scheduling. While these regulations vary from state to state, some or all of the following areas are dealt with in all state association constitutions: limitation on the number of contests to be played for a specific sport, length of season and opening and closing dates of each season, number of games per week, travel distances, and restrictions on playing teams only in the same classification (based on student population).

Interscholastic athletic league policies for scheduling vary with local league conditions. The most common league requirement is that all league members must play all other league members, usually on a home-and-away basis.

Individual schools also establish policies which must be considered in scheduling interscholastic athletic events. Schedules should be planned so that students miss a minimum number of classes for travel to the "away" games. Budget allotments are also important in schedule planning.

Other considerations in schedule making include dates for games with traditional rivals and planning the schedule so that there are the same number of home and away contests. Insofar as possible, the games should alternate between home and away.

The energy crisis has presented another factor for consideration by athletic administrators. Some school districts in larger cities have restricted or abolished out-of-town games. Schedules have been rearranged so that varsity, reserve, and girls' teams may travel in the same bus (or buses) to away games. Many school districts are scheduling outdoor interscholastic athletic contests in football, baseball, soccer, lacrosse, and track and field during the daylight hours to save energy.

SAFETY AND HEALTH SUPERVISION

One of the most important obligations of the secondary school administrator and athletic coach in interscholastic athletics is to provide effective safety and health measures for all persons concerned with the program—participants and spectators. There are many administrative controls on health and safety that may be used. One important facet of this is to teach pupils the importance of preserving health and maintaining safety.

Safety in interscholastic athletics. All sports contain an element of danger, some sports more than others. It is the danger element that appeals to most youngsters and is responsible to a large degree for the popularity of contact sports. However, it is this danger element that must be taken into consideration and controlled by every means available to the secondary school administrator.

Adequate training. No boy or girl should be allowed to participate in an athletic contest unless properly prepared to do so. Adequate conditioning of players is a responsibility which must not be taken lightly. Conditioning must be progressive, since it takes time to get the human body into the proper physiological condition for strenuous athletic competition. The well-trained coach knows that from the safety standpoint, as well as the success standpoint, he or she must get the team in the best shape possible with the least amount of injuries and illnesses. The coach should be knowledgeable in the latest advances in sports medicine, such as heat stress. Teachers of athletics should set up training and conditioning rules for the members of their squads, and should insist on adherence to them. It is not asking too much to require students to follow training rules if they expect to represent the school successfully in competitive athletics.

Adequate personal equipment. The school should sponsor only those athletic activities for which it can provide adequate equipment. It should furnish the best quality of all necessary personal equipment to players for safe participation in the activity. It is false economy to do less. This includes shoes for participants in all sports and protective equipment such as headgear and shoulder pads in football. When students purchase their own equipment, it is usually of inferior quality, since this is an additional expense to parents. Rules of most sports now specify the personal equipment to be worn by players in official contests; however, there are no such rules for practice sessions. It is the obligation of athletic coaches to see that their players are also properly uniformed at all practice sessions.

Proper playing facilities. Adequate and safe playing facilities are necessary to the athletic program. The athletic facilities of every school are unique, and each school presents certain hazards which are peculiar to that school. The school officials should be aware of these hazards and take steps to minimize the dangers they present.

Adequate maintenance should be provided to ensure that playing surfaces are kept in top condition. Such obstructions as benches, walls, stages, bleachers, drinking fountains, and stairways should be well out of the way from all playing areas. The administrator and athletic director should work in close cooperation with the maintenance personnel in assuring safe playing facilities.

Equitable competition. From the standpoint of safety, equitable competition is essential. There is no justification for the scheduling of interscholastic athletic contests with opponents of unequal strength, size, age or ability. Occasionally small schools with comparatively weak teams schedule events with larger schools out of their class for the financial remuneration involved, or large schools with powerful teams schedule games with smaller schools with poor teams as "breathers." This practice is not to be condoned.

Limiting practice periods. The length of practice periods should be limited for the health and welfare as well as safety of the students. As players become fatigued from long practice sessions, the percentage of injuries increases. Most athletic coaches agree that to get a team in condition for competition takes about three weeks of daily practice sessions lasting from one and one-half to two hours each.

Proper officiating. Once an athletic contest is in progress, the safety of the players is in the hands of the officials. Since the safety of the players is so dependent upon competent officiating, school administrators must be very careful when choosing officials who will supervise the contests. State athletic associations have taken long steps forward in recent years to provide better qualified officials by certifying officials. Officials should be chosen not only for their technical knowledge of the rules, but also for their ability to control the contest and prevent injuries.

The athletic coach and safety. The athletic coach is the key figure in the safety program. The chief school administrator and the athletic coach must work cooperatively to ensure maximum safety in the athletic program. It is recommended that when hiring athletic coaches administrators seek people who were physical education majors, because in nearly all teacher training institutions much time and consideration is given to the study of health and safety of students.

Safety for spectators. Many of the items mentioned in this chapter under contest management pertain to spectator safety. This is an exceedingly important facet from the administrative standpoint. Such safety precautions as enforcement of traffic regulations, provision of police and fire protection, of ushers, and inspection of bleachers (both temporary and permanent) are necessary for adequate protection of spectators.

For indoor contests all fire prevention rules and regulations must be enforced. It is advisable to have a qualified firefighter inspect the gymnasium at regular intervals. Some schools deem it prudent to have a firefighter present at all indoor interscholastic contests. An essential precaution is to keep all aisles open and all exits unobstructed.

Health of participants. The health of all students participating in interscholastic athletics is of major importance. The school administration and athletic personnel have the obligation of providing for the maintenance of the personal health of each participant, as well as creating a healthful environment within which to conduct the program.

The health examination. In relation to the maintenance of the health of each participant, no student should be allowed to engage in any sport without first having passed a health examination. This should not be a cursory examination, and it should include teeth, tonsils, heart, lungs, feet, and possibility of hernia.

The team physician. The team physician is the most important person in the maintenance of student health. The team physician should be hired to handle all injuries to squad personnel. It is seldom possible for high schools to have a physician attend practices, but it should be administrative policy to see that there is one in attendance at all home games. Only the physician should decide whether the physical condition of a student is such that he or she may participate in a contest or practice.

Athletic trainer. Athletic trainers make an important contribution to the physical welfare of participants in interscholastic sports as well as to the success of the team. While few high schools are able to hire a trainer, such a practice is becoming more prevalent. Some schools are employing individuals with degrees and experience in physical education and athletic training as athletic trainers to teach physical education and serve as trainers for interscholastic athletic teams. If this practice is not possible, other arrangements must be made. Most athletic coaches, particularly those who have majored in physical education, have had training which qualifies them to perform at least some athletic-training duties. When there are several coaches on the athletic staff, they may act as trainers for sports which they are not assigned to as coach. If there is one head coach and an assistant for all sports, the assistant may act as team trainer. Some duties of athletic trainers are as follows.

1. To give first-aid treatment within the bounds of the American Red Cross First Aid Manual.
2. To follow the written prescriptions of the physician in the care of the injured.
3. To keep the doctor informed of newly injured players.
4. To keep records of treatment given to each individual player.
5. To maintain a stock of all essential training supplies and equipment.
6. To tape, bandage, and massage.

Administrative policies for athletic injuries. The secondary school administrator should have definite written policies in regard to the handling of athletic injuries. Policies vary from school to school: some large high schools assume full financial responsibility for all athletic injuries, while most small schools are able to offer little or no financial aid to injured athletes. Athletic accident benefit insurance appears to be the most feasible solution to this problem.

Locker rooms. The locker rooms should be the cleanest rooms in the school. They should be rooms from which the individual derives positive environmental satisfaction. The well-planned locker room provides adequate space for students to change clothing in comfort as well as lockers sufficiently large for the storage of street clothing.

Locker-room sanitation requires daily custodial service, adequate drying facilities for equipment, and provision for the laundering of athletic costumes and towels. Cleanliness demands frequent changes of clothing for all types of athletic activity.

ATHLETIC AWARDS

The granting of awards by school authorities for successful participation in interscholastic athletics is a nationwide practice.

The National Federation of State High School Athletic Associations has waged a determined campaign to limit the amount of money spent on awards so that awards will be symbols of achievement and nothing more.

Although in most cases state associations limit the monetary value of awards, the establishment of standards for award qualifications is left to the individual schools. Hence it is up to local school authorities to determine their own policies in regard to the basis for granting awards, as well as the type of awards granted within the framework of the monetary limits set by the state association.

For best educational results the granting of awards for interscholastic athletic competition cannot be a casual, subjective procedure. Specific criteria must be established for the granting of athletic awards. When too many awards are granted, their value is decreased proportionately. When there are no definite criteria, discontent may arise.

Basis for granting awards. As stated above, the granting of awards cannot be haphazard; a definite basis must be established and followed. Bases for award granting vary from school to school. Some bases used by various high schools are

1. amount of participation,
2. recommendation of the athletic coach,
3. recommendation of the athletic coach and other school officials,
4. point system for participation in an individual sport,
5. point system based on an accumulation of points for participation in more than one sport.

In addition to one of the above, schools usually require that students receiving awards meet the academic requirement, be good school citizens, and observe all team rules.

Awards for student managers. In most high schools it is a policy to present awards to student managers for efficient service. These awards should differentiate the type of service rendered. Some schools make awards to senior managers only; others recognize juniors and sophomores as well. When awards are granted to senior, junior, and sophomore managers, they should be indicative of the student's position in the managerial hierarchy. Managers should be subject to the same eligibility and scholastic rules as members of the team they manage.

ROLE OF LOCAL NEWS MEDIA

Today every public school needs a program of public relations. Since our public schools are supported by taxation, it is the responsibility of the school to keep the public informed about its activities. Schools, both public and private, find it necessary to inform the public by every means possible to secure adequate support and cooperation. The public relations program must be well planned and carefully organized and must present the facts as accurately as possible. For a more complete discussion of this topic, see Chapter 7.

Newspapers. It is imperative that all athletic officials establish and maintain the best possible relations with the press. If a spirit of cooperation exists beween athletic administrators and newspaper people, editors and reporters are more likely to publish favorable information.

It is just as important for the athletic director and the athletic coach to establish and maintain good relations with the press as it is for the superintendent and the principal. Newspaper support, from a financial viewpoint, is invaluable to the athletic program. Schools could never afford to purchase the space they receive in the newspapers, and all they need to do to get it is maintain good relations with the sports editor.

Sports editors are a powerful force in the community in the molding of public opinion. They are often invaluable to the local high school in building and supporting an interscholastic athletic program based on the educational values inherent in the activities.

Radio and television broadcasting. Radio and television broadcasting has two main functions in relation to interscholastic athletics: (1) to publicize impending contests, and (2) to enable the public to witness interschool games. Some high schools advertise future games on radio and television, and these schools often receive free publicity from regular sports broadcasts. Both are valuable means of publicity for the school athletic program.

COMMUNITY USE OF ATHLETIC FACILITIES

In recent years there has been a movement to revive the school as the center of community life in urban areas. Everywhere today school buildings are being opened for community use during the evening hours and at other times when the regular work of the school will not be hindered.

The high school is well suited for various types of community activity, with its gymnasiums, playing fields, locker rooms, showers, workshops, music room, auditorium, kitchen, and cafeteria.

Of the various activities that may be carried on by the community in the public schools, none has more potential to serve the needs of the people than physical education and athletics. Community use of the physical education and athletic facilities should be encouraged at every opportunity.

Physical education and athletic facilities used by the community should be subject to the same rules and regulations as the rest of the school property.

CASE STUDY

The Athletic Board of Whiting High School consisted entirely of nonathletic personnel appointed by the superintendent of schools with the exception of the Athletic Director, who was an ex-officio member. During the past few years several members showed a lack of interest in this assignment. Several others, although interested, were completely devoid of any knowledge of the complexity of scheduling and conducting interscholastic contests.

Mr. Twill, the Athletic Director, confronted the superintendent with these facts and requested that a new board be appointed consisting of head coaches, the principal, and himself. The superintendent listened patiently and then exclaimed, "Send me a report giving me the advantages and disadvantages of the present board and also the one you wish to have me appoint. I shall then review the situation and let you know my decision."

1. What are the issues?
2. Assume Mr. Twill's role and prepare a report for the superintendent.
3. What principles are found in this case study?

SELECTED REFERENCES

"A Survey of Special Certification Requirements for Athletic Coaches of High School Interscholastic Teams," *Journal of Health Physical Education Recreation,* **41** (September 1970): 14, 16.

Alley, L. E. "Athletics in Education: The Double-Edged Sword," *Phi Delta Kappan,* **56** (October 1974): 102–105; and *Education Digest,* **40** (December 1974): 32–35.

Ashton, S. "Athlete's Changing Perspective: A Student View," *Journal of Health Physical Education Recreation,* **43** (April 1972): 46.

"Athletics as Academic Motivation for the Inner City Boy," *Journal of Health Physical Education Recreation,* **43** (February 1972): 40–41.

"Athletics and Education: Are They Compatible?" *Phi Delta Kappan,* **56** (October 1974): 98–146.

"Athletics and the Modern Industrial State," *Phi Delta Kappan,* **56** (October 1974): 114–115.

Athletics in Oregon K–12. Guidelines for Local School District Policies. Salem: Oregon State Department of Education, 1975.

Badner, G. "Hey, Coach! Can Betty Sue and I Get in the Game Now?" *Pennsylvania School Journal,* **123** (December 1974): 24–25.

Ballinger, J., and R. Schaffer. "What Price Coaching? Junior and Senior High Schools in Missouri," *School and Community,* **60** (December 1973): 24–25.

Barren, D. J. "Winning Edge in Coaching," *Independent School Bulletin,* **33** (December 1973): 56–57.

Blaufarb, M. "Equal Opportunity for Girls in Athletics," *Today's Education,* **63** (November 1974): 52–55.

Borozne, J., *et al. Administration and Supervision for Safety in Sports.* Sports Safety Series, Monograph No. 1. Washington, D.C.: AAHPER, 1977.

Boslooper, T. "Physical Assertiveness; Contact Sports for Girls and Women," *Journal of Physical Education Recreation,* **47** (May 1976): 35–37.

Bula, M. R. "Educating Parents About Pre-High School Competition," *Journal of Physical Education,* **69** (November 1971): 45–46.

Coppage, P. R. "Get More from Practice," *Physical Educator,* **30** (December 1973): 197–200.

Crase, D. "Negro in Sport and Physical Education: Some Considerations," *Physical Educator,* **27** (December 1970): 158–160.

———. "Athletics in Trouble," *Journal of Health Physical Education Recreation,* **43** (April 1972): 39–41.

Dannehl, W. E., and J. E. Razor. "Values of Athletics: A Critical Inquiry," *Bulletin of the National Association of Secondary School Principals,* **55** (September 1971): 59–65.

Daughtrey, Greyson, and John B. Woods. *Physical Education and Intramural Programs: Organization and Administration.* Philadelphia: W. B. Saunders, 1976.

Dunkle, M. *Competitive Athletics: In Search of Equal Opportunity.* Washington, D.C.: National Foundation for the Improvement of Education, 1976.

Engle, K. M. "Greening of Girls' Sports," *Nations Schools,* **92** (September 1973): 27–34.

Erickson, A. "Women's Lib and School Sports Can Mean Problems," *School Management,* **17** (August 1973): 33–35.

Evaluating the High School Athletic Program. Washington, D.C.: AAHPER, 1973.

Evans, M. I. "Vanishing Americans; Black Coaches," *Journal of Health Physical Education Recreation,* **44** (October 1973): 55–57.

Evans, V., and C. D. Henry. "Black High School Coach; Will He Become Extinct?" *Physical Educator,* **30** (October 1973): 152–153.

Forsythe, C. A., and I. A. Keller. *Administration of High School Athletics,* 6th ed. Englewood Cliffs, N.J.: Prentice-Hall, 1977.

Frazier, C. S. "Was the Coach Negligent?" *Athletic Journal,* **54** (January 1974): 14.

Frost, Reuben B., and Stanley J. Marshall. *Administration of Physical Education and Athletics: Concepts and Practices.* Dubuque, Iowa: W. C. Brown, 1977.

Fuzak, J., and M. B. Mitchell. "Academics vs. Athletics: Two Views." Ed. by T. A. Emmet. *College and University Business,* **55** (September 1973): 15–16.

Guidelines for Interscholastic Athletic Programs for Junior High School Girls. Washington, D.C.: AAHPER, 1972.

Haggerty, J. "The Community Athletic Program," *Community and Junior College Journal,* **46** (April 1976): 8–9, 24.

Hansan, J. F., and M. L. Green. "Coming of the Second Plague," *Physical Educator,* **32** (May 1975): 64–66.

Harding, C., and I. T. Sliger. "Student Involvement in the Administration of Sports Programs," *Journal of Health Physical Education Recreation,* **41** (February 1970): 39–43.

Hogan, J. C. "Sports in the Courts," *Phi Delta Kappan,* **56** (October 1974): 132–135.

Hutton, L. I., and J. Silkin. "Needed: Women Athletic Trainers," *Journal of Health Physical Education Recreation,* **43** (January 1972): 77–78.

Johnson, L. "Coed Sports in High School," *Journal of Physical Education Recreation,* **48** (January 1977): 23–25.

Johnson, M. L. *Functional Administration in Physical and Health Education.* Boston: Houghton Mifflin, 1977.

Johnson, T. P. "Girls on the Boys' Team: Equal Protection in School Athletics," *NASSP Bulletin,* **58** (October 1974): 55–65.

Kehres, L. "Maslow's Hierarchy of Needs Applied to Physical Education and Athletics," *Physical Educator,* **30** (March 1973): 24–25.

Knowles, L. W. "Courts Debunk Common School Sports Myths," *Nation's Schools,* **92** (September 1973): 60.

Kroll, W. "Psychological Scaling of Proposed Title IX Guidelines," *Research Quarterly,* **47** (October 1976): 548–554.

Lockhart, B. "Title IX; Prospects and Problems," *Journal of Physical Education Recreation,* **47** (May 1976): 37.

Lopiano, D. A. "Fact-Finding Model for Conducting a Title IX Self-Evaluative Study in Athletic Programs," *Journal of Physical Education Recreation,* **47** (May 1976): 26–30.

McKnight, D., and J. Hult. "Competitive Athletics for Girls: We Must Act," *Journal of Health Physical Education Recreation,* **45** (June 1974): 45–46.

Magill, R. A. "Youth Sports: An Interdisciplinary View of Readiness and Effects: Child in Sport," *Journal of Physical Education Recreation,* **48** (January 1977): 56–57.

"Mass Culture and School Sports," *Education Quarterly,* **14** (Winter 1974): 483–499.

Metz, P. R. "Course to Build Player-Coach Rapport; Athlete in Contemporary Society," *Journal of Health Physical Education Recreation,* **43** (April 1972): 50–51.

Moyer, D. G. "Department of Athletics: An Assessment," *Independent School Bulletin,* **29** (February 1970): 23–24.

Moyer, D. H. "Increasing Participation," *Journal of Physical Education Recreation,* **48** (February 1977): 36–37.

Moyer, L. J. "Women's Athletics: What Is Our Future?" *Journal of Physical Education Recreation,* **48** (January 1977): 52.

Mudra, D. "Coach and the Learning Process: Perceptual Approach to Winning," *Journal of Health Physical Education Recreation,* **41** (May 1970): 26–29.

Parsons, T. W. "What's Right About Athletics?" *Physical Educator,* **31** (March 1974): 49.

Pernice, S. "Coaches: Let Your Players Think!" *Journal of Physical Education Recreation,* **47** (September 1976): 23.

"Professional Preparation of the Administrator of Athletics," *Journal of Health Physical Education Recreation,* **41** (September 1970): 20–23.

Resick, Matthew C., and Carl E. Erickson, *Intercollegiate and Interscholastic Athletics for Men and Women.* Reading, Mass.: Addison-Wesley, 1975.

Richardson, D. E. "Preparation for a Career in Public School Athletic Administration," *Journal of Health Physical Education Recreation,* **42** (February 1971): 17–19.

Riley, B. *The Effect of Title IX of the Education Amendments of 1972 on the Administration of Girls' Competitive Athletic Programs in Selected Public High Schools of Texas.* Commerce: East Texas School Study Council, 1976.

Seidel, Beverly J., *et al. Sports Skills: A Conceptual Approach to Meaningful Movement.* Dubuque, Iowa: W. C. Brown, 1975.

Sheehan, T. J., and W. L. Alsop. "Educational Sport," *Journal of Health Physical Education Recreation,* **43** (May 1972): 41–45.

Shultz, F. D. "Broadening the Athletic Experience," *Journal of Health Physical Education Recreation,* **43** (April 1972): 45–47.

Singer, R. N. "Sport Psychology," *Journal of Physical Education Recreation,* **47** (September 1976): 24–25.

Slaughter, M. "Should Women Athletes Be Allowed to Play on Men's Teams?" *Physical Educator,* **32** (March 1975): 9–10.

Snyder, E. E., and E. Spreitzer. "Correlates of Sport Participation among Adolescent Girls," *Research Quarterly,* **47** (December 1976):804–809.

———. "Participation in Sport as Related to Educational Expectations among High School Girls," *Sociology of Education,* **50** (January 1977): 47–55.

Sprandel, D. S. "Administration in Physical Education and Athletics: A Partial Reference List," *Physical Educator,* **30** (March 1973): 17–18.

———. "Crisis in Athletic Administration?" *Physical Educator,* **31** (March 1974): 44–46.

Spreitzer, E., and M. Pugh. "Interscholastic Athletics and Educational Expectations," *Sociology of Education,* **46** (Spring 1973): 171–182.

Staffo, D. F. "Youth Sports Programs: In What Direction Are They Going?" *Journal of Physical Education,* **74** (March 1977): 88–89.

Steitz, E. S. *Administration of Athletics in Colleges and Universities.* Washington, D.C.: AAHPER, 1971.

Stern, B. E. "Cultural Crisis in American Sports; Coach-Athlete Relationship," *Journal of Health Physical Education Recreation,* **43** (April 1972): 42–44.

Stevens, G. "Use Incentives for Motivation," *Athletic Journal,* **54** (May 1974): 72–73.

Stines, R. A., *et al.* "Admissions and Athletics," *College and University,* **48** (Summer 1973): 295–298.

Stutzman, S. J., and C. McCullough. "Did DGWS Fail? Two Points of View," *Journal of Health Physical Education Recreation,* **45** (January 1974): 6.

"Trouble May Be Just Ahead for Your District if it Discriminates Against Girls in Athletics: A Special Report," *American School Board Journal,* **160** (September 1973): 19–25.

Turner, E. T. "Creativity and Coaching," *Physical Educator,* **30** (October 1973): 134–136.

Turner, M. A. *League Constitution and Bylaws for Girls' Interscholastic Programs.* Washington, D.C.: AAHPER, 1975.

Vernacchia, R. A. "Problems of Athletes: A Sociological Observation," *Physical Educator,* **32** (May 1975): 89.

Walsh, J. "Coach: A Teacher in Conflict," *Journal of Physical Education,* **70** (May 1973): 107–108.

Walter, D. "Coach and Drugs," *Physical Educator,* **30** (October 1973): 154–156.

Yost, C. P. *Sports Safety. Accident Prevention and Injury Control in Physical Education, Athletics, and Recreation.* Washington, D.C.: AAHPER, 1976.

Zeigler, E. F., and M. J. Spaeth. *Administrative Theory and Practice in Physical Education and Athletics.* Englewood Cliffs, N.J.: Prentice-Hall, 1975.

15

COMPETITIVE ATHLETIC PROGRAMS FOR GIRLS AND WOMEN

STUDY STIMULATORS

1. Should there be "separate but equal" athletic programs for girls and for boys? What are the legal ramifications of such programs?
2. Is interschool competition for women a recent innovation?
3. What organizations are leading the way to the development of a sane program of women's interscholastic sports?
4. What does the evidence show concerning the physiological or psychological damage to women who compete in vigorous sports?
5. How can girls' and women's sports be financially supported by the schools under the present structure?
6. What impact upon facilities is being made by the promotion of a complete program of interscholastic sports for girls?
7. What problems of officiating are found in women's athletics which are more easily handled in the men's program?

As to the modern feminine image, the day of Hippolyta has not yet come, but it seems to be dawning....

ELEANOR METHENY

Let her swim, climb mountain peaks, pilot an airplane, battle against the elements, take risks, go out for adventure, and she will not feel before the world . . . timidity. . . .

SIMONE DE BEAUVOIR

The history of competitive athletics for women in the United States has gone through many phases. Several factors are responsible for this chameleon-like phenomenon, not the least of which is the still popular concept that athletic prowess and femininity are incompatible. In spite of the fact that women are theoretically emancipated, many somewhat elusive forces continue to define the role of women in society along traditional, and often conservative, lines. Westervelt expresses this succinctly:

> Without question, American women have more rights and privileges than women have ever had before.... Yet there is every indication that their status, their roles, and their personal development are a matter of intense public and private concern. One gets the impression that our women are "all dressed up with no place to go."[1]

Throughout the short history of organized physical education for women in this country there has been no unanimity of opinion among women physical educators regarding the place of competi-

---

[1] Esther Manning Westervelt, "Woman as a Compleat Human Being," *Journal of the National Association of Women Deans and Counselors,* **29** (Summer 1966): 150. Reprinted by permission.

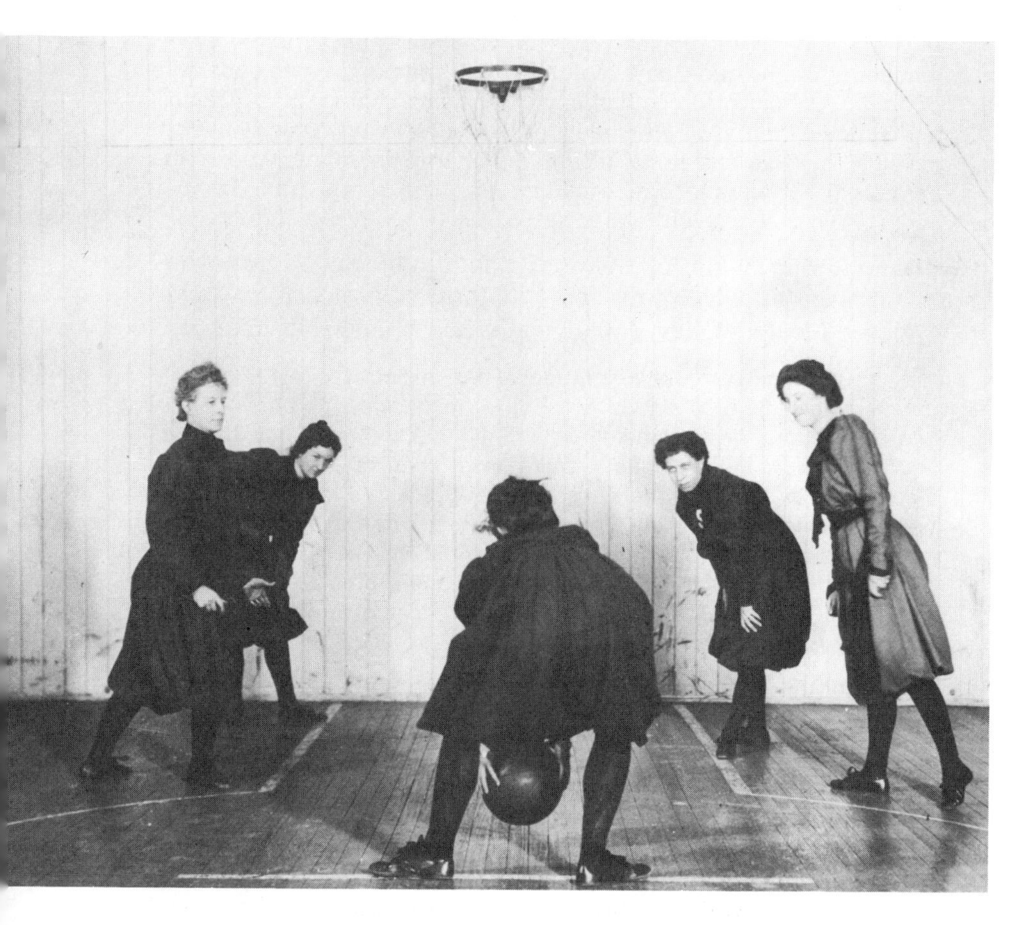

Fig. 1 Women's basketball circa 1913. (Courtesy the American Alliance for Health, Physical Education and Recreation.)

tive athletics. Perhaps the philosophy of the venerable Mabel Lee was representative of early professional leaders. In her classic, *The Conduct of Physical Education,* she indicates that she agrees with the following statement by Frederick Rand Rogers:

> Competitive sports tend to develop behavior patterns which are contrary to feminine nature. Natural feminine health and attractiveness, whether physical, emotional or social, certainly are impaired if not destroyed by the belligerent attitudes and competitive spirit the development of which intense activity inevitably fosters. One has only to postulate a female Roosevelt ["Teddy"] to reduce to absurdity the claims of those who foster the masculination [*sic*] of girls. Neither

> men nor any normal woman would embrace or willingly tolerate any tendency toward such an eventuality, yet competitive athletics will bring it about more surely than any other human behavior. . . . Games and sports for girls, by all means, of recreative types, which develop physical, psychic and social health and charm, but inter-school competition in basketball, baseball, track and field sports, and Olympic competition of whatever nature: no![2]

The following quote, by the social anthropologist James Whittington, is representative of the large majority of professional women physical educators today, and indicates how opinion has changed:

> . . . girls who show marked aptitude and a strong desire for participating in any field of endeavor should be allowed to pursue their interests without being considered unfeminine by their family, friends, and society. . . . these young women must themselves learn not to discourage or suppress their urges under pressures to "conform," to be popular, to catch a mate, to have children, and thus fulfill society's image of a woman. . . . men will have to admit that women are human beings, entitled to an identity separate from their roles as sex objects, wives and mothers. It is plain that woman cannot have a personal identity if her anatomy decides her destiny.[3]

The obvious divergence in belief as expressed in the two quotes has produced an interesting pattern of development in the history of competitive athletic programs for women, as well as heralding certain trends in future development. Interesting as well is the obvious fact that the blame for a lack of competitive athletic programs for females cannot be directed exclusively at males, a concept which some of the more radical "women libbers" have tried to perpetuate.

The emergent pattern of sports for women has gone through three distinct periods: (1) the early period, in the latter 1800s, when sports were used mostly as a means for a "respectable social encounter," conducted coeducationally, and consisted primarily of such activities as tennis, golf, archery, and croquet; (2) the middle period, the "golden decade" of 1925–1935, when not only the number of women participating increased, but also the participation extended to females outside the exclusive upper socioeconomic strata, team sports became popular, and organized sports competition was fostered largely outside schools and colleges on a noncoeducational basis; and (3) the present period, characterized by a tremendous

---

[2] Mabel Lee, *The Conduct of Physical Education* (New York: A. S. Barnes and Co., 1937): p. 69. Reprinted by permission.

[3] James Whittington, "The Nature of Woman," in the *Proceedings of the Fourth National Institute on Girls Sports,* American Association for Health, Physical Education, and Recreation, copyright © 1968, p. 15.

expansion in organized sports competition for women, conducted both within and outside the educational setting, and consisting of a wide spectrum of activities, both team and individual.[4]

HISTORICAL DEVELOPMENT

Athletic competition for girls and women in the schools of the United States probably started in 1892 with basketball at Smith College. This is indeed interesting in view of the fact that Naismith had developed the game only one year earlier! The forerunner of the present National Association for Girls and Women in Sport (NAGWS) basketball committee was formulated in 1899 at the Conference on Physical Training held at Springfield, Massachusetts. Not long after this time, other schools also entered the athletic scene by sponsoring, in addition, such activities as field hockey, tennis, swimming, and track and field.

Scott[5] traced the history of standards and policies in women's athletics by noting that the first committee of women to formulate rules was established in 1907. The present AAHPER, recognizing the value of the committee's work, established the Women's Athletic Committee in 1916–17. The charge of the committee was to constitute rules and lend assistance on any problems connected with girls' and women's sports. In 1923 the Women's Division of the National Amateur Athletic Federation was formed, and it had for its purpose the fostering of sports for all girls and women within a sound educational framework. At approximately the same time, the Women's Athletic Section, the successor to the Women's Athletic Committee, was founded as part of the American Physical Education Association (now the AAHPER). In 1940 these two groups (WAS and NAAF) merged and became known as the National Section for Women's Athletics (NSWA). Still later the Division for Girls' and Women's Sports (DGWS), an outgrowth of NSWA, was formed to recommend policy and standards as well as publish official rules for many sports.

It was natural that athletic competition for girls should extend down into the high school level, and by 1925 these programs had grown to such an extent that many undesirable practices flourished —practices which led the Committee on Athletics of the National Association of Secondary School Principals to recommend the following:

---

[4] Ellen W. Gerber *et al. The American Woman in Sport* (Reading, Mass.: Addison-Wesley, 1974), pp. 1–8.

[5] Gwendolyn D. Scott, "A Comparative Study of Standards and Policies in Athletics for Girls and Women" (Ed.D. dissertation, Case-Western Reserve University, 1963).

> The second subject which the committee believes to be worthy of your attention is the growing tendency to organize interscholastic teams among girls. Inherent evils in interscholastic competition among girls demand its suppression. These evils are so patent that they do not require much discussion. The extremely strenuous physical and mental exertion and strain are a menace to girls in the high school period. Furthermore, sooner or later, the spectacle of interscholastic contests among girls gives rise to undesirable and even morbid social influences among boys and girls, and in the community life as well.
>
> The committee therefore recommends that the National Association of Secondary School Principals throw the weight of its influence against interscholastic athletics among girls and that wherever possible state athletic associations be induced to legislate against them.[6]

As a result of this, there was a definite swing away from school-sponsored competition in most states, as well as virtual elimination of state and national championships for women sponsored by other agencies. Even the Olympic Games were affected, since there was widespread opposition to athletic participation by women.

In most states the state high school athletic association legislated against interscholastic competition for girls. Some of these same states approved play days for girls, some permitted sports days (see Chapter 13), while some barred absolutely all athletic participation.

Probably the greatest single factor in reintroducing athletic competition for women and girls was World War II. At this time women abdicated their typical roles as housewives in order to man industrial plants, thus changing the implications of femininity; fitness of the total population was stressed; and club teams and industrial teams—sponsored by agencies outside the school—flourished.

In general, women physical educators ignored the needs of the highly skilled girl, who was therefore forced to seek outlets for the expression of her skill outside the school. As might be expected, malpractices developed as untrained leadership took over, and the result was that the very evils that physical educators were trying to avoid were compounded.

The Division for Girls' and Women's Sports, which in 1957 became a section of the AAHPER, was the organization most interested in the conduct of school-sponsored athletic competition, and it took vigorous strides forward to try to ensure that all organi-

---

[6] Harry A. Scott, *Competitive Sports in Schools and Colleges* (New York: Harper Bros., 1951): p. 445.

zations interested in women's athletics worked together for the common good of the participants (organizations such as the Amateur Athletic Union, the U.S. Women's Olympic Committee, the National Collegiate Athletic Association, the National Association for Intercollegiate Athletics, the Federale Internationale Sports Union, the Collegiate Students Association, and the U.S. Gymnastics Federation). Programs were given priorities as follows: (1) the instructional program, (2) the intramural program, (3) play days and sports days, and (4) extramural competition. This stand led many people, erroneously, to conclude that DGWS was supportive of neither interschool competition for girls and women nor highly skilled participants. Such notions should have been dispelled in the policy statements of 1962, in which DGWS not only embraced a concept of opportunities in sport at all levels for girls and women, but also encouraged conducting workshops, clinics and institutes in training techniques, coaching, and sports medicine. The "mirror of time," according to Jernigan, will alone be able to measure the full impact of DGWS on women's sport.[7]

In 1969 DGWS published its *Philosophy and Standards for Girls and Women's Sports* (revised, 1972) in an attempt to pull together into one source all standards for women's athletics.[8] This reference remains of value to anyone who is responsible in any manner for the conduct of a sports program for women, since it discusses in a philosophic vein such topics as standards for the leadership of the program, types of programs advocated, pratical considerations such as financing, recruiting, scheduling and awards, and guidelines for competitive programs at various educational levels.

The number of intercollegiate athletic programs for women began to increase to a significant extent in the late 60's, and it became evident that some organization was needed to guide and control such programs. Consequently, in 1967, DGWS and the Board of Control of the AAHPER established the Commission on Intercollegiate Athletics for Women (CIAW). This Commission has since been expanded into the Association for Intercollegiate Athletics (AIAW), established by DGWS in 1971, to provide a governing body and leadership for initiating and maintaining standards of excellence in women's intercollegiate programs. AIAW presently conducts

---

[7] Sara Jernigan, "Mirror of Time: Some Causes for More American Women in Sport Competitions," *Quest,* **22** (June 1974): 82–87.

[8] Philosophy and Standards Committee, Division for Girls' and Women's Sports, *Philosophy and Standards for Girls' and Women's Sports* (Washington, D.C.: American Association for Health, Physical Education, and Recreation, revised ed., 1972).

17 national championships in 12 different sports for junior and community colleges, small colleges, and large colleges.

The *AIAW Handbook* is a periodic publication that addresses the purpose of the association, its philosophy regarding intercollegiate athletic programs for women, and the regulations that universities must follow in the conduct of such programs if they are member institutions and if they are to be eligible to participate in AIAW national championships.

NAGWS and AIAW

In March 1974 when the A.A.H.P.E.R. was reorganized into the American Alliance for Health, Physical Education and Recreation, DGWS officially disbanded in favor of the newly structured National Association for Girls and Women in Sport (NAGWS), of which AIAW is an official structure. Since NAGWS seems likely to be the dominant force behind competitive athletic programs for girls and women, it is perhaps important to understand its structural organization. The Board of Directors of NAGWS is comprised of 12 voting members, one from each of the following groups:

1. The National Coaches Associations. Such associations became operative in June 1974, and all the associations together select one of their members to serve on the Board of Directors of NAGWS.
2. NAGWS-Affiliated Boards of Officials. Presently 190 such boards are extant and together they select one representative to the Board of Directors.
3. Association for Intercollegiate Athletics for Women.
4. State High School Athletic Associations.
5. One representative from the combined group of schools which focus on club and intramural sports.
6. State NAGWS Chairmen.
7. The Student Section of NAGWS.
8. A "public representative"—a nationally prominent person interested in sports for girls and women.

An additional four voting members are the president, the president-elect, the past-president, and an at-large delegate.[9]

Because of the far-reaching effects that AIAW has already had on programs of sport for girls and women and because this organi-

---

[9] Fran Koening, "DGWS Offers More in '74," *DGWS News*. **3**:1 (Winter 1974), 1.

zation will no doubt continue to exert great influence on such programs, several of its official stances are reproduced in detail in the following pages. Figure 2 shows its "General Organization Chart," which as another example of an administrative line chart shows the interrelationships among the several subunits which together comprise the total organization. Although the AIAW is concerned with the goverance of programs for college women only, its influence extends to high school programs as well. Each of the 50 states in the United States has its own High School Athletic Association and its own set of official regulations for sports participation by girls at the secondary school level. Obviously the high schools, then, must abide by the rules in force in a particular state; however, it seems fair to judge that most such official positions were influenced to a considerable degree by AIAW philosophy and purposes.

The purposes of the AIAW are:

1. To foster broad programs of women's intercollegiate athletics which are consistent with the educational aims and objectives of the member schools and in accordance with the philosophy and standards of the NAGWS.
2. To assist member schools in extending and enriching their programs of intercollegiate athletes for women based upon the needs, interests, and capacities of the individual student.
3. To stimulate the development of quality leadership for women's intercollegiate athletic programs.
4. To foster programs which will encourage excellence in performance of participants in women's intercollegiate athletics.
5. To maintain the spirit of play within competitive sport events so that the concomitant educational values of such an experience are emphasized.
6. To increase public understanding and appreciation of the importance and value of sports and athletics as they contribute to the enrichment of the life of the woman.
7. To encourage and facilitate research on the effects of intercollegiate athletic woman and to disseminate the findings.
8. To further the continual evaluation of standards and policies for participants and programs.
9. To produce and distribute such materials as will be of assistance to persons in the development and improvement of intercollegiate programs.
10. To hold national championships and to sponsor conferences, institutes, and meetings which will meet the needs of individuals in member schools.

11. To cooperate with other professional groups of similar interests for the ultimate development of sports programs and opportunities for women.
12. To provide direction and maintain a relationship with AIAW regional organizations.
13. To conduct such other activities as shall be approved by the governing body of the Association.[10]

In its "Position Paper on Intercollegiate Athletics for Women," endorsed in May 1974, AIAW reaffirmed its philosophic stance that inner satisfactions such as enjoyment, positive self-concept, and a sense of physical well-being are the fundamental motives for athletic participation and that a complex and costly program may delimit such participation to only a select few. Consequently, the following program elements are stressed as vital:

> We believe sport is an important aspect of our culture and a fertile field for learning. The sense of enjoyment, self-confidence and physical well-being derived from demanding one's best performance in a sport situation is a meaningful experience for the athlete. These inner satisfactions are the fundamental motivation for participation in sports. Therefore, programs in an educational setting should have these benefits as primary goals.
>
> In keeping with the belief, the following program elements are vitally important:
>
> 1. The enrichment of the life of the participant is the focus and reason for the existence of any athletic program. All decisions should be made with this fact in mind.
>
> 2. The participants in athletic programs, including players, coaches, and support personnel, should have access to and representation on the policy-making group on campus and in sport governing organizations.
>
> 3. Adequate funding is necessary to provide a comprehensive program. Sufficient funds should be provided for (1) a broad spectrum of sports experiences; (b) a variety of levels of competitive experiences; (c) travel using licensed carriers; (d) appropriate housing and food; (e) rated officials; (f) well-trained coaches; (g) equipment, supplies, and facilities which aid performance and appeal to the aesthetic aspects of sport; (h) competent staff for administering and publicizing the program (i) qualified medical and training personnel; and (j) regular opportunities for social interaction with opponents.
>
> 4. Careful consideration is needed for scheduling practice sessions and games. The athletic schedule should ensure sufficient time to

---

[10] *AIAW Handbook 1977–78* (Washington, D.C.: AAHPER PRESS, 1977), p. 18. Reprinted by permission of the American Alliance for Health, Physical Education and Recreation.

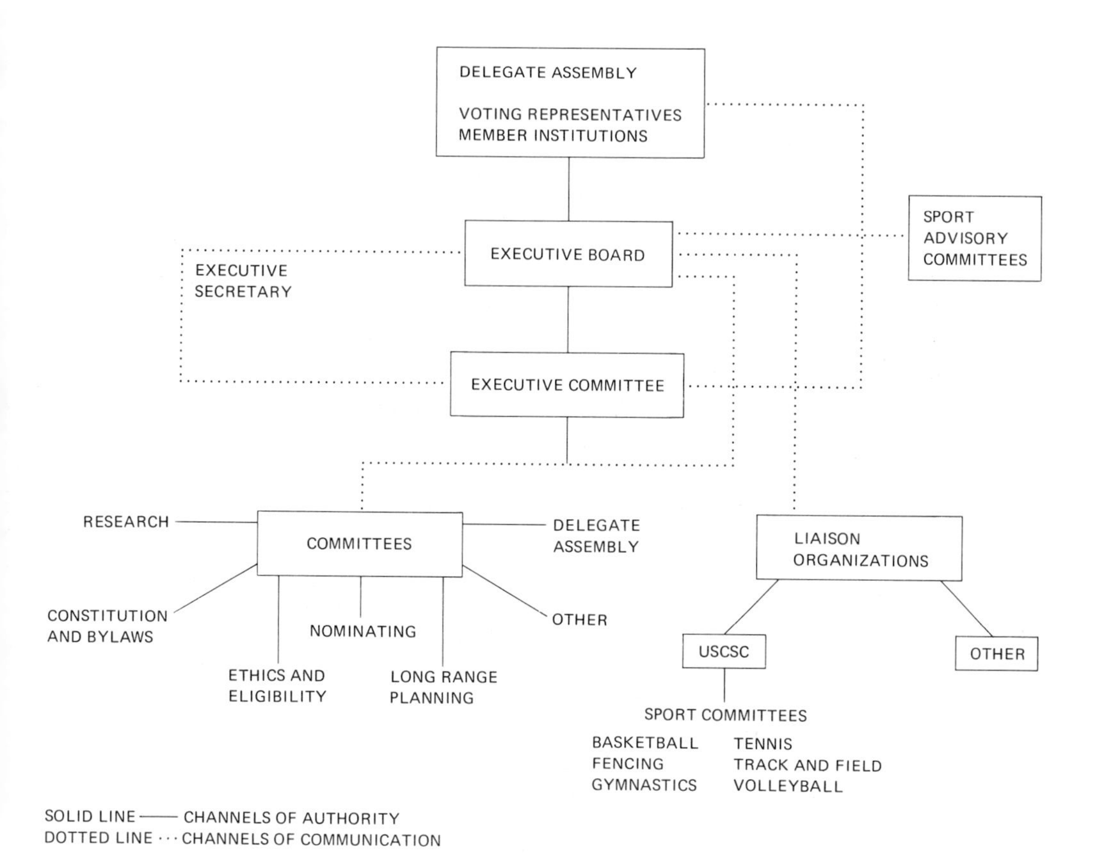

Fig. 2 General organization chart, AIAW. (*AIAW Handbook, 1977–78,* Washington, D.C.: AAHPER Press, 1977, p. 6. Reprinted by permission of the American Alliance for Health, Physical Education and Recreation.)

gain personal satisfaction from skill achievement, but should not deny the student the time to participate in other activities. Factors to be considered include: (a) equitable competition on all levels; (b) adequate pre-season conditioning; (c) appropriate spacing and length of practice sessions; (d) sufficient number of events in each sport; and (e) comparable length of seasons between sports.

5. Separate but comparable teams should be provided for women and men. In addition to separate teams, intercollegiate co-educational teams comprised of an equal number of women and men competing on opposing teams is desirable in those sports in which such teams are appropriate.

6. Athletic ability is one of the talents which can be considered in the awarding of financial aid to students. However, students should be free to choose the institution on the basis of curriculum and program. Staff time and effort should be devoted to the comprehensive program rather than to recruiting efforts.[11]

Membership in AIAW quickly grew, and some 200 member schools discussed significant issues revolving around athletic scholarships and separate teams for men and women in its historic first assembly of delegates, held in November 1973.[12] Insofar as athletic scholarships are concerned, the Assembly reversed a previous stand outlawing them by indicating that a school could grant athletic scholarships without jeopardizing its opportunity to participate in national AIAW competitions. Because of the far-reaching effects, the resolution passed by the Assembly regarding separate teams for men and women is reproduced in its entirety below:

> WHEREAS: A single team for which men and women compete to become members strongly discriminates against women due to sex-determined physiological disadvantages in strength and speed, and
> WHEREAS: A mixed (coed) team for which participants compete against members of their own sex for membership on the team and for which an equal number of males and females compete on opposing teams is not discriminatory to either sex,
> BE IT RESOLVED: There shall be separate teams for men and women. No male student may participate on a women's intercollegiate team. No female student may participate on a men's intercollegiate team. In addition to separate teams for men and women, intercollegiate mixed (coed) teams composed of an equal number of males and females competing on opposing teams are desirable in those sports in which such teams are appropriate.[13]

The rationale on which the resolution was based is also reproduced in its entirety:

> *Men not permitted on women's teams*
>
> 1. Men on women's teams prevent equality of opportunity due to the physiological differences between the male and female. There are several physiological functions which impose limitations on the female, especially in regard to strength and speed in performance.
>
> (a) The female hormone estrogen results in inhibiting the growth of muscle tissue while increasing the amounts of adipose tissue. The

---

[11] NAGWS, *AIAW Handbook* (Washington, D.C.: AAHPER Press, 1977), p. 69. Reprinted by permission of the American Alliance for Health, Physical Education and Recreation.

[12] Joan Hult, "First AIAW Delegate Assembly," *JOHPER,* **45**:3 (March 1974), 79.

[13] *Ibid.* (Reprinted by permission of the American Alliance for Health, Physical Education and Recreation.)

male hormone androgen enhances the growth of muscle tissue. The ratio of strength to weight is much greater in the male than in the female. Conditioning may enhance the development of muscle mass and minimize the amount of adipose tissue of female athletes. It should be clear, however, that physiological differences dictate that the male athlete will not only remain superior in sports requiring muscular strength and speed but will also be able to reach higher levels of training because of these factors.

(b) Maximal oxygen uptake (maximal aerobic capacity) is lower in the female than in the male. Maximal oxygen uptake is a function of both the cardiovascular and respiratory systems and is thus limited by the individual's reaction to stress variables related to these systems. An adult female has a lower maximal oxygen uptake than a male for several reasons: (1) lower level of hemoglobin and erythrocytes, (2) a smaller cardiac output and stroke volume due to smaller heart, and (3) total body mass affects maximal oxygen results. Even the well-trained woman athlete does not have the same potential for maximal aerobic capacity as the trained male athlete.

(c) Factor analysis studies make apparent the importance of the strength component in all competitive athletics, and the relative importance of the speed factor in most competitive athletics. There is an overlap in the strength and speed factors between male and female; that is to say, not all males have more strength and speed than all females. The problem lies, however, in the reality that the overlap occurs in the high end of the female distribution and the low end of the male distribution; therefore, females of above average strength cannot compete equally with males who are above average in strength. The same overlap occurs in a study of the speed factor. These facts are significant in intercollegiate competition where we are dealing with top level performance.

2. The cultural concepts of the female athletes in our society have been a factor which has affected their performance attainment in the past and the residue will continue for years to come. This is an additional disadvantage to the woman athlete who must compete with the more experienced male athlete for membership on a single team. This lack of experience is another deterrent to her athletic success on a single team composed primarily of males.

3. Without men on women's teams there is greater freedom for women to develop athletic teams which can reflect their own model, not a model of a men's intercollegiate team.

Women not permitted on men's teams

1. The policy of permitting women on men's teams is discriminatory to men. If a woman can take a man's place on his team but he can-

not take a woman's place on her team when he is superior to the woman in athletic ability, this is a discriminatory action.

2. Single teams will destroy equality of opportunity because the large majority of women will be excluded from this competition. The present policy encourages colleges and universities to avoid the responsibility of providing women's teams.

3. Programs based on the interests, needs, and capabilities of women are not possible within the context of men's intercollegiate teams which have, by tradition, been modeled for the male athlete. Growth, development, and control of top level competition for women, with its own model, is only feasible within the framework of separate women's teams.

4. Women desiring to be participants on men's teams reflect an assumption of inferiority of programs or a lack of any program. Neither of these situations should be tolerated. There must be a concerted effort to provide top level competition for female athletes and to provide teams with programs which do have equitable monies, schedules, facilities, equipment, medical care, and coaching. Excellent women's athletic teams which are designed specifically for the sex-based classification of the woman athlete can result.

Mixed (coed) teams in sports in which such teams are appropriate

1. In a mixed (coed) team setting, participants compete against members of their own sex for membership on the team; therefore, there is an opportunity for high-level competition involving members of both sexes which uses the strengths of each in a highly competitive situation. Since equal numbers of males and females compete on opposing teams, it is not discriminatory to either sex and the physiological disadvantages of females are minimized while the female advantages of balance, agility, and finesse of movement can enhance the total team play. True coed teams can lead to new strategies which are not effective in other situations and thus add to the total development of the sport.

2. The trend in our society and within the offerings of physical education programs is toward coeducational sports. This being the case, it is mandatory that we provide avenues for continued development of high-level performance opportunities within the intercollegiate setting. The mixed (coed) teams offer an enrichment and expansion of the total offerings of an athletic program; the mixed (coed) teams should be in addition to, not instead of, the two separate teams for men and women.

3. Although the purpose of the mixed (coed) teams is to enhance the total offerings of the intercollegiate programs, it might also be used as a compromise measure until separate teams for men and women are developed. While the situation of a single team composed

primarily of men is discriminatory to women athletes, a mixed (coed) team does not jeopardize the equality of opportunity or the opportunity for high-level competition for both males and females.[14]

Unlike the National Collegiate Athletic Association (NCAA), which polices its membership and tries to enforce rules, the AIAW opts for self-regulation through a commitment to its Code of Ethics, which was approved by mail vote of the AIAW membership in May 1974. Because of the obvious importance of this code, then, it is reproduced verbatim below. AIAW does have a "regulatory and enforcement scheme" based on a written report by a representative from an AIAW member institution of an infraction. *All* such written reports are investigated, and if it is found that some impropriety exists, the participation rights of member institutions or of specific student-athletes can be eliminated.

> AIAW CODE OF ETHICS The purpose of the AIAW Code of Ethics is to provide a means of assisting personnel and students of AIAW member institutions to identify ethical conduct in intercollegiate sports and to encourage those involved to pursue actions which are appropriate. The Code is not intended to be enforceable rules of conduct, the violation of which would require disciplinary action by AIAW, but rather is a guide for all concerned to apply in various aspects of sport programs. The Code of Ethics cannot be all inclusive but it does identify many areas of concern. AIAW encourages everyone involved to continue to identify and pursue conduct which promotes dignity in sport.
>
> CODE OF ETHICS FOR COACHES One of the purposes of intercollegiate athletics is to provide experiences and opportunities for players to develop socially acceptable and personally fulfilling values and characteristics. Competitive sports provide practice opportunities in making value judgments and developing social relationships which will help to determine desirable behavior and personal qualities. A coach has the unique opportunity to influence players in selecting and developing their personal values and desirable qualities. The philosophy, attitude, and behavior of the coach should exemplify quality human characteristics.
>
> The coach should recognize the uniqueness and worth of each individual and help her to develop confidence, exhibit cooperation, and make a contribution to herself and others around her. Many experiences shared by the coach and player happen under stressful competitive circumstances which require maturity and experience to cope with them. These experiences provide teachable moments in which the coach should share her good judgment and show under-

[14] *Ibid.*, pp. 79–80. (Reprinted by permission of American Alliance for Health, Physical Education and Recreation.)

standing and control which will influence the reactions of players, spectators, opponents, and the officials associated with the game. A coach also has a responsibility to provide the information and training necessary for her players to achieve the highest degree of excellence for which they have potential. She also has a responsibility to promote sports and perpetuate the understanding of sports in our society. A basic part of this is the understanding and performance of the game in the true spirit of sport.

Ethical considerations for the coach:

1. Respect each player as a special individual with unique needs, experience, and characteristics and develop this understanding and respect among the players.
2. Have pride in being a good example of a coach in appearance, conduct, language, and sportsmanship, and teach the players the importance of these standards.
3. Demonstrate and instill in players a respect for and courtesy toward opposing players, coaches and officials.
4. Express appreciation to the officials for their contribution and appropriately address officials regarding rule interpretations of officiating techniques. Respect their integrity and judgment.
5. Exhibit and develop in one's players the ability to accept defeat or victory gracefully without undue emotionalism.
6. Teach players to play within the spirit of the game and the letter of the rules.
7. Develop understanding among players, stressing a spirit of team play. Encourage qualities of self-discipline, cooperation, self-confidence, leadership, courtesy, honesty, initiative and fair play.
8. Provide for the welfare of the players by:
   (a) Scheduling appropriate practice periods,
   (b) Providing safe transportation,
   (c) Scheduling appropriate number of practice and league games,
   (d) Providing safe playing areas,
   (e) Using good judgment before playing injured, fatigued, or emotionally upset players,
   (f) Providing proper medical care and treatment.
9. Use consistent and fair criteria in judging players and establishing standards for them.
10. Treat players with respect, equality, and courtesy.
11. Direct constructive criticism toward players in a positive, objective manner.

12. Compliment players honestly and avoid exploiting them for self-glory.
13. Emphasize the ideals of sportsmanship and fair play in all competitive situations.
14. Maintain an uncompromising adherence to standards, rules, eligibility, conduct, etiquette, and attendance requirements. Teach players to understand these principles and adhere to them also.
15. Be knowledgeable in aspects of the sport to provide an appropriate level of achievement for her players. Have a goal of quality play and excellence. Know proper fundamentals, strategy, safety factors, training and conditioning principles, and an understanding of rules and officiating.
16. Attend workshops, clinics, classes and institutes to keep abreast and informed of current trends and techniques of the sport.
17. Obtain membership and be of service in organizations and agencies which promote the sport and conduct competitive opportunities.
18. Use common sense and composure in meeting stressful situations and in establishing practice and game schedules which are appropriate and realistic in terms of demands on players' time and physical condition.
19. Conduct practice opportunities which provide appropriate preparation to allow the players to meet the competitive situation with confidence.
20. Require medical examinations for all players prior to the sports season and follow the medical recommendations for those players who have a history of medical problems or who have sustained an injury during the season.
21. Cooperate with administrative personnel in establishing and conducting a quality athletic program.
22. Accept opportunities to host events and conduct quality competition.
23. Contribute constructive suggestions to the governing association for promoting and organizing competitive experiences.
24. Show respect and appreciation for tournament personnel and offer assistance where appropriate.
25. Be present at all practices and competitions. Avoid letting other appointments interfere with the scheduled team time. Provide time to meet the needs of the individual players.
26. Encourage spectators to display conduct of respect and hospitality toward opponents and officials and to recognize good play and sportsmanship. When inappropriate crowd action occurs, the coach should assist in curtailing the crowd reactions.

CODE OF ETHICS FOR PLAYERS The purpose of Intercollegiate Athletics is to provide an opportunity for the participant to develop her potential as a skilled performer in an educational setting.

As education seeks to provide ways in which each may know herself and grow emotionally, socially and intellectually, so does the intercollegiate athletic program. In addition, the participant has the opportunity to travel, represent her school and learn the art of being a team member. All this gain is not without sacrifice, for the player may lose some individual rights and privileges as she accepts the policies of the program when she becomes a member of the team.

Ethical considerations for the player:

1. Maintain personal habits which enhance healthful living.
2. Objectively acknowledge one's own strengths and weaknesses. Recognize that each person has her own strengths and weaknesses—praise the strengths and help to strentghen weaknesses.
3. Value one's personal integrity.
4. Respect differing points of view.
5. Strive for the highest degree of excellence.
6. Willfully abide by the spirit of the rules as well as the letter of the rules throughout all games and practices.
7. Uphold all standards and regulations expected of participants.
8. Treat all players, officials and coaches with respect and courtesy.
9. Accept victory or defeat without undue emotion.
10. Graciously accept constructive criticism.
11. Respect and accept the decisions of the coach. When ethical decisions are questionable, the participant should direct her questions to the coach in private and follow appropriate channels to voice her concerns.
12. Be willing to train in order to achieve one's full potential.
13. Respect the achievements of the opponent.
14. Extend appreciation to those who have made the contest possible.
15. Be grateful for the opportunity afforded by the intercollegiate program and be willing to assist in program tasks as evidence of this gratefulness.
16. Assist in promoting positive relations among all participants who are striving to achieve athletic excellence.
17. Exhibit dignity in manner and dress when representing one's school both on and off the court or playing field.
18. Respect the accomplishments of one's teammates.
19. Expect fans to treat officials, coaches and players with respect.

20. Recognize and value the contribution of each team member.
21. Keep personal disagreements away from practices and contests.
22. Keep the importance of winning in perspective with regard to other objectives.
23. Contribute to the effort to make each practice a success.
24. Exert maximum effort in all games and practices.
25. Seek to know and understand one's teammates.
26. Place primary responsibility to the team rather than to self.
27. Refrain from partaking of drugs which would enhance performance or modify mood or behavior at any time during a season unless prescribed by a physician for medical purposes.
28. Refrain from partaking of alcoholic beverages while representing one's school.

CODE OF ETHICS FOR ADMINISTRATORS The purpose of the women's intercollegiate program is to provide competition for highly skilled women who have come to the institution for both educational and athletic opportunities. The initial guidance and example must come from the chief administrator of the athletic program. The primary aim of the administrator is to foster ethical practices of behavior which will accomplish and fulfill goals of wholesome and desirable experiences for all individuals in the program.

Ethical considerations for the administrator:

1. Hire coaches or assign coaching duties to personnel who are qualified and interested in the particular sport.
2. Insist that players and coaches abide by and ahere to the rules and regulations set forth by organizations of which the institution is a member.
3. Strive to obtain the services of a full-time Athletic Trainer and Team Physician.
4. Encourage coaches to become knowledgeable in the prevention and immediate care of athletic injuries.
5. Ultimately be responsible for the health and safety of all participants in the intercollegiate program by:
   (a) Assuring that health forms are completed for all players prior to participation.
   (b) Assuring that some form of medical insurance covers each player for the duration of a season.
6. Reflect support of the intercollegiate program to both players and coaches through personal actions and, when possible, through presence at athletic events.

7. Strive to obtain adequate funds for the intercollegiate program and disperse such funds to the various sports in a fair and equitable manner. There should be no designation of major and minor sports.
8. Make provisions for the budgeting of qualified officials.
9. Seek approval for the use of adequate facilities for practices and competition and assure that teams are supplied with quality equipment.
10. Strive to gain release of class time and/or compensation for personnel who have coaching duties; and to seek approval for the hiring of additional personnel if the size of the program warrants.
11. Keep university administrative personnel informed of problems, issues, and accomplishments of the intercollegiate program in order to maintain or create greater understanding between the university and athletic administrations.
12. Strive to obtain and/or retain a cooperative working relationship with personnel associated with the men's athletic program.
13. Constantly be aware of changes in policy and rules of the organizations with which the institution is affiliated.
14. Attend, when possible, meetings, workshops, conventions, etc., in order to obtain greater insight into the operating procedures of intercollegiate organizations.
15. Provide for student input when formulating policies and procedures regarding intercollegiate participation.
16. Continually evaluate existing policies regarding operation of the intercollegiate program and, with input from coaches and players, initiate action to improve and strengthen the program.

CODE OF ETHICS FOR OFFICIALS It is the responsibility of the official to enforce the letter and spirit of the rules in order to maintain the quality of competition necessary to achieve the goal of excellence, as well as to protect the health and welfare of each participant.

The official commands respect by her appearance, voice and actions. It is her attitude toward questions, criticisms, and varying situations and the manner in which she exhibits control which ultimately influences the tone and atmosphere of the game.

Courtesy, respect, and understanding breed a similar attitude, among coaches, players, and spectators. The official serves in the capacity of an arbitrator; the successful fulfillment of this role lies in the promotion of quality competition through a thorough knowledge of the game, an attitude of impartiality, and the creation of a positive atmosphere. In this sense, the attributes of the official become a very vital and indispensable aspect of every game situation.

Ethical considerations for the official:

1. Maintain the highest standards of honesty and integrity, making decisions without deference to team, score, spectators or home facility.
2. Maintain an objective view, keeping the game within the spirit of the rules without imposing one's own philosophical beliefs upon the participants.
3. Maintain consistency in interpreting and enforcing the rules.
4. Exhibit a thorough knowledge of the rules and a willingness to interpret rules and clarify decisions.
5. Seek to maintain the differences between the philosophy of NAGWS and that of other organizations by interpreting and enforcing the rules properly.
6. Exhibit alertness in reacting to the immediate situation without interjecting her own personal feelings.
7. Exhibit concern for the player's welfare by correcting those situations which involve actions detrimental to the welfare of participants.
8. Maintain a friendly and communicative attitude toward players, coaches, and spectators.
9. Fulfill role as an arbitrator by recognizing and controlling the tempo of the game and the feelings of the spectators.
10. Maintain a sense of composure in respect to players, coaches, and spectators.
11. Avoid repeated assignments and tournament games which involve a direct affiliation with coaches, players and/or a specific team.
12. Always wear the proper uniform and be neatly and appropriately attired.
13. Consistently seek to improve one's own abilities by attending rules discussions and interpretation clinics.
14. Recognize and seek to fulfill her role in the development of player's, coach's, and specator's attitudes toward sport.
15. Provide opportunity for players to react honestly concerning the rules by acknowledging those infractions in which it may be difficult for an official to determine fair play.

CODE OF ETHICS FOR SPECTATORS Winning is often so important that some people have lost sight of the educational values inherent in athletics. If the full benefit of athletics as an educational tool is to be utilized, colleges and universities must immediately concern themselves with spectator sportsmanship.

The playing of the game should be regarded by the spectators as an art, and should be appreciated and enjoyed as such. Respect for all players, coaches, and officials, regardless of their own team loyalty, is essential for raising the standards of good sportsmanship.

Ethical considerations for the spectators:

1. Recognize the official as a person of integrity and qualification, and respect the decisions accordingly.
2. Refrain from creating disturbances which would be detrimental to the flow of the game and/or to the safety of the participants involved.
3. Refrain from harrassment, profane language or ostentatious behavior in respect to players and coaches.
4. Become familiar with the rules of the game in order to enjoy it more and to understand the decisions made by the officials.
5. Exhibit respect for the local policies and regulations regarding the usage of athletic facilities.
6. Exhibit team loyalties and support without negative action toward their opponents or officials of the game.

Flagrant violations of the Codes of Ethics at National Championships which are reported to the Ethics and Eligibility Committee shall be communicated to the individual responsible for the women's athletic program or the appropriate administrator in the institution in violation via a letter. Disciplinary action shall be deferred to that institution.[15]

PRESENT STATUS

It is an undeniable fact that competitive athletic programs for girls and women are dramatically increasing in number and scope. As the public, government officials, school administrators, and physical educators become more educated in such areas of concern as the physiological, sociological, and psychological aspects of competition for women, they accept the premise that there is nothing inherently wrong with a well-conducted program of athletics and that, in fact, the practice of neglecting the highly skilled girl is an undemocratic and even a discriminatory one. Consequently, they press for the introduction or extension of such a program.

A legal precedent was set for equal athletic programs for girls and women by Title IX of the Education Amendments Act of 1972, Public Law 92–318, passed by Congress on June 23, 1972, which states:

---

[15] *AIAW Handbook 1977–78* (Washington, D. C.: AAHPER Press, 1977), pp. 34–39. Reprinted by permission of the American Alliance for Health, Physical Education and Recreation.

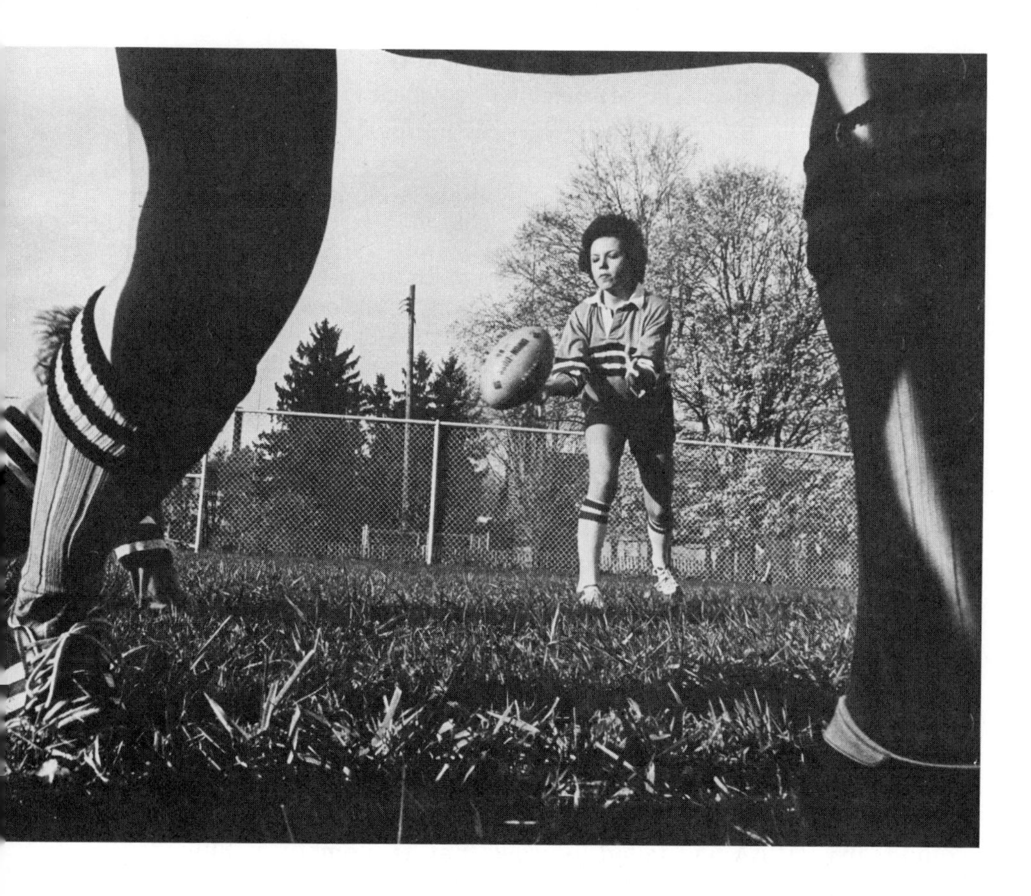

Fig. 3 Title IX has increased opportunities for women to participate in sports. (Courtesy of Indiana University News Bureau.)

> No person in the United States shall, on the basis of sex, be excluded from participation in, be denied the benefits of, or be subject to sex discrimination under any education program or activity receiving Federal financial assistance.[16]

The Act empowered the Department of Health, Education and Welfare to issue regulations for implementing the Act, and the Office of Civil Rights was given the task of writing specific regulations, which took effect in July 1975. Speaking specifically to athletic programs, the regulations state that competitive athletics are defined as

---

[16] Marjorie Blaufarb, "Opportunity Knocks Through Title IX," *AAHPER Update* (April 1974), p. 1. Reprinted by permission.

> . . . all athletic teams operated by a recipient [an institution receiving Federal financial assistance], selection for which is based upon competitive skill, including all training, coaching, and other activities related thereto. . . .[17]

Insofar as the operation of competitive athletic programs are concerned, the regulations also state:

> [recipients] shall not discriminate therein on the basis of sex in the selection of sports or levels of competition, provisions of equipment or supplies, scheduling of games and practice times, travel and per diem allowance, award of athletic scholarships, opportunity to receive coaching and instruction, assignment of coaches and instructors, provisions of locker room, practice, or competitive facilities, provision of medical facilities and services, publicity, or otherwise.[18]

There has been much confusion about, and probably much misinterpretation of, Title IX, its implementation, and its probable effects. The National Collegiate Athletic Association, for example, submitted legal objections to the regulations and asked for their withdrawal because "no existing record indicates Congress had any intention of applying Title IX to athletics when it passed the legislation." [19] NCAA based its stand that athletics should be excluded from this legislation on the fact that "no athletic program receives any Federal financial aid in any form." [20] However, in what was called a "decisive victory for women," U.S. District Court Judge Earl E. O'Connor dismissed the lawsuit in January 1978 on the grounds that NCAA had failed to prove that its member institutions or their athletic programs would be "injured" by the regulations of Title IX.[21] It would seem that one direct result of this ruling will be to force into total compliance those institutions that perhaps have used delaying tactics.

Many present interscholastic and intercollegiate athletic programs for women are still, by definition, *extramural* in nature. As was explained in Chapter 13, the term "extramurals," much used in women's physical education, simply means that although two schools are competing against each other the players are not *varsity* players and thus the program is informally organized and conducted. Whereas "varsity" connotes a group of highly skilled,

---

17 *Ibid.*, p. 3.

18 *Ibid.*

19 *N.C.A.A. News.* **11**:4 (March 15, 1974). 1.

20 *Ibid.*

21 Anne C. Roark, "Court Rejects NCAA Challenge to Ban on Sex Bias in Sports," *Chronicle of Higher Education,* **15** (January 16, 1978): 1.

selected players who receive extra coaching for the purpose of playing a prearranged schedule of contests, the school team in extramural competition for girls and women is usually a "club" team which "cuts" no one from its roster, which receives a very limited amount of coaching, and which schedules a minimal number of games only a week or two in advance.

Competitive athletic programs for girls and women, whether varsity or extramural in nature, are increasing in numbers and in scope at a phenomenal rate. Such growth is bound to focus greater attention on the role and status of the female and the psychological, physiological, cultural, and legal barriers, real or imagined, to her participation in athletics.

THE FEMININE ROLE

Just as the female had to fight for political and professional emancipation, so, too, she has had to fight for the physical right to be fit and to compete in athletics. The women's liberation movement strongly asserts that a woman's anatomy should not determine her destiny. Although there is evidence that the traditional role of the female is changing, if for no other reason than that discrimination against women is now illegal, there is still much emotional debate about femininity and other qualities of "ladies" and their relationship to athletic competency. Much research has been directed toward seeking answers to time-honored beliefs concerning physiological, psychological and social limitations of the female. As this research continues to disprove such limitations, athletic programs are extended; and as the programs continue to expand so too does the research. Since much work has been done on disproving the negative effects of athletics, the scope of the research should be broadened to include investigations of the positive effects of the program. As Gendel states:

> In the debates about women and physical exertion, competitive sports, and Olympic participation, the emphasis has been chiefly on proving that no *harm* will be done. What is needed is more information on what *good* might be accomplished were these activities recommended. The "good" being more than the physical exuberance, camaraderie and well-being experienced by participants. The "medical" advantages which may be present should be explored more fully and explained.[22]

[22] Evalyn S. Gendel, "Women and the Medical Aspects of Sports," *Journal of School Health*, **37** (November 1967): 429.

More scientific studies need to be undertaken in all facets of competition, and evaluation needs to be a continuous process. The findings of research studies regarding some of the more significant issues are discussed briefly below.

Physiological Aspects

No doubt the aspect of athletic competition that has most concerned women physical educators and members of the medical profession is the physical effect on the participants. Many studies in this area have concluded that menstrual and child-bearing characteristics are not significantly affected by participation in athletics. Erdelyi's research showed that

1. participation in active competitive sport does not disturb the onset of the menarche;
2. athletes generally have shorter, easier labors with normal deliveries;
3. competitive sports participation during adolescence has no untoward effect on the development of the bony pelvis of the female;
4. female athletes do not show signs of masculinization even after years of participation, although some female athletes have male characteristics in their body build and musculature *before* their sports careers;
5. the *performance* of the female athlete may be affected during different stages of the menstrual cycle.[23]

Erdelyi's study and others show that in all biological characteristics other than those dealing with the unique procreation function of the female, "differences between the sexes appear to be relative rather than categorical."[24] This general conclusion is corroborated by the American Medical Association in a position paper written in 1973 by the Committee on the Medical Aspects of Sports. The statement is reproduced in its entirety below since it not only supports the fact that active participation by the female is medically desirable but also supports the position of NAGWS that girls should have programs of athletics separate from boys' programs.

---

[23] Gyula J. Erdelyi, "Gynecological Survey of Female Athletes," *Journal of Sports Medicine and Physical Fitness*, **2** (September 1962): 174–179.

[24] Eleanor Metheny, "Sports and the Feminine Image," *Gymnasion*, **4** (Winter 1964): 17.

FEMALES IN CONTACT AND NON-CONTACT SPORTS

Girls Participating in Exercise and Sports Competition

The Committee on the Medical Aspects of Sports reiterates the beneficial aspects of sports and exercise participation for girls and women. The female's participation in such programs previously was discouraged in alignment with societal and cultural stereotypes, which considered such participation a departure from the traditional role of the female and a detraction from her femininity. Much to the contrary, physiological and social benefits are to be gained by girls and women through physical activity and sports competition. In many cases, vigorous physical activity improves the distinctive biological functions of the female.

Usually, dysmenorrhea is unaffected by sports participation or subsides as a result of such participation. Exercise can also improve regulation of the menstrual cycle. Following active sports involvement of international caliber, female athletes have experienced a greater number of complication-free pregnancies and greater ease of delivery than recorded for a normal but less physically active control group. These specific benefits often accrue to female athletes quite apart from the normal physiological benefits to both males and females from regular exercise or sports participation, including improvements in muscle tone and strength, increased joint range of motion, and improvement in a host of cardiovascular parameters. Thus, there is no medical or scientific rationale for restricting the normal female from participating in vigorous non-contact sports, and many reasons to encourage such participation. Physical activity and sports programs can contribute significantly to their personal fulfillment and healthful living.

Girls Participating in Non-Contact Sports with Boys

In recent years, athletic associations have recognized the value of girls' competing in sports. Indeed, girls' high school sports participation has increased 175 percent over the last two years. Girls themselves and their representatives have also requested participation on boys' teams in non-contact sports. Where no comparable girls' program exists, or where limited staff and facilities do not permit sports programs for both boys and girls, this interim measure is a desirable solution for selected sports. However, it is in the long-range interest of both male and female athletes that they have their own programs. During preadolescence there is no essential difference in the work capacity between boys and girls, except that girls reach their maximum work capacity sooner than boys. Females also sustain their flexibility over a much longer period of time than do males. However, following puberty boys uniformly surpass girls in all other athletic performance characteristics mainly because of a higher lean body weight to adipose tissue ratio. Thus, only the exceptional girl will have

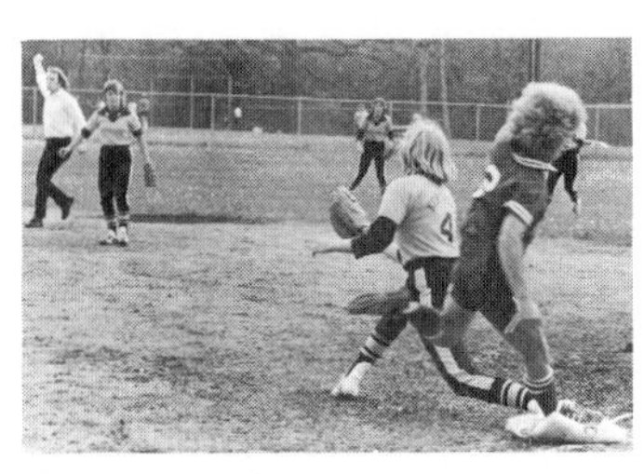

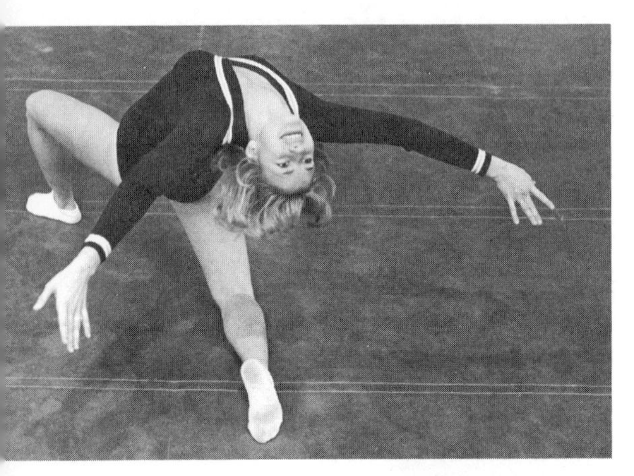

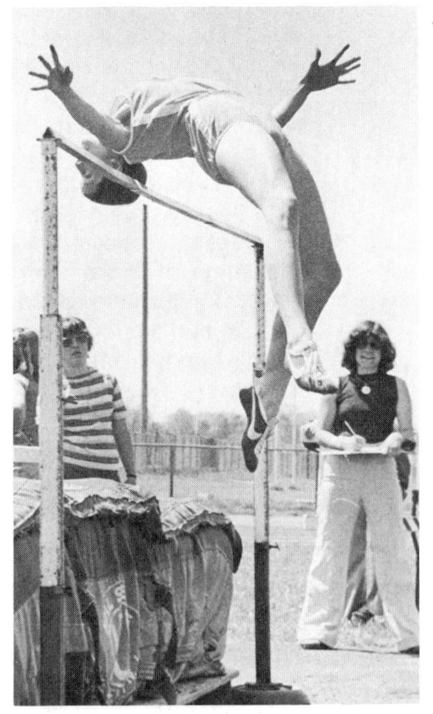

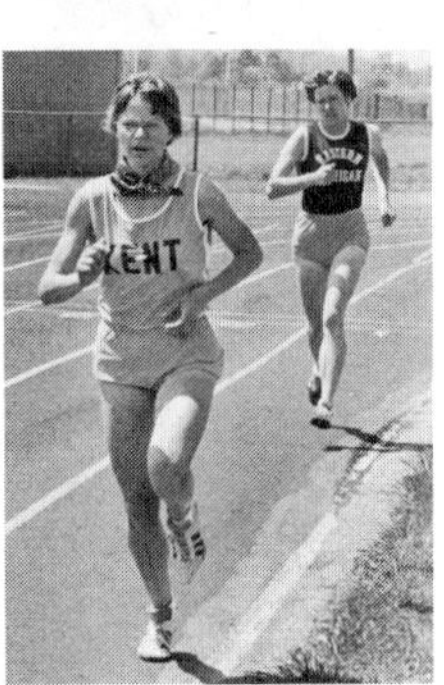

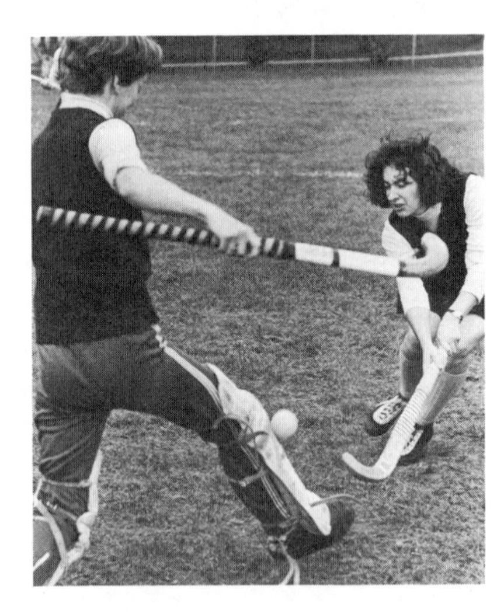

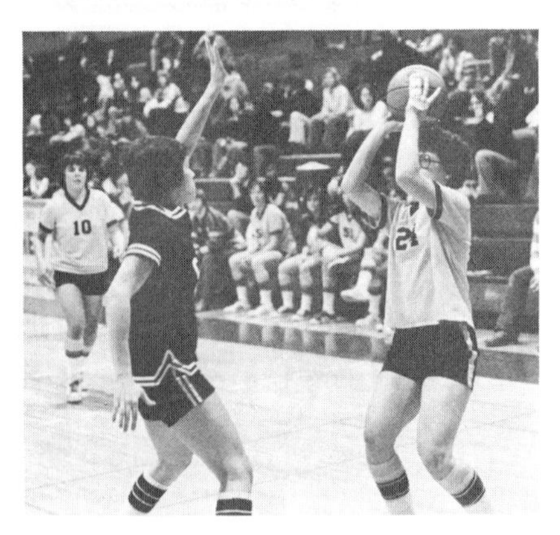

Fig. 4 Individual and team sports for women. (Courtesy the Office of Sports Information Director, Kent State University.)

the necessary ability to make and compete on a boys' team. If girls demand equal rights to compete on boys' teams, boys are likely to request the same rights in return. Since boys are generally superior to girls in most athletic performance measures, boys will win a majority of the positions on girls' teams, which will result in the virtual elimination of girls' programs.

Girls Participating in Contact Sports on Girls' Teams

The classification "contact sports" includes sports that involve minimal frequency and force of body contact (i.e., basketball), as well as those that involve maximal frequency and force (i.e., football). Thus, contact sports vary tremendously in their trauma potential. Basketball and girls baseball, for example, are often classified as contact sports, but their contact is really much less in nature and extent than the contact involved in ice hockey or football. Indeed, girls already participate and have participated for some time both in numbers and extent in a host of the less "physical" contact sports. The real issue concerns whether it is medically advisable for girls to participate in the more vigorous contact sports such as ice hockey and football.

It has already been established that there is no physiological reason to restrict females from such programs and many reasons to endorse and encourage such involvement. In essence, the limiting factor in making such a judgment becomes one of determining whether females are more susceptible to injury because of their biological makeup than are boys who engage in similar activities. The frequency and severity of injuries to boys in contact sports such as football is known. If healthy girls are not likely to be injured more frequently or more severely than boys, restricting them from participating in such sports is not justified.

Fracture rate is a useful severity index of the trauma potential of a specific sport. Unfortunately, valid sports injury data for comparison rates of injury between males and females is scant. Girls do experience more fractures than do men while skiing. The principal factors appear to be less strength, less skill and lesser bone density. However, the gravity-assisted momentum generated while skiing downhill is a major contributing factor in these injuries. In contact sports such as football and ice hockey, there is no gravity-assisted momentum. Thus, girls with their lesser muscle mass (than boys) in relation to proportionate body size will not generate the same momentum, and potential trauma forces upon body contact will be much less. Girls' lesser muscle mass makes it unlikely that they would experience as many fractures as do boys.

This issue parallels one that developed in the recent past regarding the advisability of preadolescent boys playing tackle football. They, too, had lesser muscle mass and bone density than more skeletally mature youths. Medical authorities had every reason to believe that such youths would experience an increased rate of fracture and more serious fractures of the epiphyseal plate (secondary growth centers) of the long bones. This concern was largely dispelled by a study of over 5,000 youths that showed that fractures were rare in these youths and that epiphyseal fractures were even more rare. Apparently, these youths lacked the aggressiveness or strength necessary to deliver a blow sufficient enough in magnitude to cause a fracture. A similar situation prevails with girls participating in contact sports.

The Committee on the Medical Aspects of Sports maintains that it is very unlikely that girls competing in contact sports will sustain more injuries than boys engaged in similar activities, and could conceivably suffer fewer injuries because of their more limited strength to generate momentum.

The other feature of contact sports for girls that makes considerations different than those in the same sports for boys is the protective equipment required. Since breast tissue is susceptible to injury in contact and non-contact sports, appropriate and adequate protection should be provided and its use encouraged.

Thus, the Committee on the Medical Aspects of Sports on medical considerations endorses the concept of contact sports for girls, on girls' teams when they are provided the same safeguards that apply to boys' contact sports programs, namely, an annual medical examination, adequate conditioning, proper coaching, fair officiating, and proper equipment and facilities.

Girls Competing in Contact Sports on Boys' Teams

Here the Committee will confine its remarks to the vigorous contact sports such as football and ice hockey, where the frequency and severity of collision forces is substantial.

Since girls are at a distinct disadvantage to boys in such sports because of their lesser muscle mass per unit of body weight and bone density, it is advisable on medical grounds that they not participate in such programs. The differential between the weight of boys and girls opposing each other would be substantial. Even by matching competitors according to weight, the girls are still exposed to potentially greater injury, since the ratio of adipose tissue to lean body weight varies considerably between the two sexes to the disadvantage of girls. Therefore, the Committee is opposed to contact sports such as football and ice hockey for girls on boys teams on the medical issue involved that such participation with its inordinate injury risk jeopardizes the health and safety of the female athlete, outweighing the benefits of such participation.[25]

[25] Committee on the Medical Aspects of Sports, American Medical Association, "Females in Contact and Non-Contact Sports," 1973. (Endorsed by DGWS, 1973.)

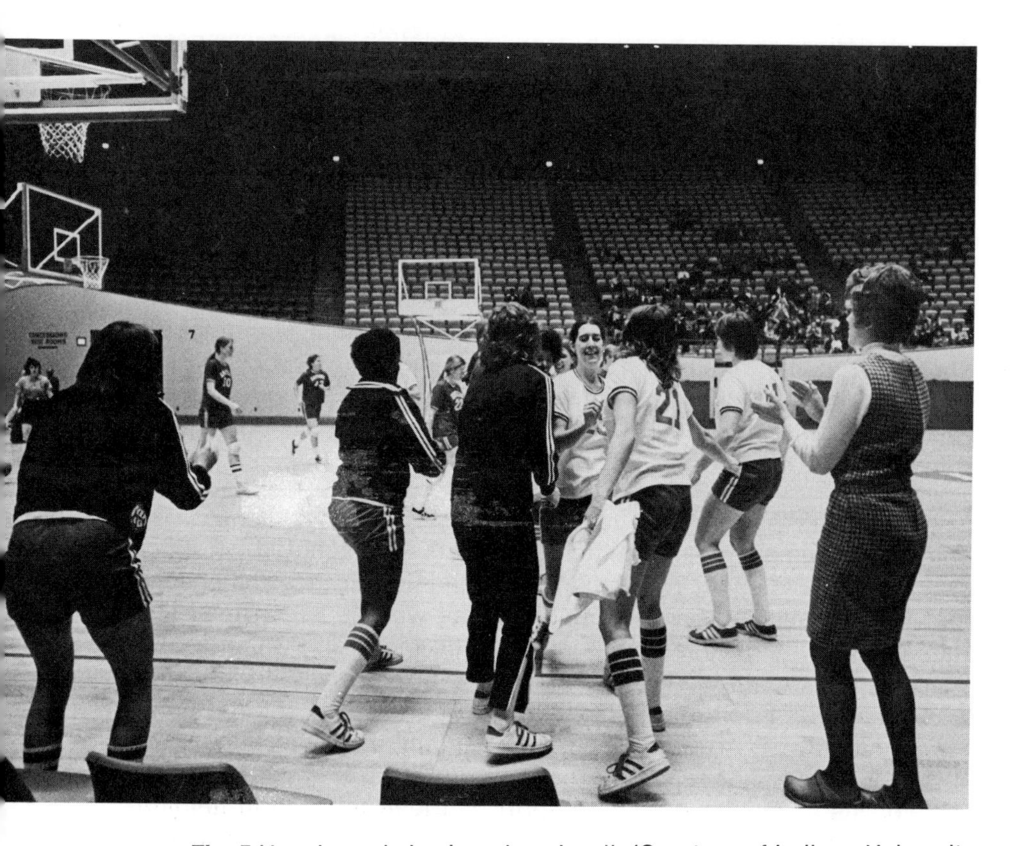

Fig. 5 Happiness is having played well. (Courtesy of Indiana University News Bureau.)

Psychological Aspects

Whereas maleness and femaleness are rather clear biological facts, masculinity and feminity are basically learned. However, it is hoped that theorists will begin to focus on *human* behavior rather than on masculine or feminine behavior.

The psychological studies that have been done tend to focus only on the two areas of emotion and personality. Although much more research on the effects of competition is needed in these areas, thus far studies indicate that generally girls are more emotional than boys (a factor which according to many psychiatrists is an advantage in emotional stability). Such emotionalism is due to sociological environment rather than physiological make-up. Girls who participate in competitive athletics exhibit such personality characteristics as extroversion, accommodation, aggressiveness, cooperation, and self-confidence. While these traits are valuable in athletic competition, not all of them are wholly acceptable for the female in the eyes of society at large. However, as society tends increasingly to accept athletic participation for girls and women, the female athlete will have no need eventually to concern herself with society's standards; instead of concentrating on how to be a "feminine athlete," she can focus on "how to be." [26] If it is true, as research studies tend to suggest, that women display lower self-confidence than men across almost all achievement situations, it would seem that researchers need to define more precisely the variables that influence a woman's perception of self-confidence. For without self-confidence, a focus on *being* and *self* is doomed to failure.

Socio-Cultural Aspects

Culturally, women's participation in sports is accepted so long as it conforms to society's concept of femininity. However, this concept varies considerably internationally, as well as within the confines of the United States, and seems to be more diversified in the more complex cultures. For example, "... in the black community, the woman can be strong and achieving in sport and still not deny her womanness." [27] The concepts of femininity and masculinity are obviously culturally defined. Perhaps the growing number of sports sociologists and philosophers of sport can lead the way in helping to determine what these concepts *ought* to be in a democratic society. Once determined, the leadership in women's athletic programs can encourage the athletic girl to develop whatever "feminine" qualities are deemed desirable in her pursuit of excellence.

Legal Aspects

One of the most succinct yet comprehensive publications which deal with the legal implications of competitive athletic programs for women is that prepared by the Project on the Status and Education of Women of the Association of American Colleges, *What Constitutes Equality for Women in Sport?* [28] This publication outlines some of the issues related to equal opportunity for women in sport, gives examples of some situations that may need reassess-

---

[26] Dorothy V. Harris (ed.), *DGWS Research Reports, Women in Sports,* Vol. II. (Washington, D.C.: A.A.H.P.E.R. Press, 1973): p. 31.

[27] M. Marie Hart (ed.), *Sport in the Socio-Cultural Process,* 2d ed. (Dubuque, Iowa: W. C. Brown, 1976): p. 441.

[28] Project on the Status and Education of Women, *What Constitutes Equality for Women in Sport?* (Washington, D.C.: Association of American Colleges), 1974.

ing, and discusses some of the proposed alternatives for action. Although its primary thrust, as the title implies, is on what legally constitutes equality in such phases of an athletic program as facilities, equipment, financing, administrative structure, single-sex teams vs. mixed teams, conditions of employment for women, and affirmative action to motivate participation by women, the educational value of sport and attitudes toward women in sport are also treated. In essence, issues of concern to people interested in sport, no matter what their specific orientation may be, are thoughtfully addressed from a research viewpoint as well as from an ideological perspective. Perhaps the legal ramifications of the entire picture of athletic programs for women are best summarized in the following quote:

> Some institutions have been reluctant to change policies and practices mandated by athletic conference or association rules, even though they have a discriminatory impact. Such regulations, however, *do not* alter the obligation of an institution to provide equal opportunity to women and men under federal law. It is becoming increasingly likely that, because of pressure on institutions to have nondiscriminatory policies, athletic associations and conferences will be forced to change their rules and regulations.[29]

Geadelmann, in an equally comprehensive publication, reviewed court cases on sex discrimination in athletics and summarized them as shown in Table 1. An Ohio federal judge, in the most recent decision in a court case of this kind, ruled that an Ohio High School Athletic Association regulation barring girls from playing on mixed-sex teams is unconstitutional (see Fig. 6). The decision was based on the Fourteenth Amendment, equal protection rights, rather than on Title IX. However, the judge dismissed the pleas of the OHSAA that its regulations were in compliance with Title IX, with the opinion that the regulations of Title IX are also unconstitutional.[30] If this decision is upheld, one wonders whether the parents of a girl who is injured, because of the physical differences between the sexes, while playing on a mixed-sex team can successfully sue the sponsoring school on the basis of the American Medical Association's view about the dangers of such participation (see p. 412). One wonders, too, whether as women gain "equality," they lose freedom. It would seem that if females' demands to play on male teams are granted in great number by the courts, the inherent uniqueness of women's sports may be lost.

---

[29] *Ibid.*, p. 1.

[30] "Judgment on Decision by the Court," *Ohio High School Athlete*, **37** (February 1978): 193–197.

Table 1 Summary of Court Cases on Sex Discrimination in Athletics

Case	Court	Date	Nature	Ruling	Special Notes
Hollander vs. *Connecticut Interscholastic Conference, Inc.*, No. 11 49 27 Superior Court, New Haven County Conn.	Superior Court New Haven County	March 29, 1971	High school girl wanted to participate on boys' cross-country and track team. None for girls. Individual suit.	In favor of defendants	Cited position of General Assembly of Conn. to "show solicitude for women" and safeguard them "where aspects of physical involvement are concerned." Said that to allow girls to compete with boys would remove incentive for boys and nullify the challenge to win and the glory of achievement.
Gregorno vs. *Board of Ed. of Asbury Park* No. A-1227-70 App. Div., Ap. 5, 1971	Superior Court, New Jersey	April 5, 1971	Female requested participation on boys' tennis team. No team for girls.	In favor of defendants	Court used the psychological well-being of the girl as rationale for exclusion. Appeal court did not find this decision to be unreasonable or arbitrary.
Reed vs. *Nebraska Act. Assoc.*, 341 F. Supp. 258 (1972)	U.S. District Court D. Nebraska	April 12, 1972	Girl wanted to play on boys' golf team. None provided for girls. Individual suit.	Prelim. injunction granted to allow girl to participate	"Her right is the right to be treated the same as boys unless there is a rational basis for her being treated differently" (p. 262 at 5). "If the program is valuable for boys, is it of no value for girls?"
Harris vs. *Illinois High School Assn.*, Civil No. S-Civ. 72–25	U.S. District Court S.D. Illinois	April 17, 1973	High school girl wanted to participate on varsity (boys) tennis team. None for girls. Individual suit.	In favor of defendants	Court said that there is no "right" to participate in interscholastic competition. "Classification by sex is not inherently suspect in this instance." Bylaws merely prohibiting mixed competition are not arbitrary and capricious. Classification by gender is "perfectly rational."

Brenden vs. *Ind. School District,* 342 F. Supp. 1224 (1972)	U.S. District Court D. Minnesota	May 1, 1972	Brenden wanted to be on boys' tennis team, St. Pierre on the cross-country skiing and distance running teams. None provided for girls. Individual suit.	In favor of the girls	Girls' outstanding ability was a real factor in the decision. Implied favoring separate programs but stated these girls were exceptional.
Brenden vs. *Ind. School District,* 477 F. 2d 1292 (1973)	U.S. Court of Appeals 8th Circuit	April 18, 1973	Ind. School District made the appeal.	Affirmed the District Court Decision	Court rejected arguments that physiologically and psychologically girls would be at a disadvantage in mixed competition and declared, "their schools have failed to provide them with opportunities for interscholastic competition equal to those provided for males with similar athletic qualifications. Accordingly, they are entitled to relief" (p. 1302).
Bucha vs. *Illinois High School Assoc.,* 351 F. Supp. 69 (1972)	U.S. District Court N.D. Illinois E.D.	Nov. 15, 1972	Girls wanted to be on boys' swim team—objected to restrictions applicable to girls which were not applied to boys' sports programs. Class action.	In favor of defendants	Girls' program did exist—differing regulations upheld on basis of physiological and psychological differences between males and females. Quoted testimony from *Brenden.*

Table 1 (cont.)

Case	Court	Date	Nature	Ruling	Special Notes
Haas vs. *South Bend Comm. School Corp.*, 289 N.E. 2d 495	Supreme Court of Indiana	Nov. 27, 1972	Girl wanted to play on boys' golf team. Individual suit.	In favor of girl	"Until girls' programs comparable to those maintained for boys exist, the difference in athletic ability alone is not justification for the rule denying 'mixed' participation in non-contact sports." The fact that the records of one sex are superior to the other is not sufficient evidence—for constitutional purposes an investigation would have to focus on the *causes* of any differential in M-F Performance.
Morris vs. *Michigan Board of Education,* 472 F. 2d 1207 (1973)	U.S. Court of Appeals 6th District	January 25, 1973	Two girls wanted to play on boys' tennis team. Individual suit.	Prelim. injunction granted. Subsequent to the injunction, the Michigan legislature passed a bill allowing females to participate in all non-contact sports	Court of appeals changed the injunction to apply only to non-contact sports.

Ritacco vs. *Norwin School District,* 361 F. Supp. 930 (1973)	U.S. District Court W.D. Pennsylvania	August 3, 1973	Girls wanted to try out for the boys' tennis team rather than the girls' tennis team. Class action.	Rule did not invalidly and unfairly discriminate. Girl had graduated and was no longer a member of the class.	"Sound reason dictates that 'separate but equal' in the realm of sports competition, unlike that of racial discrimination, is justifiable and should be allowed to stand. . . ." (p. 932)
Gilpin vs. *Kansas State High School Act. Assoc. Inc.,* 377 F. Supp. 1233 (1974)	U.S. District Court D. Kansas	May 22, 1974	Girl wanted to be on cross-country team. Individual suit.	Ruled in favor of girl	Court implied ruling might have been otherwise had a separate team existed for girls. As it was, there was *no opportunity* for a talented girl whereas all boys regardless of talen had the opportunity.
Commonwealth of Pennsylvania vs. *Pennsylvania Interscholastic Athletic Assoc.,* Pa. Cmwlth, 334 A 2d 839	Commonwealth Court of Pennsylvania	March 19, 1975	Commonwealth filed suit against athletic assoc., maintaining rule forbidding mixed competition was unconstitutional under the State ERA.	Rule declared unconstitutional	"The existence of certain characteristics to a greater degree in one sex does not justify classification by sex rather than by particular characteristic." (p. 843) ". . . it is apparent that there can be no valid reason for excepting these two sports (football and wrestling) from our order in this case." (p. 843)

Table 1 (cont.)

Case	Court	Date	Nature	Ruling	Special Notes
Darrin vs. *Gould,* State of Washington, No.43276	Supreme Court, State of Washington	September 25, 1975	Two Darrin girls wanted to play on the high school football team. Action challenging a state athletic association rule excluding girls. Class action.	In favor of girls. Said the association rule discriminated on the basis of sex which was in violation of the state's ERA	Court said, "the overriding compelling state interest as adopted by the people of this state in 1972 is that 'equality of rights and responsibility under the law shall not be denied or abridged on account of sex.'" Court cited an agreement with the rationale used in the Pennsylvania case (above).
Carnes vs. *Tenn. Secondary School Athletic Assn.,* 415 F. Supp. 569 (1976)	U.S. District Court E.D. Tennessee	May 10, 1976	Female high school senior seeking prelim. injunction against TSSA prohibiting enforcement of a rule prohibiting mixed partic. in contact sports, of which baseball is so named and in which plaintiff seeks partic.	Prelim. injunction granted	Court questioned reasoning for TSSAA rule in that the rule permits males highly prone to injury to play while preventing highly fit females from playing. Court also questioned if baseball could reasonably be classified a contact sport. Stated that to deny Carnes participation would result in an irretrievable loss for her.

Cape vs. *Tennessee Sec. School Athletic Assn.*, 424 F. Supp. 732 (1976)	U.S. District Court E.D. Tennessee	Nov. 24, 1976	Female high school junior claimed that the application of six-player half-court basketball rules which allow only forwards to shoot is a deprivation of her right to equal protection of the laws guaranteed by the Fourteenth Amendment. Also claimed right to relief under Title IX.	Rules declared to be in violation of the Equal Protection Clause of the Fourteenth Amendment	Rational basis test applied. Court stated, "... when a state chooses to deny a significant educational experience to a class of its citizens solely because of sex, and no rational justification for such different treatment can be found, the Constitution requires that such distinction be voided." Court said half-court rules are based on underlying assumption that "female athletes are weaker, less capable, and more awkward," generalizations which are "archaic and overbroad." Rules are under-inclusive in that weak males are not provided for. For most situations Title IX is not interpreted as granting a private right of action. If so, plaintiff first required to exhaust administrative remedies available under Title IX.

Patricia L. Geadelmann, "Court Precedents," in *Equality in Sport for Women* (Washington, D.C.: A.A.H.P.E.R Press, 1977), pp. 72–75. Reprinted by permission of the American Alliance for Health, Physical Education and Recreation.

JUDGMENT ON DECISION BY THE COURT CIV 32 (7-63)

United States District Court

FOR THE
SOUTHERN DISTRICT OF OHIO

CIVIL ACTION FILE NO. C-3-6-205

YELLOW SPRINGS EXEMPTED VILLAGE
SCHOOL DISTRICT BOARD OF EDUCATION, et al.,

vs. Plaintiffs,

JUDGMENT

OHIO HIGH SCHOOL ATHLETIC ASSOCIATION, et al.,

Defendants.

This action came on for (hearing) before the Court, Honorable Carl B. Rubin, United States District Judge, presiding, and the issues having been duly (heard) and a decision having been duly rendered,

It is Ordered and Adjudged that defendants' motion are hereby Denied and the Board's motion is Granted insofar as it alleges violations of the Fourteenth Amendment by the Association, the Ohio Board of Education, and Robert Holland and the individual Ass'n defendants, and is Granted insofar as it alleges violations of Section 1983 by the individual State defendants and the individual Assn. defendants. The defendants are enjoined from continuing to enforce or maintain Assn. Rule 1 § 6, or from enforcing any rule which bars physically qualified girls from participating with boys in interscholastic contact sports. The defendants are further enjoined from disciplining, imposing sanctions, or otherwise penalizing the Morgan Middle School, any official thereof, its basketball team, any member thereof, or its coach because of participation on said team by females. Award of costs and attorney fees will await submission of motion by plaintiff with appropriate supporting documents.

Dated at Dayton, Ohio, this
ninth day of January, 1978.

JOHN D. LYTER
Clerk of Court

BY: Carole A. Makley
Carole A. Makley, Deputy

IN THE UNITED STATES DISTRICT COURT
FOR THE SOUTHERN DISTRICT OF OHIO
WESTERN DIVISION

YELLOW SPRINGS EXEMPTED
VILLAGE SCHOOL DISTRICT
BOARD OF EDUCATION, et al.,

vs. Plaintiffs

NO. C-3-76-205

OHIO HIGH SCHOOL ATHLETIC
ASSOCIATION, et al.,

Defendants

Fig. 6 A recent legal decision.

It seems probable that the next few years will see even more dramatic changes in women's athletic programs than have evolved over the past decade. Such changes almost invariably give rise to legal problems, some of which were discussed earlier in this chapter. In the attempt to provide programs for girls commensurate with those for boys, it is imperative that the responsibility, training, and experience of coaches and administrators of female teams be evaluated carefully so that the best possible leadership is provided and thus negate any unnecessary encroachment of the American legal system into the world of school-sponsored sport.

In summary, then, the era of little or no competition for girls and women is a thing of the past. It is hoped that all agencies that sponsor competitive programs for girls and women—whether within the framework of a school system or not—will cooperate with one another so that the good of the participant is the paramount concern.

ADMINISTRATIVE PROBLEMS

Chapters 14 and 16 deal with administrative problems encountered in interscholastic programs for boys. Although in many cases the discussion is also relevant to the program for girls, several somewhat unique considerations warrant further treatment.

Finances

Programs that depend on gate receipts as their sole means of survival are less than desirable. Too often the public that pays to see a sports contest demands a winner. This fosters an overemphasis on winning, which in turn tends to negate the educational values of the program. At the same time, in an era in which schools are faced with severe financial problems, almost all so-called extracurricular programs are faced with the threat of extinction if they are not self-supporting.

Hard-core reality, then, forces a look at the possible ways in which programs can be financed. Recommendations concerning complete subsidy of all athletic programs (for boys as well as for girls) by board of education monies, student fees, and the like are still extant. However, a practical concept which recognizes the severe limitations of such financing may have to override the more theoretical considerations. This may dictate, for example, a limited number of contests, a geographical limitation in scheduling, and limitations on the sizes of the squads for both boys' and girls' programs. It appears that some of the financial hardship with which athletic programs for girls and women have struggled will be eased by the implementation of Title IX, which mandates that schools receiving federal funds make affirmative efforts to provide necessary equipment and supplies for girls' and women's teams. Regardless, the necessity for gate receipts should be kept to a minimum in order to prevent undue pressure to win being placed on both coaches and athletes.

Facilities

Specialized facilities in which to conduct athletic programs are quite expensive. Therefore, the typical school has a minimum of such areas. One of the biggest administrative problems in the entire field of physical education and athletics is that of trying to schedule all the activities which need these specialized facilities at times which can be justified educationally. It is not unusual to find that a girls' team at a particular school is forced to practice very early in the morning or that one of the boys' teams in a nonrevenue sport, such as indoor track, does likewise. Or perhaps one or the other of these teams practices very late in the evening. Since educationally, such procedures cannot be justified, as discussed in Chapter 13, and since, legally, such practices are now prohibited by Title IX, administrators must choose among some of the following alternatives:

1. to convince the public of the need for more facilities (this is not as difficult to do if the public is also allowed use of the facilities, as for example in a school-community swimming pool),
2. to schedule *all* activities so that everyone shares both desirable and undesirable times,
3. to cancel some of the activities, and thus revert to the justly criticized practice of using expensive facilities, time, and coaching for a very small minority of the total school population.

Coaching and Officiating

All recommended standards for the girls' and women's program stress the use of qualified women coaches and officials whenever possible. Again, the reality is that this practice is not always possible because such qualified women are simply not available. The profession of physical education, then, needs to recruit future women teachers more vigorously, and teacher-training institutions need to emphasize coaching and officiating techniques to a greater extent. As a matter of fact, many such institutions are now offering courses of study to females which lead to certification as athletic coaches or athletic trainers. In addition, greater efforts to utilize the talents of former women physical educators who have left the profession might pay dividends. Among the male coaching ranks the prolific use of workshops and clinics which utilize successful coaches, trainers, and officials as teachers and consultants seems

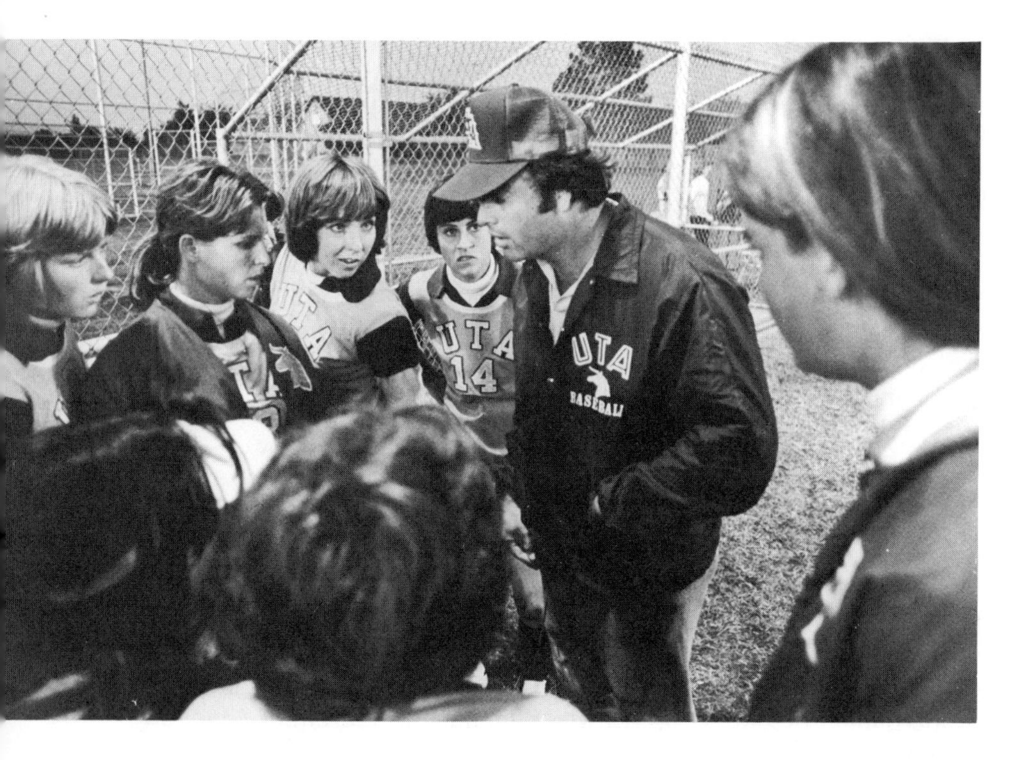

Fig. 7 Getting ready for competition. (Courtesy of UTA New Service, James Russell.)

to have paid great dividends. Although females in the athletic realm are beginning to sponsor similar in-service opportunities, the number of them is limited. Until the time that such avenues become more universally available, perhaps females would be well advised to enroll in appropriate male-oriented sports clinics.

NAGWS is attempting to solve the officiating problem by working cooperatively toward joint ratings with such groups as the U. S. Field Hockey Association. A noted accomplishment along this line is the formulation of the National Gymnastics Rating Committee which comprises representatives from NAGWS and AAU as well as from the U. S. Gymnastics Federation.

In situations in which qualified women coaches and officials are not available, it seems wiser to use qualified men than unqualified women. In fact, it is educationally unsound *not* to take advantage of the greater experience and expertise of the male coaches, whether in a coaching or an advisory capacity. The use of male coaches in these positions is not an uncommon practice, particularly in some sections of the country, but in such cases the use of women educators as chaperones at all times cannot be advocated too strongly. A recent article by Griffith[31] pointed up the importance of such a procedure by noting that in Iowa the second greatest proportion of dismissed male teachers were discharged for reasons of immorality. Of these, almost 50 percent were male coaches of girls' basketball teams who were dismissed because of "improper relationships with members of their girls' basketball teams" and in each case "the single most important factor that was missing was adequate supervision of the girls by adult women sponsors."

Leadership

Leadership is the key to an effective, educational athletic program. It is hoped that women physical educators, after studying all facets of competitive athletic programs, will come forward and keep such programs within sane boundaries. Women physical educators cannot abrogate this responsibility, for it seems safe to predict that competitive sports programs for girls are going to grow regardless of the quality of leadership. Bowen summarized the entire situation cogently:

> With the expanding competitive sports program for girls and women, it is imperative that the proper leadership comes forward. The program will grow whether the best of women's leadership assumes responsibility for it or not. Some of the "evils" of the program for boys and men have developed because of a failure on the part of men of wisdom and leadership ability to accept their obligation in the early development of these programs. Likewise, the reluctance to accept the leadership role and the grave responsibility it carries could produce serious problems for women.
>
> Such leadership is sure to involve decisions which will not be popular. However, failure to assume the responsibility and to stand aside and allow others to take over does not carry with it the right to deplore unsound practices. If women do not more actively develop the high level competitive program for the superior athlete they must accept responsibility for any program, however bad, which arises under one leadership.[32]

---

[31] L. H. Griffith, "An Overlooked Problem in Girls' Interscholastic Basketball," *School Activities,* **39** (December 1967): 3–4.

[32] Robert T. Bowen, "A Man Looks at Girls' Sports," *Journal of Health Physical Education Recreation,* **38** (November–December 1967): 43. Reprinted by permission.

THE FUTURE OF COMPETITIVE ATHLETIC PROGRAMS FOR GIRLS AND WOMEN

Felshin posits a triple option insofar as the future for women in sport is concerned: (1) The Apologetic, in which rationalizations for participation in sport are developed by women who have chosen to be involved despite the view that sport is the "idealized socialization of masculine traits"; (2) The Forensic, in which, because of changes in the socio-legal structure of society, certain "logical imperatives" for sport are defined; and (3) The Dialectic, in which, based on a "feminist-humanist" assumption, the "model of sport" that is dependent on a "harsh competitive" is rejected.[33] Felshin concludes in a distinctly existential vein:

> The shape of sport in the future is not easy to predict. Faith in the dialectic of women and sport implies the development of new and more humanistic modes for social interaction, behavior, and motivation. It also means that women must explore their options; they must be encouraged to try and to be whatever they are impelled to seek; for it is self that is sought, and no apology is required.[34]

There are some who would say that Felshin's dialectic is not a valid, attainable option. For example, in a description of women's programs in basketball at the college level, Hannon asserts:

> The bottom line is this: women's basketball is women's athletics right now, at least on the college level. And it has a chance to become the third women's sport—following the lead of tennis and golf—to capture a substantial share of the public's entertainment dollar and to attract big television money.
>
> This is startling because women's basketball is hardly a polished game. Nonetheless, in six years it has progressed from intramural status to the brink of over-emphasis. It has its own weekly Top 20 and full-ride scholarships, and by all indications it is headed down the same rocky road of recruiting violations and other abuses that the men's game has traveled. In short, the game may be young, but it is already in trouble. Recruiting in many places is similar to the Oklahoma land rush; the talent is out there for the taking, and fewer and fewer coaches and administrators seem concerned about how they go about getting it. Women are switching schools "to play on a national champion." Meanwhile the AIAW, which does not require that transfer students lay off a year before becoming eligible—as the NCAA discovered long ago was necessary—staunchly defends their "right to seek a better education."

---

[33] Jan Felshin, "The Triple Option . . . for Women in Sport," *Quest*, **21** (January 1974): 36–40.

[34] *Ibid.*, p. 40.

> Worse still, these actions are being undertaken in cavalier fashion; the coaches involved are laughing at the rules and at the AIAW's inability to enforce them. The problem is that half of the AIAW membership wants to run a sophisticated physical-education program for college women; the other half wants to get involved in the business of big-time sports. Half of the AIAW leadership is too naive to believe that the above examples of wrongdoing are taking place on a wide scale; the other half is too busy trying to get a piece of the action to worry that the sport is sitting on a powder keg.
>
> "We've plunged in so quickly that we already may have gone too far," says Emily Harsh, the women's athletic director at Vanderbilt. "The men are trying to back out of the same situation the women are nearing. It's a shame. One coach sees another coach get a player and figures it must've been crooked. She thinks she's got to do it, too, or she'll get behind. Then the ball begins to roll. There seems no end to it."[35]

It should be remembered that the quote above appeared in a popular magazine rather than in a research article; perhaps, therefore, some of the contentions were not as well documented as they should have been. However, the administrative ramifications of this quote, *if true,* are legion. There must be "an end to it" if sports are to survive in an *educational* setting!

CASE STUDY

Snyder High School, which has always had a fine intramural program for girls, is now moving toward total compliance with the regulations of Title IX, including a varsity program for girls. Whereas in the past the girls needed gymnasium space only two days per week, they now need space five days per week for their varsity program alone. Ms. Wilson, the coordinator of the intramural and the varsity programs for girls, is thoroughly convinced that each program is important and that neither should be sacrificed for the sake of the other.

The problem of inadequate facilities in which to conduct both boys' and girls' programs is a serious one, and it is compounded by the fact that the new boys' varsity basketball coach, Mr. Welch, was informed when he was employed that he is expected to win at least 75 percent of his games. Naturally, Mr. Welch is reluctant to give up any time in the gym, which he considers is rightfully his, and he is demanding that he be allowed to use the complete gym facility every day from 3:00 to 5:30 P.M. He justifies his demand on the basis that he is the only coach who has been specifically told that he must win.

---

[35] Kent Hannon, "Too Far, Too Fast," *Sports Illustrated,* **48** (March 20, 1978): 34–45. © 1978 Time, Inc. Excerpted by permission.

Ms. Wilson and Mr. Jones, the coordinator of the boys' intramural program as well as the varsity wrestling coach, are adamant that Mr. Welch not be permitted exclusive use of "prime time." In fact, they state if he receives such permission, they will file a class action suit against the school, charging noncompliance with Title IX regulations.

1. What are the essential issues in this case?
2. What solutions are possible?
3. What principles evolve from a case of this type?

SELECTED REFERENCES

AAHPER. *Equality in Sport for Women.* Washington, D.C.: The Association Press, 1977.

Balazs, Eva. "Psycho-Social Study of Outstanding Female Athletes," *Research Quarterly,* **46** (October 1975): 267–273.

Blaufarb, Marjorie. "Opportunity Knocks Through Title IX." *AAHPER Update* (April 1974), pp. 1–3.

Bowen, Robert T. "A Man Looks at Girls' Sports," *Journal of Health Physical Education Recreation,* **38** (November-December 1967): 42–44.

Craig, W. L. "Implementing Title IX in Secondary Schools," *NASSP Bulletin,* **61** (January 1977): 56–61.

Coakley, Jay J. *Sport in Society.* St. Louis, Mo.: C. V. Mosby, 1978.

Deatherage, Dorothy, and C. Patricia Reid. *Administration of Women's Competitive Sport.* Dubuque, Iowa: W. C. Brown, 1977.

DGWS. *Philosophy and Standards for Girls' and Women's Sports* (rev. ed.). Washington, D.C.: AAHPER Press, 1972.

———. "Sports Programs for Girls and Women: A DGWS Position Paper." *Journal of Health Physical Education Recreation,* **45**: 4 (April 1974): 12.

"The Difference of Woman and the Difference It Makes—A Symposium," *The Great Ideas Today.* Chicago: William Benton, Publisher, 1966.

Dunkle, Margaret, and Bermice Sandler. *Sex Discrimination Against Students: Implications of Title IX of the Education Amendments of 1972.* Washington, D.C.: Association of American Colleges, 1975.

Eitzen, D. S., and G. W. Sage. *Sociology of American Sport.* Dubuque, Iowa: W. C. Brown, 1978.

Erdelyi, Gyula J. "Gynecological Survey of Female Athletes," *Journal of Sports Medicine and Physical Fitness,* **2** (September 1962): 174–179.

Felshin, Jan. "The Triple Option . . . For Women In Sport." *Quest,* XXI (January 1974): pp. 36–40.

Gendel, Evalyn S. "Women and the Medical Aspects of Sports," *Journal of School Health,* **37** (November 1967): 427–431.

Gerber, Ellen W., et al. *The American Woman in Sport.* Reading, Mass: Addison-Wesley, 1974.

Griffith, L. H. "An Overlooked Problem in Girls' Interscholastic Basketball," *School Activities,* **39** (December 1967): 3–4.

Hannon, Kent. "Too Far, Too Fast," *Sports Illustrated,* **48** (March 20, 1978): 34–45.

Harris, Dorothy V. (ed.). *Research Reports: Women in Sports.* Vol. I. Washington, D.C.: AAHPER Press, 1971.

———. *Research Reports: Women in Sports.* Vol. II. Washington, D.C.: AAHPER Press, 1973.

———. *Women and Sport: A National Research Conference.* State College, Penn.: The Pennsylvania State University, 1972.

Hart, M. Marie (ed.). *Sport in the Socio-Cultural Process.* Dubuque: W.C. Brown, 1972.

Hoepner, Barbara J. (ed.). *Women's Athletics: Coping with Controversy.* Washington, D.C.: AAHPER Press, 1974.

Hult, Joan. "First AIAW Delegate Assembly," *Journal of Health Physical Education Recreation,* **45**: 3 (March 1974): 79–80.

Kelley, Barbara J. "Implementing Title IX," *Journal of Physical Education and Recreation,* **48** (February 1977): 27–28.

Koenig, Fran. "DGWS Offers More in '74." *DGWS News,* **3**: 1 (Winter 1974): 1.

Lee, Mabel. *The Conduct of Physical Education.* New York: A.S. Barnes, 1937.

Lockhart, B. (ed.). "Title IX, Prospects and Problems: A Symposium," *Journal of Physical Education and Recreation,* **47** (May 1976): 23–37.

Loy, John, Barry McPhersen, and Gerald Kenyon. *Sport and Social Systems.* Reading, Mass.: Addison-Wesley, 1978.

Metheny, Eleanor. "Sports and the Feminine Image," *Gymnasion,* **4** (Winter 1964): 17–20.

Miller, Donna Mae, and Kathryn Russell. *Sport: A Contemporary View.* Philadelphia: Lea and Febiger, 1971.

NAGWS. *AIAW Handbook 1977–78.* Washington, D.C.: AAHPER Press, 1977.

National Education Association. *Combating Discrimination in Schools: Legal Remedies and Guidelines.* Washington, D.C.: The Association Press, 1973.

Project on the Status and Education of Women. *What Constitutes Equality for Women in Sport?* Washington, D.C.: Association of American Colleges, 1974.

Roark, Anne C. "Court Rejects NCAA Ban on Sex Bias in Sports," *Chronicle of Higher Education,* **15** (January 16, 1978): 1.

Schnee, R. G. "Frying Pan to Fire: School Advocacy of Title IX," *Phi Delta Kappan,* **58** (January 1977): 423–424.

Scott, Gwendolyn D. "A Comparative Study of Standards and Policies in Athletics for Girls and Women." Ed.D. dissertation. Case-Western Reserve University, 1963.

Scott, Harry A. *Competitive Sports in Schools and Colleges,* New York: Harper Bros., 1951.

Stutzman, Sandra, Charles McCullough, and Fran Koenig. "Did DGWS Fail: Two Points of View." *Journal of Health Physical Education Recreation,* **45**: 1 (January 1974), 6–10.

Talamini, John T., and Charles H. Page (eds.). *Sport and Society.* Boston: Little, Brown, 1973.

Ulrich, Celeste. *The Social Matrix of Physical Education.* Englewood Cliffs, N.J.: Prentice-Hall, 1968.

U.S. Department of Health, Education and Welfare. *Final Title IX Regulation Implementing Education Amendments of 1972.* Washington, D.C.: U.S. Government Printing Office, 1975.

Westervelt, Esther Manning. "Woman as a Compleat Human Being," *Journal of the National Association of Women Deans and Counselors,* **29** (Summer 1966): 150–155.

Women's Board, U.S. Olympic Development Committee and Division for Girls' and Women's Sports, American Association for Health, Physical Education, and Recreation. *Proceedings, First National Institute on Girls' Sports.* Washington, D.C.: AAHPER, 1965.

———. *Proceedings, Second National Institute on Girls' Sports.* Washington, D.C.: AAHPER, 1966.

———. *Proceedings, Third National Institute on Girls' Sports.* Washington, D.C.: AAHPER, 1967.

———. *Proceedings, Fourth National Institute on Girls' Sports.* Washington, D.C.: AAHPER, 1968.

16

MANAGEMENT OF INTERSCHOLASTIC ATHLETIC CONTESTS

STUDY STIMULATORS

1. What details should be attended to prior to a home contest?
2. What is the role of the student manager in a home contest?
3. How should cheerleaders be chosen? What functions do they perform?
4. What arrangements must be made for news media?
5. What financial arrangements are necessary to conduct a sound interscholastic program?
6. What details are necessary in planning for games away from home?

. . . management, however wise its genius may be, can do nothing without the privileges which the community affords.

W. L. MacKENZIE KING

The administration of interscholastic contests involves a myriad of details and the cooperation of many persons. The school principal usually delegates the responsibility and authority for administering athletic contests to the athletic director or the business manager for athletics. In this chapter we will discuss methods for handling the many details of interscholastic contests.

MANAGEMENT OF HOME CONTESTS

The importance of careful planning and efficient management of home interscholastic athletic events cannot be overestimated. At such events the school is the host not only to local students and adults but also to visitors from other communities. The school administration must exert every possible effort to make the contest attractive and well organized. Since a majority of boards of education have not seen fit to finance interscholastic athletics, most schools charge admission fees. The school authorities are obligated to those who support the team and purchase tickets to present an efficiently planned sports contest. However, the school official in charge should constantly keep in mind that first consideration goes to the participants and students of the school.

Efficient management of interscholastic contests is a necessity. The size of the school has no bearing on this. Small schools do not have as many details to handle, but items that are necessary for the management of interschool contests should be administered to the best of the ability of those in charge.

In the discussion of the various facets of contest management, the reader should remember that assignment of responsibility for the various details of the program varies with local conditions. The superintendent, principal, athletic director, athletic coach, and student manager are responsible for different duties in different size schools.

A check list of the many details involved in contest management should be used. This administrative procedure has proved to be invaluable.

Contracts for athletic contests. It is a fundamental rule of athletic administration that no interscholastic athletic contest be engaged in without an official contract. All contracts should be made on official state association athletic contest contract forms. No one should sign the contract except the principal of the high school or a designated faculty representative. The individual charged with this duty should be certain that all such contracts are in proper order and the conditions of each contract noted and executed. The school official designated to handle the financial aspects should arrange to pay the representative of the visiting school, according to contract terms, at half-time or immediately after the contest.

Eligibility lists. It is standard practice for schools that engage in interscholastic athletics to exchange lists of those students eligible to participate prior to the contest. This is usually done within three days to a week before the contest. Eligibility list forms are usually distributed by the state high school athletic association to all member schools. The local school is almost always required to send a list of eligible participants for every sport the member school participates in to the state athletic association office. The school principal or superintendent is required to sign this eligibility list; therefore, he or she must be sure that these lists are correct.

The contest officials. Most state high school athletic associations provide member schools with standard official contract blanks. These blanks help school personnel and officials to understand their obligations. Officials' contracts are usually made in triplicate. The official retains one, the school administrator or athletic director keeps one for the files, and the visiting school receives the third copy. One way for administrators to be sure of getting the officials they know are competent is to hire early. Lists of registered officials for each sport are maintained by the state association for the guidance of school administrators.

The selection of competent officials is vital to the success of interschool athletic contests. An inexperienced official, one who is unfamiliar with the rules of the game or the mechanics of officiating, or is incompetent in handling participants, can do great harm to the athletic program. Most state high school athletic associations now require that officials in all sports be registered with the state associations to be eligible to officiate in interscholastic athletic contests.[1]

Many state high school athletic associations, in the interest of better officiating, sponsor officials' clinics for each sport in various sections of the state; here they work on interpretation of rules and the mechanics of officiating. In Ohio, for example, there are many such local groups. Every registered official in this state is required to belong to such a group and to attend at least four meetings during the season of the sport in which he or she is registered. The local associations frequently work out agreements with high school conferences to supply them with officials for all their athletic contests.

Officials' contracts should be checked at least a week ahead of time, and a reminder should be sent to each official giving the date, time, and place of the game, as well as the official or officials with whom he or she will work. Administrators should remember that officials are guests of the school. A student manager should be assigned to meet the officials as they arrive and to escort them to a private dressing room. It is best to pay officials before the contest or at half-time, since this allows them to leave at their convenience after the contest. Payment should be made by check.

Parental permission. No student should be permitted to engage in an interscholastic athletic contest without written parental permission. Standard forms should be used. While some schools require permission for every contest, in most cases the granting of permission prior to the beginning of the season is sufficient. The procuring of parental permission slips not only is a good public relations endeavor but also acquaints the parents with the school policy regarding athletic injuries. However, this does not preclude local school athletic associations from being sued in case of injury to a student, particularly if negligence is suspected on the part of members of the school faculty. All signed parental permission slips should be kept on file in the principal's office.

Physician in attendance at all athletic contests. No interscholastic contest should be played unless a physician is in attendance. This policy is frequently violated and may subject the school administration to liability for neglect. When possible, a team physician should be employed.

Faculty representation at athletic contests. No interscholastic contest should be played unless a member of the faculty is present. In some cases the athletic coach fulfills this requirement.

Insurance. In 1930 the State of Wisconsin inaugurated the first statewide scheme of athletic injury coverage for high school players. Some state high school athletic associations followed suit, but most associations have abandoned insurance programs. If the state association does not maintain an insurance program, the school should secure athletic insurance from a reliable insurance company.

Student managers. Student managers are essential to the efficient operation of the interscholastic athletic program. They should be selected for their interest, willingness to work, and ability to assume responsibility. The senior manager has a large responsibility as supervisor of the duties of the rest of his or her staff. By the time the senior manager attains this position, he or she is well acquainted with the details necessary for the successful operation of a team and can be an invaluable aid to the athletic coach and faculty manager. The student manager plan offers excellent opportunities for leadership and followership. Numerals are often presented to assistant managers, with the senior manager and the assistant receiving varsity letters for three years of work. Policies on the selection of managers and the system of awards should be in written form for the information of all students.

Among the various duties of student managers are the following:

1. to meet visiting teams, provide them with information, show them their locker room, provide towels and other materials they may desire;
2. to meet officials, escort them to their dressing room, furnish towels and other materials they may need;
3. to keep facilities and equipment for practice and competition in good condition;
4. to care for the personal equipment of players by issuing it, checking it in, having it cleaned, mended, and stored;
5. to aid the coach by keeping score, keeping time, taking roll, collecting and filing information about competitors, making

performance charts on individual players, and keeping the coach informed on amount and condition of equipment.

Personal equipment. The member of the faculty or the student manager responsible should have a check list for all personal playing equipment and other equipment necessary for the contest. This will aid the coach in that all equipment will be available at the proper place and time.

Visiting team courtesies. From an educational standpoint it is vitally important that the visiting team and its supporters be treated as guests and not as adversaries. Their visit to the community for an athletic contest should be a pleasant one.

It is important to send pertinent information to the visiting school at least a week ahead of the contest. This information should include admission prices, number of complimentary tickets it is to receive, the place the team will dress, directions for getting there, arrangements for the band, half-time ceremonies, the names of the officials, and the color of jersey to be worn by the home school. A wise administrative procedure is to have the above information printed on a form to be sent to visiting schools as a matter of routine.

Before, during, and after the contest, the visitors should be afforded fair and respectful treatment. A student manager should be assigned to the visiting team to direct them to their dressing room and to take care of any needs they might have.

Reserve games. Contests between reserve players should receive the same careful planning and attention to detail as the varsity games. The same precautions are taken for the health and safety of the players, including good personal equipment, a physician in attendance, and competent officiating.

When reserve contests are played preliminary to varsity contests, the game should be started sufficiently early to ensure that the varsity game will start on time. The reserve game as a preliminary to varsity games has become most common in basketball. Many schools have adopted the policy of playing all reserve contests in football and baseball on days other than those on which the varsity contests are held.

Publicity. Publicity for interscholastic athletic contests should emphasize the educational values of the activities rather than concentrate on increasing attendance at games. It is essential to inform the public of the educational objectives of athletics. The amount of time, energy, and money devoted to publicizing interscholastic athletics depends on such factors as size of the school, seating capacity, and interest in the program.

There are many media available for the advertising of interschool sports. Among them are posters, school newspapers, daily newspapers, radio, television, motion pictures, game programs, windshield stickers, signs, billboards, school annuals, direct mail, talks by athletic coaches, bulletin boards, handbills, leaflets, window displays, and school assemblies.

One member of the faculty should be in charge of all publicity. This person should plan and coordinate the various methods of publicizing the program. All news released pertaining to the activities or the personnel of the teams should be cleared with the coach of the sport involved. It is vital to establish and maintain good relationships with the local press. Whatever methods are used to publicize the interscholastic program should be within the bounds of reason and good judgment.

Ticket sales. Since interscholastic athletics are partially or totally financed by gate receipts in most secondary schools, efficient business-like methods of selling tickets and handling receipts should be initiated.

Season tickets should be offered to students and members of the community. These can be offered at a lower price and a good sale assures the school of a fund for operation of the program early in the season. There should be advanced sales of tickets for individual contests at the school during certain announced hours and at designated places in the community. The final method of disbursement is via the ticket booth at the time and scene of the contest. Only adults should be ticket sellers.

One faculty member should be in charge of the sale of tickets and the handling of receipts. When the size of the school warrants it, a staff of assistants should be appointed. All persons who handle money should be bonded. All records of tickets released and sold should be made in duplicate. When an agreement has been made with the visting school, a supply of tickets should be allotted to them for advanced sale. There should be a definite written policy agreed upon by the athletic council or by those in authority in regard to complimentary tickets, which should be kept to a minimum.

Condition of stadium, bleachers, gymnasium. While the maintenance of the athletic facilties is essentially the duty of the custodial staff, it is important that the administration keep close watch on the work of this group to assure that the facilities are ready for a contest. When temporary bleachers are erected, it is vitally important that these bleachers be safe for occupancy. They should be inspected by the municipal building authorities and their stamp of approval should be placed upon them before they are used.

Public address system. The public address system, when manned by an experienced announcer, is an excellent aid to the enjoyment of the game by the spectators; it is also extremely useful in case of emergency. The public address announcer should be a mature person with good judgment and emotional stability.

Scoreboards. Scoreboards are necessary equipment at practically all interschool contests. Electric scoreboards add to spectator enjoyment and are recommended. It is not necessary to spend large sums for an elaborate scoreboard.

Police protection. Police protection is essential at all public gatherings of appreciable size. Interscholastic athletic contests are no exception. The presence of police officers at interschool games is felt by some to be a denunciation of these contests. However, this is not so, and these public servants are necessary for the safety of all concerned. These law officers aid in directing traffic, supervising parking, and controlling the crowd. The city and state police departments are generally willing to cooperate by dispatching special details of officers for athletic contests.

Crowd control. Crowd control has become a major administrative problem for persons responsible for the conduct of interscholastic athletic contests. Football and basketball games present the most problems; however, crowd control may be a factor in other sports as well.

Successful crowd control requires cooperation among school and community groups, such as the school administration, faculty, student body, parents, press, radio and television personnel, and law enforcement agencies. Written policy statements for crowd control and procedures for their implementation should be developed by representatives from the above listed groups. The policies and procedures should be comprehensive enough to provide for any situation.

Smith has developed a list of successful procedures for preventing major crowd control problems:

I. Game Site Operation

A. Design and Layout

1. Plan for traffic flow—pedestrian, car, buses and parking area.
2. Have the ticket windows far enough away from the admission gates or planned so that pre-game ticket holders do not get tied up at ticket windows.
3. Separate players, officials and coaches from crowd with proper fencing.
4. Have proper crowd, traffic and field area lighting.
5. Have directional signs and select colors as to their reflective and visual qualities—BE PLAIN AND SIMPLE.
6. Plan for position stations for ushers and police so that they are helpful and do not block or congest crowd flow.
7. Keep up maintenance, especially painted areas. (Run down facilities invite vandalism.)

B. Crowd Control—(Have a uniformed police *service,* not a police *force.*)

1. Pre-game Meeting
   a. Go over security plan, procedures, duties and responsibilities so that everyone knows what to do in case of emergency.
   b. Do not open crowd gates until police are on their posts.
   c. Have ushers identified by arm band, cap, etc. Their duties should be to collect confetti, horns, etc. Do not have objects that can be thrown around sold at or near the field such as apples, bottled pop, etc.
2. Game
   a. Have police on posts and moving around their area.
   b. Cover parking lots.
   c. Have a closed room where you can talk to people involved in difficulty. Don't get in a shouting contest with troublemakers in front of a crowd.
   d. Have uniformed police remove troublemakers. Don't try it yourself as most people may not know you.
3. Post-game
   a. Have auxiliary police walk out with crowd.
   b. Have plenty of well marked exits.
   c. Have regular police direct traffic flow and clear out site.
   d. Have police in parking lots moving around.
   e. Have squad cars with radio at the field and cruising the area.

4. Safety for the Player and the Spectator
   a. Have a doctor present.
   b. Have permanent ushers trained in first aid (police *are* trained).
   c. Have access to an emergency phone.
   d. Have ambulance service.
   e. Have a stretcher.
   f. Have oxygen tanks at hand.
   g. Have a Red Cross aid station (especially with large crowd and many participants—example: Junior Olympics).

II. Attitudes

A. Coaches
1. Most instrumental person in crowd control.
2. Gentlemanly professional attitude (well dressed also).
3. Knowledge of rules.
   a. Lake Erie League Rules Clinics with officials present.
   b. State Rules Interpretation Meetings.
4. Actions on sidelines with players (no gestures, grabbing, pushing, etc.—arm on shoulder in fatherly attitude fine). Shouting at officials is out.

B. Players
Fair play and good clean competition.

C. Cheerleaders
When to cheer and when not to cheer.

D. Bands
At the pre-game time have raising of the flag and the National Anthem. (How many other places than athletics today do this?)

E. Officials
1. Should have knowledge of rules.
2. Have pre-game officials meeting.
3. Run the game in a business-like manner. (In just one game a poor official can ruin everything you have tried to build over a period of years.)
4. Do not have gestures of a nature that will antagonize a crowd.
5. Do not have more than two games in a season with the same team.

F. Spectators
1. Knowledge of the rules (booklet—"Football for Feminine Fans").
2. Fair Play—"Home of Good Sports."
3. Encourage faculty to attend contests (don't sit in one tight group).[1]

---

[1] Rex Smith, "Successful Procedures for Preventing Major Crowd Control Problems," *Texas Coach* (October 1970): pp. 38–39.

Code of Ethics for Spectators. Rules of good conduct for spectators are part of the total crowd control plan. The staff of the North Carolina High School Athletic Association has developed a "Code of Ethics for Spectators" which spells out key concepts to improve spectator control. The code is as follows.

> Believing that sportsmanship is a by-product of a spirit of tolerance and good will and the centering of attention on the good qualities of all involved, and
>
> Believing that my conduct is an important part in the school athletic program, I pledge myself to act in accordance with these principles.
>
> As an athletic spectator I will:
>
> 1. EXEMPLIFY the highest moral character, behavior, and leadership so as to be a worthy example.
> 2. MAINTAIN and exhibit poise, self-discipline, and restraint during and after the contest.
> 3. CONDUCT myself in such a manner that attention is drawn not to me, but to the participants playing the game.
> 4. REGULATE my actions at all times so that I will be a credit to the team I support, knowing the school gets the praise or blame for my conduct since I represent my school the same as does the athlete.
> 5. SUPPORT all reasonable moves to improve good sportsmanship.
> 6. TREAT the visiting team and spectators as guests, being courteous and fair.
> 7. AVOID actions which will offend the individual athlete.
> 8. ACCEPT the judgment of the coach.
> 9. HONOR the rights of the visitors in a manner in which I would expect to be treated.
> 10. RESPECT the property of the school.
> 11. DISPLAY good sportsmanship by being modest in victory and gracious in defeat.
> 12. PAY respects to both teams as they enter for competition.
> 13. APPRECIATE the good plays by both teams.
> 14. SHOW sympathy for an injured player.
> 15. REGARD the officials as guests and treat them as such.
> 16. DIRECT my energy to encouraging my team rather than booing the officials.
> 17. BELIEVE that the officials are fair and accept their decisions as final.

18. LEARN the rules of the games in order to try to be a more intelligent fan.
19. CONSIDER it a privilege and duty to encourage everyone to live up to the spirit of the rules of fair play and sportsmanship.
20. REALIZE that privileges are invariably associated with great responsibilities and that spectators have great responsibilities.[2]

Ushers. Ushers are essential at athletic contests. Besides helping individuals to find their seats, they can aid in controlling unruly spectators. Varsity letter winners, members of school clubs, boy scouts, or other organizations may serve as ushers. Ushers should be distinguished by badges, hats, or some other device. When possible they should be in uniform. Frequently an adequate ushering staff can be obtained by giving volunteer ushers free admission to the contest; at other times it may be necessary to pay for such service. A school official should be responsible for the securing and supervising of the ushers.

Concessions. Concessions may be handled by the school athletic association or other school organizations, or the concession rights may be sold to a commercial firm. If the concessions are handled by a school group, a faculty member should be in charge. Board of health permits are usually necessary and should be obtained before the season starts. High standards of cleanliness and business-like methods should be demanded of whoever handles the concessions.

Programs. Programs are a source of information and another aid to spectator enjoyment of athletic contests. Game programs range from one-page listings of names and numbers of the contestants to elaborate multipage publications with paid advertisements, photographs, stories and statistics. The one page is frequently distributed free of charge, while the more comprehensive programs are usually sold. The simple program distributed free of charge to the spectators appears to be more suitable and in keeping with the proper spirit of secondary school athletics. The contest program is another one of the details for which a specific faculty member should be responsible.

Cheerleaders. Cheerleaders are usually selected after tryouts held by a member of the faculty, a faculty committee, or the student body. Regardless of the method of selection, care should

---

[2] North Carolina High School Athletic Association, "A Code of Ethics for Spectators," *Texas Coach* (November 1969): p. 45.

be exercised in obtaining the best possible group, for cheerleaders are important not only in creating enthusiasm for the team among students, but also in helping to set the tone of the crowd for good sportsmanship and courtesy. The composition of the cheerleading squad varies from school to school; some institutions have all boys; others, all girls; and still others, both. The cheerleaders should be neatly and sensibly uniformed. Suitable awards, generally in the form of school letters, are granted to upperclass students who perform as cheerleaders in a satisfactory manner. A member of the faculty, preferably a physical education teacher, should supervise the activities of this group.

Bands. School bands have become an accepted part of the interscholastic athletic scene, particularly at football games. Definite seats should be allotted for the home school band and the visiting school band if it attends. The band director or directors, as the case may be, should be informed of the flag-raising ceremony details, as well as the time allotted for pregame and half-time entertainment.

Half-time entertainment. If half-time entertainment is to be presented at football, basketball, or other interscholastic athletic contests, the administration should make certain that it is well planned and under the directorship of responsible persons. There is no justification for a mediocre performance before the public. Besides school bands, some of the more common forms of half-time entertainment are physical education class demonstrations, drill team exhibitions, Dad's Day, Mom's Day, and homecoming celebrations.

Press, radio, and television. Members of the press and radio, and television broadcasters should be provided with suitable working facilities. These people are a source of free publicity. All official employees of newspapers, radio and television stations should be furnished with complimentary passes to the games.

Scorers, timers, judges. Arrangements should be made to obtain competent persons for these important jobs for the contests that require them. In basketball, for example, the scorer and timer are important officials. It is recommended that faculty members be used for these jobs. Some schools have adopted the policy of paying two members of the faculty to assume these duties at all games.

Financial report. A complete financial report should be made on every interscholastic athletic contest. This report should include receipts from ticket sales and concessions, and all expenditures. Standard forms for this report should be adopted. If this report is made by any faculty member other than the school superintendent or principal, each of these school officials should receive a copy for his or her information and use.

Contest data. All data pertaining to specific athletic contests should be filed in one place, preferably the principal's office. Pertinent papers include such things as all correspondence, and game and officials' contracts.

MANAGEMENT OF AWAY CONTESTS

Detailed planning is as essential for contests that are played away from home as it is for those that take place at home. Trips should be conducted in an orderly fashion. The school official in charge of the trip should use a check list of all details essential to the efficient planning of the trip.

Trip personnel. The list of team members, student managers, and other school personnel who will make the trip should be posted at least three days in advance.

Trip schedule. For short trips, when the team returns home the same day, the departure time as well as the expected time of return should be posted. For overnight or longer trips, each member of the party should receive a mimeographed sheet of information. The information sheet should include time and place of departure, time and place of all meals, location of hotel, time of all interim transportation, any free time the squad may have, departure and arrival times on the return trip, and miscellaneous instructions, such as the handling of personal uniforms and equipment. In secondary schools few overnight trips should be scheduled.

Tickets. Arrangements should be made with the host school for a block of tickets to be sold in advance for those students and adults who wish to accompany the team.

Contest details. The trip will proceed more smoothly if all details pertaining to the contest are known prior to departure. The official in charge of the trip should have information in regard to time and place of the game, location of the dressing room, officials, band arrangements, cheerleader and manager arrangements, price of admission and complimentary ticket regulations.

Eligibility records. The eligibility of all players should be checked before they are taken on a trip. The person in charge of the trip should have copies of the eligibility requirements of both schools in his possession for ready reference.

Game contract. The school official supervising the trip should have in his or her possession a copy of the game contract. This will aid in having all financial transactions proceed according to the terms of the contract.

Parental permission. Most school officials assume that parental permission granted at the beginning of the season for participation in an interscholastic sport is sufficient for all contests. However, some administrators deem it prudent to require written parental approval for each individual trip. This procedure is an added indication to parents that the school is interested in the welfare of their child. The validity of written parental permission in releasing a school from liability in case of an accident is questionable.

Transportation. The arrangement of suitable transportation is one of the most important items in planning for games away from home. School buses are a useful vehicle for transporting teams; however, the laws of some states prevent the use of school buses for transportation of personnel for interscholastic contests, or they require special bonding for such purposes. When school buses are not available, buses should be chartered from a reliable public transportation company. If the money required to hire bus transportation is not available, private cars may be used, provided they are sufficiently insured and that they are driven by adult, licensed drivers. In any case team members should be required to go and return from the game as a group.

If the trip is made by bus, only the team members, managers, athletic coaches, and school officials should be permitted to travel in the official party. It is strongly recommended that when weather conditions make driving hazardous, contests should be canceled.

Finances for the trip. The school official in charge of conducting the trip should withdraw sufficient money from the school athletic treasury to pay all necessary expenses on the trip. An itemized expense account should be kept and submitted to the chief school administrator. It is suggested that large items such as transportation and hotel bills be paid by check. The money or check received from the host school for the contract guarantee should not be used to finance the trip, but should be deposited directly in the athletic treasury.

Equipment. Student managers should be responsible for assembling, packing, and loading all necessary equipment for the contest other than the players' personal playing equipment, which should be the responsibility of each player. Duffel bags should be tagged with names prior to loading. The same procedure should be followed on the return trip.

Band. When the school band accompanies the team on a trip, careful planning is as essential for this group as for the squad. Band trip details are similar to those for athletic teams. The band should be impressed with the fact that they are representatives of the school and should conduct themselves accordingly. The host school should be notified sufficiently in advance that the band is attending the contest, so they can make plans to seat them and include them in the program. The band director should coordinate all plans with the athletic director and principal in planning the trip.

Trip data. All data pertaining to specific trips should be filed in one place, preferably the principal's office; home game data should be kept there too. This information is valuable in planning future trips.

CASE STUDY

The entire athletic program of Hoyt High School depended on the revenue obtained during the football season. Mr. Weaver, the athletic director, was becoming increasingly concerned about the drop in the level of support for this sport, particularly since the team had a series of winning seasons.

In a staff meeting called for the purpose of attacking this problem, two solutions were brought forth. One solution was to raise the price of both season and game tickets by about 25 percent. The other solution was to cut down on the number of complimentary tickets that were being allotted to different groups. A cursory examination showed that approximately one-third of all adults were attending games on complimentary passes. The holders of these passes included the press and their friends, parents of the players, members of the booster clubs, and some influential alumni.

The staff agreed that they should not raise the price of tickets since they were already priced above the average high school ticket and just slightly below that of a local college. The group was left with the problem of limiting the number of complimentary tickets given out.

1. What are the issues involved?
2. What solutions should be considered?
3. What principles or guides should evolve from this problem?

SELECTED REFERENCES

Atterbom, H. A. "Sports Officiating," *Journal of Physical Education Recreation,* **47** (October 1976): 23–24.

Bucher, Charles A. *Administration of Health and Physical Education Programs, Including Athletics.* St. Louis, Mo.: C.V. Mosby, 1971.

———. *Administrative Dimensions of Health and Physical Education Programs, Including Athletics.* St. Louis, Mo.: C.V. Mosby, 1971.

Bula, M.R. "Competition for Children: The Real Issue," *Journal of Health Physical Education Recreation,* **42** (September 1971): 40.

———. "Educating Parents About Pre-High School Competition," *Journal of Physical Education,* **69** (November 1971): 45–46.

"Changes in the NATA Educational Program for Athletic Trainers," *Journal of Health Physical Education Recreation,* **44** (October 1973): 10.

"Crowd Control at Athletic Events," *Journal of Health Physical Education Recreation,* **40** (April 1969): 27–31.

Dannehl, W.E., and J.E. Razor. "Values of Athletics: A Critical Inquiry," *Bulletin of the National Association of Secondary School Principals,* **55** (September 1971): 59–65.

Daughtrey, Greyson, and John B. Woods. *Physical Education and Intramural Programs: Organization and Administration.* Philadelphia: W. B. Saunders, 1976.

Davies, G.J. "Checklist for the Athletic Trainer on Game Day," *Athletic Journal,* **53** (April 1973): 82–83.

Delforge, G., and R. Klein. "High School Athletic Trainers Internship: University of Arizona," *Journal of Health Physical Education Recreation,* **44** (March 1973): 42–43.

Dick, E. "Spectator Sports: Opportunity or Nightmare?" *Bulletin of the National Association of Secondary School Principals,* **55** (May 1971): 185–188.

Engle, R. L. "Sports Officiating: An Aid to Coaching," *Physical Educator,* **33** (October 1976): 129–130.

Erickson, A. "Women's Lib and School Sports Can Mean Problems," *School Management,* **17** (August 1973): 33–35.

Fagan, C.B. "Players Brawls Must be Eliminated," *Physical Educator,* **29** (May 1972): 59.

Forsythe, Charles E., and Irvin A. Keller. *Administration of High School Athletics.* Englewood Cliffs, N.J.: Prentice-Hall, 1972.

Frost, Reuben B., and Stanley J. Marshall. *Administration of Physical Education and Athletics: Concepts and Practices.* Dubuque, Iowa: W. C. Brown, 1977.

Fuoss, D. E., and R. J. Troppmann. *Creative Management Techniques in Interscholastic Athletics.* New York: Wiley, 1977.

Fuzak, J., and M.B. Mitchell. "Academics vs. Athletics: Two Views." Ed. by T.A. Emmet. *College and University Business,* **55** (September 1973): 15–16.

Harding, C., and I.T. Sliger. "Student Involvement in the Administration of Sports Programs," *Journal of Health Physical Education Recreation,* **41** (February 1970): 39–43.

"High School Interscholastic Teams," *Journal of Health Physical Education Recreation,* **41** (September 1970): 14, 16.

Horyza, L. "Are Officials Really Necessary?" *Journal of Physical Education Recreation,* **48** (February 1977): 33.

Johnson, M. L. *Functional Administration in Physical and Health Education.* Boston: Houghton Mifflin, 1977.

Johnson, T.P. "Courts and Eligibility Rules: Is a New Attitude Emerging," *Journal of Health Physical Education Recreation,* **44** (February 1973): 34–36.

Moyer, D.G. "Department of Athletics: An Assessment," *Independent School Bulletin,* **29** (February 1970): 23–24.

Mudra, D. "Coach and the Learning Process: Perceptual Approach to Winning," *Journal of Health Physical Education Recreation,* **41** (May 1970): 26–29.

"Professional Preparation of the Administrator of Athletics," *Journal of Health Physical Education Recreation,* **41** (September 1970): 20–23.

Razor, J.E. "Game Management," *Athletic Journal,* **51** (April 1971): 66–67.

———. "Variables in Crowd Control," *Athletic Journal,* **52** (November 1971): 30.

Resick, Matthew C., and Carl E. Erickson, *Intercollegiate and Interscholastic Athletics for Men and Women.* Reading, Mass.: Addison-Wesley, 1975.

Richardson, D.E. "Preparation for a Career in Public School Athletic Administration," *Journal of Health Physical Education Recreation,* **42** (February 1971): 17–19.

Schurr, Evelyn L., and J.A. Philipp. "Women Sports Officials," *Journal of Health Physical Education Recreation,* **42** (November 1971): 71–72.

Schwank, W.C., and S.J. Miller, "New Dimensions for the Athletic Training Profession: A Curriculum for Athletic Trainers," *Journal of Health Physical Education Recreation,* **42** (September 1971): 41–43.

Seidel, Beverly J., *et al. Sports Skills: A Conceptual Approach to Meaningful Movement.* Dubuque, Iowa: W. C. Brown, 1975.

Smith, G. "Violence and Sport," *Journal of Health Physical Education Recreation,* **42** (March 1971): 45–47.

Spreitzer, E., and M. Pugh. "Interscholastic Athletics and Educational Expectations," *Sociology of Education,* **46** (Spring 1973): 171–182.

"Trouble May be Just Ahead for Your District if it Discriminates Against Girls in Athletics: A Special Report," *American School Board Journal,* **160** (September 1973): 19–25.

Wilson, H., and M. Albohm. "Women Athletic Trainers," *Journal of Health Physical Education Recreation,* **44** (May 1973): 57.

INDEX